Mastering
ACLS

Mastering
ACLS

Springhouse
Springhouse, Pennsylvania

STAFF

Publisher
Judith A. Schilling McCann, RN, MSN

Creative Director
Jake Smith

Executive Editor
Kate Jackson

Clinical Manager
Joan M. Robinson, RN, MSN, CCRN

Clinical Editors
Kate McGovern, RN, BSN, CCRN (clinical project manager); Joanne M. Bartelmo, RN, MSN; Patricia Kardish Fischer, RN, BSN; Collette Bishop Hendler, RN, CCRN

Editors
Brenna H. Mayer (senior associate editor), Cynthia C. Breuninger, Ty Eggenberger, Stacey Ann Follin, Kevin Haworth, Jacqueline Mills, Julie Munden, Kirk Robinson

Copy Editors
Jaime L. Stockslager (supervisor), Kimberly Bilotta, Scotti Cohn, Tom DeZego, Heather Ditch, Shana Harrington, Carolyn Petersen, Pamela Wingrod

Designers
Arlene Putterman (associate design director), Mary Ludwicki (book designer), Susan L. Sheridan (design project manager), Joseph John Clark, Donna S. Morris

Illustrator
Judy Newhouse

Projects Coordinator
Liz Schaeffer

Electronic Production Services
Diane Paluba (manager), Joyce Rossi Biletz

Manufacturing
Patricia K. Dorshaw (manager), Otto Mezei (book production manager)

Editorial Assistants
Beverly Lane, Beth Janae Orr, Elfriede Young

Indexer
Manjit Sahai

Printed in the United States of America.

MACLS – D N O S A J
03 02 01   10 9 8 7 6 5 4 3 2 1

Library of Congress Cataloging-in-Publication Data

Mastering ACLS.
    p. ; cm.
    Includes bibliographical references and index.
    ISBN 1-58255-107-3 (alk. paper)
    1. CPR (first aid) 2. Cardiac resuscitation. 3. Cardiovascular emergencies.
    [DNLM: 1. Cardiovascular Physiology. 2. Advanced Cardiac Life Support—methods. 3. Educational Measurement—methods. 4. Heart Arrest—therapy. WG 202 M423 2001]
I. Springhouse Corporation
RC87.9 . M375 2001
616.1′025—dc21   2001020927

Contents

Contributors and consultants

Patricia L. Eltz, RN, MSN, CEN
Community Health Educator
Pottstown (Pa.) Memorial Medical
Center

Carol A. Knauff, RN, MSN, CCRN
Clinical Educator
Grand View Hospital
Sellersville, Pa.

Mary P. Reilly, RN, BSN
Dictionary Technical Advisor
Clinical Data Management
Wyeth Ayerst Pharmaceuticals
Radnor, Pa.

Ruthie Robinson, RN, MSN, CCRN, CEN
Nursing Instructor
Lamar University
Beaumont, Tex.

Mary A. Stahl, RN,CS, MSN, CCRN
Clinical Nurse Specialist
Saint Luke's Hospital
Kansas City, Mo.

Foreword

Cardiac disease is the leading cause of death in the United States and many foreign countries. Our ability to successfully treat patients with cardiac disease and other forms of critical illness has grown significantly during the past 40 years. We've witnessed the development of cardiopulmonary bypass, intra-aortic balloon pump counterpulsation, pacemakers, pulmonary artery catheters, cardioversion and defibrillation technology, endovascular therapies, and thousands of new medications. In just 40 years, emergency and critical care has grown dramatically in complexity at an astounding rate. It doesn't seem likely that things will slow down in the near future.

Health care providers working in emergency and critical care practice settings learn early that the high-tech demands of their environments make it necessary for them to adopt two essential values: teamwork and practice standardization. The result? Interdisciplinary teams within these settings work together to support the needs of their patients, and team members provide efficient, effective, and smoothly orchestrated care — in the midst of the most challenging, chaotic clinical scenarios — because they have carefully assigned functions and roles. As the science governing the care of critically ill patients continues to evolve, these providers agree that a standardized approach to patient management improves patient outcomes and maximizes team performance.

The American Heart Association's Advanced Cardiac Life Support (ACLS) program is also driven by these two essential values. Experienced ACLS providers function within collaborative, highly effective interdisciplinary teams and are armed with state-of-the-science knowledge and skill to support critically ill patients in various extreme states. Although ACLS certification remains a minimum entry standard for practitioners in most emergency and critical care practice settings, accomplishment heralds acceptance to a level of practice that recognizes excellence in highly skilled care delivery.

Mastering ACLS was designed to help readers attain ACLS certification, using a framework that highlights the value of team care and standardized practice. From fundamental skills to ACLS in action, this book offers both content and practice tests to help readers attain this goal. Furthermore, the user-friendly format of *Mastering ACLS* cuts through complex material and concepts in a manner that enhances learning and application.

The journey to ACLS certification marks the start of a new career pathway for many providers. Attaining ACLS certification opens the door to the world of emergency and critical care, enabling practice that meets the needs of highly vulnerable patients.

For those who practice in emergency and critical care, the years ahead will dramatically challenge us with more new technology, medications, care techniques, and procedures. Given the lesson of the past 40 years, one thing is certain as we look to the future: Tomorrow's successful emergency and critical care practitioners will embrace a personal commitment to lifelong learning. Start that journey into the future today by *mastering ACLS.*

***Anne W. Wojner,** RN, PhD(c), CCRN*
President, Health Outcomes Institute, Inc.
The Woodlands, Tex.
Assistant Professor of Neurology
University of Texas Medical School
Houston

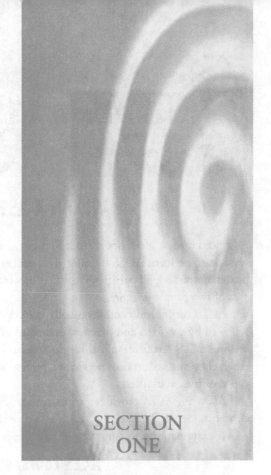

SECTION
ONE

Overview

About ACLS

What is ACLS?

Advanced cardiac life support (ACLS) presents a systematic approach to resuscitative efforts. ACLS training gives rescuers a coordinated way to approach desperately ill patients, regardless of whether the response team consists of two people or more.

ACLS certification courses usually involve 6 to 8 hours of coursework followed by a written and practical examination. Health care professionals seeking ACLS certification include doctors, registered nurses, advanced emergency medical services personnel, professionals in the dental and surgical care areas, and others.

Mastering ACLS provides a concise, thorough guide to learning ACLS concepts. (See *ACLS core concepts.*) It also provides study strategies for the ACLS examination and a preview of how the examination works.

ACLS courses

A typical ACLS course takes place over 2 days in a classroom in a hospital, university, or other teaching setting. It involves lectures on ACLS concepts and hands-on practice involving simulated ACLS situations.

A certification card is issued to those who successfully complete the ACLS course. It doesn't provide a license to perform any of the techniques discussed or reviewed. The ability to perform a technique (such as endotracheal intubation or insertion of an I.V. catheter) is determined by the person's professional scope of practice and licensure within the state.

Recertification in ACLS is a shorter process, typically involving one-half day of review followed by the examination. The renewal period is determined by each American Heart Association chapter — typically it's every 2 years.

One doesn't need a doctorate to qualify to be an instructor. An ACLS instructor typically has successfully completed the ACLS course, expressed a desire to teach, showed exemplary understanding of the core concepts, and followed a formal process to become an instructor.

ACLS core concepts

Here are core concepts and skills needed for ACLS certification.

General skills

For all devices and procedures, you should know:
- indications
- precautions
- proper use.

For every medication, know:
- why to use it
- when to use it
- how to use it
- what to watch for.

Airway management

You should be practiced in and knowledgeable about performing endotracheal intubation. You also should know alternative ventilation techniques, such as bag-valve mask and transtracheal catheter ventilation.

Early management

You should know how to manage the first 30 minutes of emergencies resulting from such causes as:
- acute myocardial infarction
- cardiac arrest associated with trauma
- cardiac arrest involving a pregnant patient

- drowning and near-drowning
- electrocution and lightning strike
- hypothermia
- possible drug overdose
- stroke.

Electrical therapy

You should be able to safely use electrical devices, such as an automated external defibrillator and a conventional defibrillator.

Emergency conditions

You should be able to identify indications for ACLS, such as asystole, pulseless electrical activity, and ventricular fibrillation. You should also be able to quickly institute the proper treatment for the identified indication.

I.V. and invasive techniques

You should be familiar with I.V. and invasive therapeutic techniques such as peripheral I.V. line insertion.

Pharmacology

You should know the action, indication, dosages, and precautions for the major drugs used during ACLS, such as adenosine and lidocaine.

Study strategies

The ACLS examination demands preparation and dedication. The test assesses both knowledge of ACLS concepts and the ability to apply those concepts to high-pressure emergency situations. Still, as a trained health care professional, you should view the ACLS examination as just another step in your professional development. With effective studying and preparation, you'll feel a sense of confidence about the examination.

There are many different study strategies that can help you prepare. Not all strategies are appropriate for every student. For most, a combination of strategies will help them learn ACLS and maintain an enthusiasm for the material.

Key points

Study tips
- Use a combination of study strategies to help you learn.
- Create a guide of "know well" and "needs review."
- Create a study schedule.
- Use additional materials to maintain motivation.

Creating an effective study space

Effective use of time is important when preparing for the ACLS examination, but so is effective use of space. Many people study in places that aren't conducive to concentration, so they often waste time. Look for a study space that:
■ is located in a quiet, convenient place, away from normal traffic patterns
■ contains a solid chair that encourages good posture
■ uses comfortable, soft lighting that allows you to see clearly without straining your eyes
■ has a temperature between 65° and 70° F (18.3° and 21.1° C)
■ contains flowers or green plants, familiar photos or paintings, or other elements that will give you a sense of comfort.

Determining strengths and weaknesses

ACLS training focuses on a broad range of skills, from airway management to pharmacology to leadership during emergency situations. Chances are, you feel more familiar with some areas than with others. One good way to begin your study preparation is to look at the list of ACLS core concepts provided in this chapter. Then, on a sheet of paper, create two columns. Title one column "Know well." Title the other "Needs review."

Now go through the list of ACLS core concepts, placing each in either the "Know well" or "Needs review" column, depending on how confident you feel about the material. Don't worry if one column becomes longer than the other. This will provide an initial guide to how much time you should allot to each topic.

Remember, you'll still study the topics listed in the "Know well" column; you just don't need to spend *as much* time on those topics as on those with which you are less familiar.

Setting a schedule

Most people can identify a period in the day when they feel most alert. If you feel most energized in the morning, for example, set aside blocks of time in the morning for topics that need a lot of review. Then you can use the evening, the time when you feel less alert, for topics that need less review. If the opposite is true, plan your schedule accordingly.

With that in mind, set up a basic schedule for studying. Using a calendar or organizer, determine how much time you have until you plan to take the ACLS examination. Fill in the remaining days with specific times and topics to study. For example, you might schedule I.V. techniques for a Wednesday afternoon and electrical therapy for a Friday morning.

Keep in mind that you shouldn't study all day. Set aside time for normal activities. Also, know your own study capabilities and set realistic goals.

Virtual studying

Many Internet sites offer materials that can help you prepare for the ACLS examination. For example, several sites offer ACLS simulators, in which you can practice your ACLS skills on virtual patients. Sites like these offer immediate feedback as well as a fun approach to studying. Some sites to try include *netmedicine.com, heartinfo.com, embbs.com,* and *acls.net.* These sites also offer links to other sites that are helpful for ACLS candidates. Remember, however, that ACLS information and recommendations may change, so check to see when a site was last updated before relying on it too heavily.

In addition, many professional sites (such as the American Medical Association, the American Heart Association, and various other nursing and medical sites) offer material to help you research and understand specific concepts and provide up-to-date information on the changing field of health care.

You'll feel better about yourself — and your chances of passing the ACLS examination — when you meet your goals regularly. (See *Creating an effective study space.*)

Creative studying

Even the most determined student needs a change of pace occasionally to maintain motivation. For example, studying with a partner or group can be an excellent way to energize your studying. Working as partners allows you to test one another and give encouragement and motivation. When choosing a partner, it's important to select someone with similar goals, motivation level, and knowledge; otherwise, you can waste valuable time chatting or reviewing basic material.

Audiovisual tools can also provide a welcome addition to your study routine. Flash cards, flowcharts, drawings, and diagrams all provide images that can enhance retention. Even the process of creating these materials will help you learn. (See *Virtual studying.*)

If you understand and retain information more effectively by hearing rather than seeing, consider recording key ideas using a handheld tape recorder. Like flash cards, tapes are portable and perfect for those short study periods during the day.

The ACLS examination

The ACLS examination includes both a written and a practical section. The written examination is issued by the American Heart Association and contains 30 to 50 questions, depending on the version used. It's written in a multiple-choice format, with questions similar to those provided in this textbook.

To pass the written section of the examination, you must answer 84% of the questions correctly. You may take the examination a second time at a later date if you didn't pass the written section and you and the instructor feel it's necessary. The written portion of the examination takes approximately 1 hour. The test is given in standard format; no computerized form presently exists.

The practical section of the examination follows the written section. You'll have the opportunity to participate in established case scenarios, including a typical Megacode situation. A Megacode is a realistic re-creation of a situation in which a team approach may be used. Every team member will have a chance to enact roles (such as leader, person in charge of the airway, medication provider, and cardiopulmonary resuscitation provider) and will then be expected to carry out all necessary steps of that role in a precise, thorough manner. This section of the test may take 5 to 10 minutes for each role, depending on the case scenario.

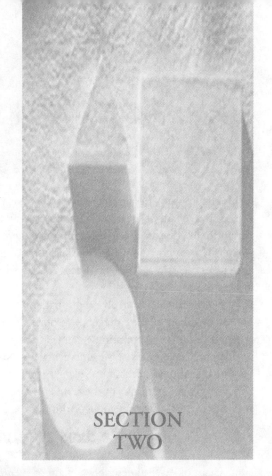

SECTION
TWO

ACLS core concepts

CHAPTER TWO

Know the essentials

This chapter provides an overview of the basic principles of ACLS. It discusses the "chain of survival," a phrase used by the American Heart Association to describe an effective community response to a cardiovascular emergency. It also shows how basic life support (BLS) differs from ACLS and discusses the primary and secondary ABCD surveys — the approach that forms the basis of ACLS.

Successful ACLS involves both patient care and effective organization of the members of the emergency response team. This chapter discusses the phased-response organization system, which provides a general organizing principle for members of the emergency response team and charts the events that should occur at every emergency situation, from anticipation of an emergency to critique of the team's performance after the event. It also reviews the use of treatment algorithms as tools for learning ACLS.

The chain of survival

The chain of survival describes a chain of events — each interdependent — that plays a crucial role in helping a person survive cardiac arrest. This series of events is referred to as a chain because each link must be strong for the process to work on a consistent basis. If one link is weak or missing, poor survival rates will result even if the rest of the emergency cardiac care system is excellent.

The four links in the adult chain of survival are:
- early access
- early cardiopulmonary resuscitation (CPR)
- early defibrillation
- early ACLS.

Early access: The first link
Early access consists of the events that occur from the patient's collapse to the arrival of emergency medical services (EMS) personnel. The more quickly EMS personnel arrive, the greater the patient's survival rate. Early access aims to bring EMS personnel to the scene as quickly as possible.

Early access involves these steps:
- Someone quickly identifies the patient's collapse and activates the system.

■ An EMS response team is rapidly summoned, usually by telephone. In the United States, this typically occurs via a 911 call.

■ Dispatchers quickly recognize a potential cardiac arrest and guide an EMS team to the patient.

■ EMS personnel arrive quickly with all of the necessary equipment (defibrillator, oxygen, and airway management equipment).

■ EMS personnel correctly identify a cardiac arrest and initiate treatment.

Early CPR: The second link

Bystander CPR (an attempt to provide CPR by a person who isn't part of the organized emergency response system) is the second link in the chain of survival. Even with an effective emergency response system, a delay between the patient's collapse and the arrival of EMS personnel may be inevitable. Therefore, early CPR forms the next link in the chain of survival, bridging the gap between the patient's collapse and the arrival of EMS personnel with defibrillation equipment.

Many studies have confirmed the value of bystander CPR and have shown that CPR is most effective when started immediately after a patient collapses. Bystander CPR seems to have the greatest impact on the survival rates of infants and children.

New approaches to teaching CPR, including simplified curricula, practice-while-watching and practice-after-watching videos, and emphasis on regular practice have been shown to increase CPR skill retention. The growing use of computer software and the Internet to practice skills may also contribute to improving the quality of bystander CPR.

Early defibrillation: The third link

If performed correctly, early defibrillation is the link in the chain of survival most likely to improve the patient's survival rate. (See *Which link is most important?* page 10.) This link is typically performed by EMS personnel equipped with automated external defibrillators (AEDs).

AEDs are computerized, low-maintenance defibrillators that analyze the patient's heart rhythm to determine if a shockable rhythm is present. If the AED detects a shockable rhythm, it charges and then prompts the rescuer to press a button to deliver the shock.

Because AEDs have evolved into user-friendly devices, large numbers of people can be trained in their use. Programs that equip firefighters, police personnel, and airplane personnel with AEDs and train them in their use have all shown promising results. Because early defibrillation is so important, any program that safely shortens the time between collapse and defibrillation can have a significant impact on patient survival rates.

Which link is most important?

Individuals preparing for the ACLS examination often ask, "Which link in the chain of survival is most important?" Because early defibrillation is ultimately the only way to reverse cardiac arrest resulting from ventricular fibrillation, it's often deemed the most important link in the chain of survival.

The whole is greater than the individual parts

This response, however, fails to recognize that the overall effectiveness of an emergency cardiac care system can't be measured by its individual parts. A strong survival rate will occur only if the entire system works together. Therefore, no single link in the chain of survival is most important. Each link is as important as the next because failure of one link inevitably weakens the link that follows it.

Early ACLS: The fourth link

Early ACLS, performed by professional personnel, forms the fourth and final link in the chain of survival. After defibrillation has occurred, early ACLS, including advanced airway control and administration of rhythm-appropriate I.V. medications, is the next step in patient care.

EMS systems should provide a minimum of two responders trained in ACLS for all emergencies. Studies have shown that an ideal response team consists of two members trained in ACLS supported by two members trained in BLS.

BLS vs. ACLS

The skills involved in BLS form an important introduction to ACLS. A thorough understanding of the principles of BLS will prepare you to learn the more advanced skills ACLS demands.

BLS involves CPR and airway management and includes such skills as closed-chest compressions and the abdominal thrust. BLS interventions can be performed by any trained person who reaches a patient before ACLS-certified personnel. These interventions, such as checking for breathing, beginning ventilations, checking for signs of circulation, and beginning CPR, form an important bridge between the patient's collapse and the initiation of ACLS.

In some ways, ACLS is simply an advanced version of BLS. ACLS adds more sophisticated interventions to BLS, such as intubating, initiating I.V. access, and giving medications. However, both BLS and ACLS emphasize the same elements: airway, breathing, and circulation.

Primary ABCD survey

ACLS provides a systematic approach to caring for patients in respiratory and cardiac emergencies. Although it's important to master the individual skills necessary for performing ACLS (such as giving chest compressions and initiating I.V. access), mastery of ACLS involves much more than being able to perform individual skills. Only by understanding ACLS's systematic approach will you be able to use those skills effectively in an emergency situation.

ACLS employs a two-pronged approach: a primary ABCD survey followed by a secondary ABCD survey. You should employ this approach with all potential cardiac arrest patients and at all major decision points during a difficult resuscitative effort.

The primary ABCD survey focuses on basic CPR and defibrillation. It includes:
- **A**irway — Open the airway.
- **B**reathing — Ventilate the patient.
- **C**irculation — Perform chest compressions.
- **D**efibrillation — Defibrillate ventricular fibrillation (VF) and ventricular tachycardia (VT).

Airway

As in all emergency care situations, the A in ABCD survey stands for airway. After assessing the patient and determining that he is unresponsive, you should call for help. Then, your first step in a primary ABCD survey is to open the patient's airway. (See *Preliminary actions,* page 12.)

To open the airway, open the mouth using the chin-lift maneuver of basic CPR. Then inspect the upper airway for obstruction. If an obstruction is present, remove it using two fingers covered with gauze or a piece of cloth.

Breathing

The B in ABCD survey stands for breathing. First assess the patient's breathing using the "look, listen, and feel" technique of basic CPR. Look to see if the chest is rising while you listen for air passing from the patient's mouth; also try to discern if you feel breath on your cheek. It's important to assess breathing at this point because an unresponsive patient may still be breathing or may have begun breathing after the airway has been opened. If so, continued maintenance of an open airway may be your only required action at this point.

When you confirm breathlessness in the patient, insert an oropharyngeal airway and begin ventilations with a pocket face mask. Provide two

Key points

Understanding primary ABCD survey steps
- Assess the patient — call for help.
- Establish a patent airway.
- Ensure breathing.
- Assist circulation.
- Deliver shocks.

Preliminary actions

Although opening the airway is the first step in the primary ABCD survey, it isn't actually the first action taken in an emergency situation. When confronted with a possible cardiac arrest, you should:
- assess unresponsiveness
- call for help
- position the patient
- position the rescuer (yourself).
  After you've taken these steps, you can begin the primary ABCD survey.

rescue ventilations in 2 to 4 seconds. Allow 1 to 2 seconds between ventilations to give the patient time to exhale.

Circulation

The C in ABCD survey stands for circulation. As with breathing, the first step here is assessment. Check for a pulse at the carotid artery on the side closest to you. This pulse check should last for 5 to 10 seconds because the pulse may be slow, irregular, weak, or rapid and, therefore, difficult to detect.

If there is no pulse, perform closed-chest compressions using BLS techniques:
- Kneel with your knees apart for a wide base of support.
- Using the hand closest to the patient's feet, locate the lower margin of the rib cage and move along it until you feel the xiphoid process.
- Your middle finger and index finger should remain over the xiphoid process as you place the heel of your other hand on the sternum, next to the index finger.
- The first hand should come up off of the xiphoid area and be placed directly over the top of the other hand. Fingers should be interlaced or straight out.
- Your elbows should be locked and your shoulders should be directly over the patient. Your body will now act as a fulcrum as you apply chest compressions.
- Chest compressions should be given with the weight of the upper body and at a depth over the sternum of 1½″ to 2″ (3.5 to 5 cm).
- Give 15 compressions and 2 breaths for both one- and two-person CPR until the airway is secured. For two-person CPR, one team member performs the compressions while the other performs rescue breathing. After the airway is secured with a cuffed endotracheal (ET) tube, the ratio can be changed to 5 compressions to 1 ventilation.

In ACLS, you're expected to demonstrate how to perform CPR; however, most ACLS courses don't offer certification in BLS.

Defibrillation

The ABC approach to emergency care is familiar to many health care professionals; however, the primary ABCD survey of ACLS adds an important step: defibrillation. Defibrillation must occur as soon as possible; a person in VF, for example, has almost no chance of survival if defibrillation doesn't occur within 10 minutes of collapse. That means you should move quickly and efficiently through the ABC portion of the survey and proceed to defibrillation as promptly as possible.

Current ACLS training emphasizes the use of AEDs for defibrillation. All AEDs operate using four steps:
- Power — Turn the AED on.
- Attachment — Attach the AED to the patient.
- Analysis — Place the AED into analyze mode to detect a shockable rhythm.
- Shock — Press the shock button when indicated.

Repeat these steps until VF or VT is no longer present. (If no AED is available, follow steps for using a manual defibrillator. Specific guidelines for using defibrillators and AEDs are provided later in the text.)

Secondary ABCD survey

After completing the primary ABCD survey, move immediately to the secondary ABCD survey. The secondary survey employs the same basic concepts but with more in-depth interventions and assessments. It includes:
- **Airway** — Perform ET intubation.
- **Breathing** — Assess bilateral chest movement and ventilation.
- **Circulation** — Gain I.V. access, determine the heart rhythm, and give medications appropriate to that rhythm.
- **Differential diagnosis** — Search for, find, and treat reversible causes of the arrest.

Airway

The first step of the secondary ABCD survey focuses on the patient's airway. Reassess the airway to check that it hasn't become blocked.

The patient should then be intubated to make sure that the airway remains clear. Although noninvasive ventilation techniques may be adequate, only ET intubation provides definitive airway management.

Breathing

In the breathing section of the secondary ABCD survey, you should assess the patient's breathing status using more sophisticated techniques than

Key points

Understanding secondary ABCD survey procedure
- Reassess the airway.
- Intubate as soon as possible.
- Check for bilateral chest sounds; confirm tube placement.
- Perform interventions to deliver medications, identify heart rhythm, and monitor blood pressure.
- Determine what caused the event.

those used in the primary survey, such as confirming ET tube placement by physical examination and a secondary confirmation device such as an end-tidal carbon dioxide (CO_2) detector. Physical examination includes observing for equal chest movement and auscultating for bilateral breath sounds. A portable chest X-ray should be done as soon as possible. Secure the ET tube to prevent dislodgement and confirm oxygenation and ventilation with an end-tidal CO_2 monitor and an oxygen saturation monitor. Make any necessary adjustments to ensure that the patient is breathing adequately, including removing the tube and, when necessary, starting over.

Circulation

The circulation component of the secondary ABCD survey involves several interventions ultimately designed to identify arrhythmias and determine and deliver appropriate medication to the patient. As one person obtains I.V. access, another attaches monitor leads, identifies heart rhythm, and measures blood pressure.

After I.V. access is obtained and the heart rhythm is identified, decide which medication to administer to help restore heart rate and rhythm. Then determine other treatments that may be necessary.

Differential diagnosis

In the secondary ABCD survey, D stands for differential diagnosis. You need to consider such potentially reversible causes as hypovolemia, hypoxia, acidosis, hyperkalemia, hypokalemia, hypothermia, drug overdose, cardiac tamponade, tension pneumothorax, coronary thrombosis, or pulmonary thrombosis. Even if you've succeeded in restoring the patient's normal rhythm, cardiac arrest can recur if the underlying cause isn't identified and treated.

Phased-response approach

The primary and secondary ABCD surveys provide an overall structure for patient care before, during, and after a cardiopulmonary emergency. Similarly, the phased-response approach lends an overall structure to the management of the emergency response team and guides the team through all phases of an emergency, from preparation to postemergency evaluation.

The phased-response approach has seven phases. In an actual emergency, one phase may slightly overlap with the next, but the phased-response approach serves as a guide when the team must refocus its activities on a different aspect of the emergency. The phases are:
- anticipation
- entry
- resuscitation

Key points

Phased-response approach steps
- Prepare the scene.
- Make contact with the patient.
- Cover the basics of primary and secondary ABCD surveys.
- Maintain the patient's condition.
- Inform the family.
- Transfer the patient to an appropriate facility or unit.

- maintenance
- family notification
- transfer
- critique.

Anticipation

The anticipation phase involves the rescuers' preparations as they move to the scene of a possible cardiac arrest or await the arrival of a patient with possible cardiac arrest. Steps that occur during this phase include gathering the team, agreeing on a leader, delineating duties, preparing and checking equipment, and positioning the rescuers.

Entry

In the entry phase, the team makes first contact with the patient. Steps to perform during this phase include obtaining entry vital signs, transferring the patient in an orderly manner from BLS personnel to the ACLS team (if applicable), obtaining and evaluating arterial blood gas levels and other laboratory values, gathering a concise history, and repeating vital sign assessment.

Resuscitation

The basics of the resuscitation phase have been covered in the primary and secondary ABCD surveys. During this phase, the team leader needs to keep the team focused on the basics of airway, breathing, and circulation. Effective communication is key during this phase, and team members should state vital signs every 5 minutes or in response to any change in the monitored parameters. Team members should also state when procedures and medications are completed.

Maintenance

The maintenance phase begins when vital signs have stabilized. During this time, team members need to maintain the patient's condition by focusing on the ABCs and staying ready for any renewed problems.

Family notification

During this phase, members of the team inform the family of the patient's condition. Whether you're bearing good news or bad news, this notification must be done with honesty, sensitivity, and promptness. If the family members are present, they may wish to observe the resuscitation as these may be the final moments for the patient. If they do, a professional must remain with the family to direct them where to stand, to answer questions, and to explain procedures. The professional can also watch for signs of acute discomfort in the family members and end the observation.

Transfer

In the transfer phase, the resuscitation team transfers the patient to a team of equal or greater expertise. You should transfer the patient and all relevant information in a concise, complete, and well-organized manner.

Critique

Every emergency situation should finish with a critique of the team's performance. It's important to carry out this phase in a constructive, honest, and useful manner. Frequently, these critiques are done during debriefing exercises away from the crisis situation. This critique allows for honest self-assessment, identification of areas for self-improvement, and reflection on positive and negative outcomes as well as the opportunity to defuse feelings in dealing with volatile situations.

Treatment algorithms

The American Heart Association uses treatment algorithms as educational tools for learning ACLS. Algorithms are flowcharts that can serve as memory tools for carrying out the steps involved in a number of different emergency situations.

It's important to remember that real-life patient care rarely corresponds exactly to any particular algorithm. Therefore, algorithms provide a useful guide but can't replace a flexible, thorough understanding of patient care. Throughout the text, you'll be introduced to the ways in which algorithms are put together to function as a unit and how they work in various clinical scenarios to ensure that nothing is missed in the treatment of the individual.

CHAPTER THREE

Airway management

The major function of the respiratory system is gas exchange. During gas exchange, air is taken into the body on inhalation (inspiration) and travels through respiratory passages to the lungs. Oxygen (O_2) in the lungs replaces carbon dioxide (CO_2) in the blood, and the CO_2 is expelled from the body on exhalation (expiration).

When an interruption in respiratory function takes place, the entire body becomes compromised. Brain damage occurs within 5 minutes, and brain cell death occurs within 10 minutes. Therefore, maintaining a patent airway and restoring respiratory function are vital to ACLS success. This chapter briefly describes the anatomy of the airways to help you understand how to maintain a patent airway. It then describes techniques for positioning the patient and establishing an open airway and discusses the devices designed to help you control the airway, ventilate the patient, and provide oxygenation.

Conducting airways

The conducting airways allow air into and out of the structures of the lungs. The conducting airways include the upper airway and the lower airway. (See *Structures of the respiratory system,* page 18.)

Upper airway
The upper airway consists of the nose, mouth, pharynx, and larynx. The upper airway allows air to flow into and out of the lungs. It warms, humidifies, and filters inspired air and protects the lower airway from foreign matter.

Upper airway obstruction occurs when the nose, mouth, pharynx, or larynx become partially or totally blocked. Upper airway obstruction can stem from trauma, tumors, or foreign objects.

Lower airway
The lower airway consists of the trachea, right and left mainstem bronchi, five secondary bronchi, and bronchioles. The lower airway facilitates gas exchange. Each bronchiole descends from a lobule and contains terminal bronchioles, alveolar ducts, and alveoli. Terminal bronchioles are anatomic dead spaces because they don't participate in gas exchange. The alveoli are the chief units of gas exchange.

Key points

Basics of conducting airways
■ The upper airway consists of the nose, mouth, pharynx, and larynx.
■ The upper airway warms, humidifies, and filters inspired air.
■ The lower airway consists of the trachea, right and left mainstem bronchi, five secondary bronchi, and bronchioles.
■ The lower airways facilitate gas exchange.
■ Upper and lower airway obstruction occurs when a structure becomes partially or totally blocked.

Structures of the respiratory system

Becoming familiar with the airway structures will help you manage your patient's airway efficiently and effectively in an emergency situation. This illustration features structures located in the upper and lower airways.

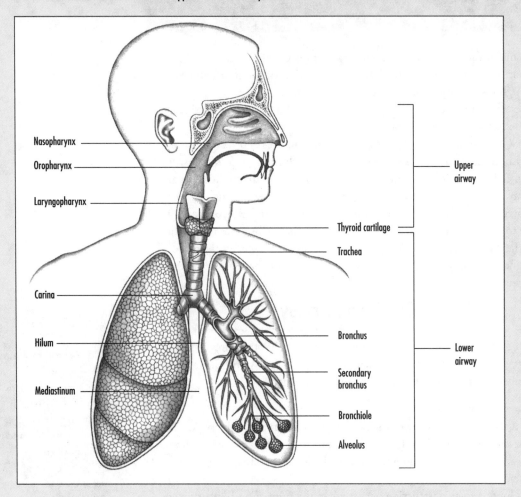

Like the upper airway, the lower airway can become partially or totally blocked as a result of inflammation, tumors, foreign bodies, or trauma.

Proper positioning

When you approach a patient in possible cardiopulmonary compromise, the first step in airway management is proper positioning of both the rescuer and the patient. Without proper positioning, it's difficult to assess the patient's breathing and to ensure a patent airway.

The rescuer should be at the patient's side, at about the level of the patient's upper chest. From this position, the rescuer can perform both rescue breathing and chest compressions.

For effective ACLS, the patient must be in a supine position and on a firm, flat surface. You may encounter a patient lying face down or on his side. If that's the case, roll the patient as a unit so that his head, shoulders, and torso move simultaneously. Take care to avoid twisting the patient's body. After the patient is in a supine position with the arms along the body, you can begin to assess breathing.

Opening the airway

A patient's airway can become obstructed or compromised by vomitus, food, edema, his tongue or teeth, or saliva. The most common cause of airway obstruction is the tongue. That's because muscle tone decreases when a person is unconscious or unresponsive, which increases the potential for the tongue and epiglottis to obstruct the pharynx.

Begin by assessing the patency of the airway. Look to see if there are any foreign bodies visible in the airway. Check to see that the chest rises with inspiration and falls with expiration. Wheezing; suprasternal, supraclavicular, or intracostal retractions; or cyanosis may all signify airway obstruction.

Then open the airway using either the *head-tilt, chin-lift maneuver* or the *jaw-thrust maneuver.* Use the head-tilt, chin-lift maneuver to relieve an upper airway obstruction that's caused by the patient's tongue or epiglottis (see *Using the head-tilt, chin-lift maneuver,* page 20). If the head-tilt, chin-lift maneuver is unsuccessful or if there's a suspected neck injury, use the jaw-thrust maneuver (see *Using the jaw-thrust maneuver,* page 20).

After one of these maneuvers is successfully performed, address foreign body airway obstruction by removing the foreign object by using subdiaphragmatic abdominal thrusts (adult) or chest thrusts (pregnant or pediatric patient), performing a finger sweep or, if the foreign body is seen, using forceps or suction, if available. After the airway is opened, the patient may begin breathing spontaneously. If so, deliver supplemental O_2 in the most effective but least invasive manner possible.

If spontaneous breathing doesn't occur, you must initiate rescue breathing until an invasive airway can be inserted.

Key points

Opening an airway
- *Most common cause of airway obstruction:* the tongue
- *Upper airway obstruction caused by the patient's tongue or epiglottis:* Use the head-tilt, chin-lift maneuver.
- *Neck injury (or if the head-tilt, chin-lift maneuver is unsuccessful):* Use the jaw-thrust maneuver.
- *Foreign body airway obstruction:* Remove the foreign object with subdiaphragmatic abdominal thrusts (adult) or chest thrusts (pregnant or pediatric patient).

Using the head-tilt, chin-lift maneuver

In many cases, the muscles controlling the patient's tongue will be relaxed, causing the tongue to obstruct the airway. If the patient doesn't appear to have a neck injury, use the *head-tilt, chin-lift maneuver* to open his airway.

To accomplish this, first place your hand closest to the patient's head on his forehead. Then apply firm pressure — firm enough to tilt the patient's head back. Next, place the fingertips of your other hand under the bony portion of the patient's lower jaw, near the chin. Then lift the patient's chin, making sure to keep his mouth partially open (as shown at right).

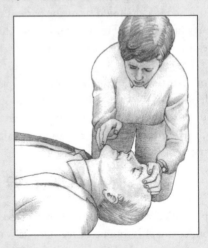

Avoid placing your fingertips on the soft tissue under the patient's chin because this may inadvertently obstruct the airway you're trying to open.

Using the jaw-thrust maneuver

If you suspect a neck injury, use the *jaw-thrust maneuver*. Kneel at the patient's head with your elbows on the ground. Rest your thumbs on the patient's lower jaw near the corners of his mouth, pointing your thumbs toward his feet. Then place your fingertips around the lower jaw. To open the airway, lift the lower jaw with your fingertips (as shown at right).

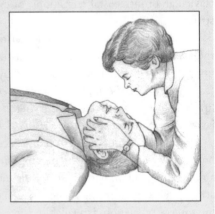

Airway devices and techniques

If manual steps such as the head-tilt, chin-lift maneuver aren't sufficient to open the patient's airway, you may need to use an airway device. The devices described here are invasive. Typically, they are used with an unconscious patient who has no gag reflex because insertion stimulates the gag reflex, placing the conscious patient at risk for aspiration. When these devices prove necessary in the conscious patient, administer sedation before insertion.

Invasive airway devices and techniques include endotracheal (ET) intubation, esophageal-tracheal combitube (ETC), laryngeal mask airway (LMA), nasopharyngeal airway, oral airway, pharyngotracheal lumen airway (PTLA), and transtracheal catheter. If these techniques are unsuccessful or inappropriate, a surgical cricothyroidotomy may be necessary.

Always observe standard precautions when performing any procedure that places you at risk for contact with blood or body fluids.

Endotracheal airway

An ET airway involves the insertion of a tube through the mouth or nose into the trachea to obtain or maintain a patent airway. It's considered the gold standard of invasive airway control in unconscious patients.

An ET airway prevents aspiration and allows oxygenation and ventilation of the patient. To ease insertion, a pharmacologic agent may be used if the patient is conscious or has an intact gag reflex.

An experienced practitioner can accomplish ET intubation quickly with direct vision in awake or apneic persons. However, this should only be performed by those trained and experienced in the procedure, with each attempt lasting no longer than 30 seconds. Between unsuccessful attempts, make sure that the patient is ventilated with a bag-valve mask.

Indications
- Cardiopulmonary arrest
- Respiratory distress
- Persistent apnea
- Accidental extubation of a patient unable to maintain adequate spontaneous ventilation
- Obstructive angioedema (edema involving the deeper layers of the skin, subcutaneous tissue, and mucosa)
- Upper airway hemorrhage
- Risk of increased intracranial pressure
- Laryngeal and upper airway edema
- Absent swallowing or gag reflexes
- Situations in which noninvasive ventilatory efforts are unsuccessful

Equipment needed
- Laryngoscope, comprised of handle (where batteries for light source are housed) and blade (curved or straight) with bulb
- ET tube of proper size and type; for average adult males, use size 8 mm; for average adult females, use size 7.5 mm; also have handy ET tubes that are 0.5 mm and 1 mm smaller than the selected size for cases in which the size chosen by the rescuer is inappropriate for the patient; tubes with low-

Key points

Understanding the endotracheal airway
- Insertion of a tube through the mouth or nose into the trachea to obtain or maintain a patent airway
- Considered the gold standard of invasive airway control in unconscious patients
- Prevents aspiration and allows oxygenation and ventilation
- May require a pharmacologic agent for insertion if the patient is conscious or has an intact gag reflex

Intubation procedure
- Assess respiratory status.
- Hyperventilate with bag-valve mask and 100% O_2.
- Administer medication for relaxation or paralysis (if necessary).
- Visualize larynx using laryngoscope.
- Insert endotracheal tube.
- Confirm placement.
- Secure tube.

pressure cuffs are used in patients older than age 8; uncuffed tubes are used for children age 8 and younger (the anatomy of their trachea provides a natural cuff)
■ Stylet of appropriate size for tube to facilitate proper tube insertion; plastic-coated (may be lubricated with water-soluble lubricant) for ease of insertion into the tube; must end ½" (1.3 cm) before it reaches the distal end of the tube
■ 10-ml syringe to inflate tube cuff
■ Magill forceps to assist with tube placement or to remove foreign matter from airway
■ Water-soluble lubricant
■ Suction device (both rigid and soft devices should be available)
■ Bag-valve mask and O_2 source
■ Oral airway or bite block
■ Tape or tube holder
■ Extra laryngoscope batteries and bulbs
■ Limb restraints
■ Equipment to assist with proper placement detection (pulse oximeter or CO_2 detector and stethoscope)

Procedure
Begin by assembling the equipment and checking it for proper functioning. To ensure that the laryngoscope is operational, attach the blade and snap it to a right angle to test the light. Select the proper size and type of blade, either the straight (Miller) blade or the curved (Macintosh) blade, according to the size of the patient. The practitioner's preference may also play a role. Inflate the tube cuff to detect air leaks, and check the tube lumen for patency, keeping it in its sterile wrapper until it's used. Check that the adapter fits snugly into the ET tube's proximal end.

Next, prepare the patient:
■ Assess respiratory status and color.
■ Place the patient's head in the sniffing position to align the airway and visualize the larynx. (See *Essential anatomic landmarks.*)
■ Hyperventilate using a bag-valve mask and 100% O_2.
■ Administer a pharmacologic agent as required:
  – sedative to induce sleep and relax patient
  – paralytic agent to block tracheal reflexes (gag, swallow)
  – topical anesthesia for local dulling of irritation-induced reflexes.
■ Apply wrist restraints, if appropriate, to prevent accidental extubation.
■ Remove the patient's dentures, if present.
  Now begin the procedure to insert the tube:
■ Hold the laryngoscope in your nondominant hand.
■ Hold the ET tube in your dominant hand.

Essential anatomic landmarks

Locate the landmarks shown here when inserting an endotracheal tube through the oral cavity. These landmarks will help you ensure proper tube placement.

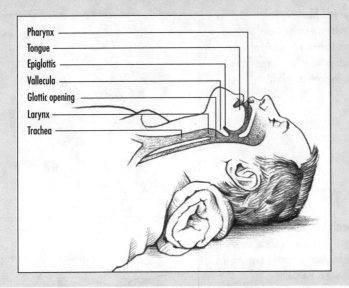

Pharynx
Tongue
Epiglottis
Vallecula
Glottic opening
Larynx
Trachea

■ Insert the lubricated blade into the right side of patient's mouth, and advance it midline to the base of tongue.

■ After visualizing the arytenoid cartilage, lift the epiglottis directly with the straight blade or indirectly by inserting the curved blade into the vallecula. (See *Varying technique with blade type,* page 24, and *Structures seen during direct laryngoscopy,* page 25.)

■ Expose the larynx by pulling the handle of the laryngoscope in the direction toward which it points (90 degrees to the blade); don't cock the handle (especially with the straight blade) because doing so may fracture teeth.

■ Lift forward and upward to expose the glottis.

■ Insert the ET tube to the right of the laryngoscope and into the trachea, passing through the cords.

■ If you can visualize the arytenoid cartilage but not the glottis, have another person apply cricoid pressure or use a curved stylet to direct the tube anteriorly. (See *Applying cricoid pressure,* page 26.)

■ Remove the laryngoscope while holding the tube in place.

■ Look for tube depth marks between the 19- and 23-cm marks at the front teeth.

■ Attempt to ventilate the person using the bag-valve mask with an adapter attached to the ET tube.

Varying technique with blade type

You need to vary your laryngoscope technique during intubation depending on the type of blade used.

Curved blade

If you use a curved blade, apply upward traction with the tip of the blade in the vallecula. This displaces the epiglottis anteriorly.

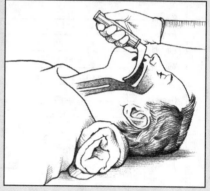

Straight blade

If you use a straight blade, elevate the epiglottis anteriorly, exposing the opening of the glottis.

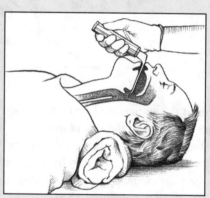

Now assess for placement. Check that:
- the chest rises and falls with each ventilation
- breath sounds are equal in both upper and lower lobes
- condensation is present on the inside of the ET tube
- end-tidal CO_2 measurement indicates a lack of CO_2, confirming that the tube is in the esophagus
- chest X-ray shows tube placement about ¾″ (2 cm) above the carina.

When proper position is confirmed, inflate the cuff using 15 to 20 cc of air. For proper cuff inflation, stop when audible air leaks are eliminated (too much pressure will harm the tracheal mucosa or the lumen of the ET tube). Insert an oral airway or a bite block to prevent occlusion of the airway caused by the patient biting and clamping the tube.

Structures seen during direct laryngoscopy

Locating anatomic structures with a laryngoscope is key to successful intubation. This illustration shows the anatomic structures of the larynx.

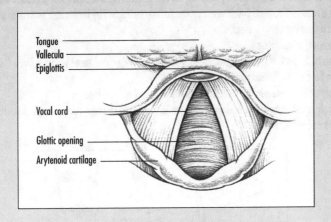

Tongue
Vallecula
Epiglottis

Vocal cord

Glottic opening
Arytenoid cartilage

Now stabilize the ET tube using tape or ties, and secure it so that it's immobile. If you're using tape:

■ Tear about 2′ (60 cm) of tape, split both ends in half about 4″ (10 cm), and place it adhesive-side up on a flat surface.

■ Tear another piece of tape about 10″ (25 cm) long and place it adhesive-side down in the center of the 2′ piece.

■ Slide the tape under the patient's neck and center it.

■ Bring the right side of the tape up and wrap the top split end counter-clockwise around the tube; secure the bottom split end beneath the lower lip.

■ Bring the left side of the tape up and wrap the bottom split piece clockwise around the tube; secure the top split above the upper lip.

If you're using ties:

■ Cut about 2′ (60 cm) and place it under the patient's neck.

■ Bring both ends up to the tube and cross them at the bottom of the tube near the lips.

■ Bring the ends to the top of the tube and tie an overhand knot.

■ Bring the ends back to the bottom of the tube, tie another overhand knot, and then secure it with a square knot (right over left, left over right).

Reconfirm tube placement after you've finished securing it. Following ET intubation, reverify tube placement every 5 to 10 minutes by noting bilateral breath sounds and continuing end-tidal CO_2 readings. If necessary,

Applying cricoid pressure

Also called the Sellick maneuver, the cricoid pressure technique involves applying pressure to the patient's cricoid cartilage. This displaces the trachea posteriorly, compressing the esophagus. It prevents gastric inflation, thereby reducing the risk of vomiting and aspiration. It's contraindicated in a conscious patient. Cricoid pressure should only be applied by health care professionals when a third rescuer is present.

To apply cricoid pressure:
■ Locate the patient's thyroid cartilage with your index finger, and then slide your index finger to the base of the thyroid cartilage.
■ Palpate the prominent horizontal ring, which is the cricoid cartilage.
■ Apply firm but moderate backward pressure to the cricoid cartilage using the tips of your thumb and index finger.

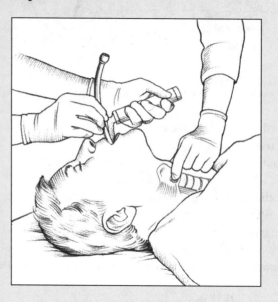

use the ET tube to remove secretions with tracheal suctioning (See *Tracheal suctioning.*)

Special considerations
■ Needs to be inserted with caution in patients with epiglotiditis (usually performed in the operating room) due to the potential for laryngospasm and complete airway obstruction
■ Not ideal intubation method for anyone with suspected cervical spine injury
■ Awake or uncooperative patients may need a short-acting muscle relaxant while you maintain the airway with a bag-valve mask or cricothyrotomy

Tracheal suctioning

Tracheal suctioning involves the removal of secretions from the trachea. It's performed by inserting a catheter through the mouth, nose, tracheal stoma, and tracheostomy tube or endotracheal (ET) tube. This procedure helps maintain a patent airway to promote optimal exchange of oxygen (O_2) and carbon dioxide. It's performed as frequently as the patient's condition warrants. Tracheal suctioning calls for strict aseptic technique.

Equipment required

- O_2 source
- Portable or wall-mounted suction system
- Connecting tube
- Suction catheter kit or a sterile suction catheter, one sterile glove, one clean glove, and a disposable, sterile solution container
- Sterile water or normal saline solution
- Handheld resuscitation bag

Procedure

When preparing to perform tracheal suctioning:
- Check all equipment for proper functioning.
- Attach suction canister and tubing to wall or portable system.
- Set suction between 80 and 100 mm Hg (this amount is adequate to clear the airway without causing tissue trauma); suction catheter should be half the diameter of the ET tube.
- Open the suction kit or catheter.
- Put on sterile gloves.
- Fill sterile container with sterile water or normal saline solution, per facility policy.
- Deliver three to six breaths with the handheld resuscitation bag to preoxygenate the patient, or set the ventilator on 100% O_2 for suctioning (if available).

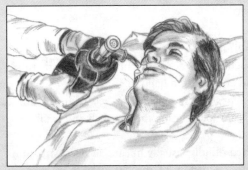

To perform tracheal suction:
- Remove the catheter from the kit.
- Manipulate the connecting tubing and attach the catheter to the tubing.

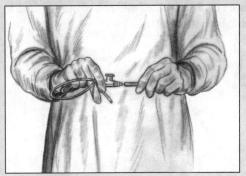

- Hold the catheter with your dominant hand while placing the thumb of your other hand over the control valve.

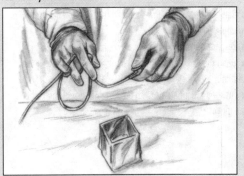

- Dip the catheter tip in the sterile solution and suction a small amount of solution through the catheter.

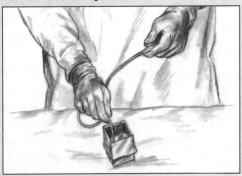

(continued)

Tracheal suctioning *(continued)*

■ Place the catheter into the tube without engaging suction, with the ET tube firmly positioned, and gently advance it until resistance is felt.

■ Suction the patient for 10 to 15 seconds: Pull the catheter back about 1 cm, slowly rotate and withdraw it, and use your thumb to intermittently occlude the vent.

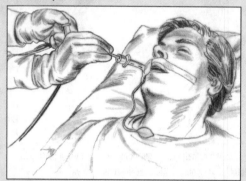

■ Deliver breaths with the handheld resuscitation bag between attempts.

■ Reconnect the patient to the O₂ source.

■ Clean the catheter and tubing by aspirating sterile saline solution.

■ Ensure a patent airway and properly dispose of the catheter and gloves.

Key assessment tips

■ Observe the patient for signs of anxiety, and calmly explain what's occurring.

■ Maintain ET tube integrity during suctioning.

■ Report respiratory distress immediately.

Special considerations

■ Interrupting ventilation causes decreased lung volume, which may cause hypoxemia and lead to cardiac arrest.

■ Suctioning may stimulate the gag reflex and cause vomiting, so maintain ET tube cuff inflation to prevent aspiration.

■ Prolonged suctioning (more than 15 seconds) may cause hypoxia and can lead to cardiac arrest.

■ Suctioning may stimulate the cough reflex, which can cause an increase in intracranial pressure (ICP), constricting blood flow to the brain.

■ Suctioning may increase ICP, hypertension, and tachycardia; produce cardiac arrhythmias; or stimulate a vagal response. Monitor the patient closely.

■ Suctioning may cause feelings of suffocation in the patient (be sure to calmly reassure him).

■ Suctioning may introduce bacterial infection into the airway.

■ Overzealous suctioning or improper technique may cause tracheal trauma.

■ Suctioning must be limited in patients taking anticoagulants (observe for blood in the secretions).

Esophageal-tracheal combitube

The ETC, or esophageal-tracheal double-lumen airway, is a plastic tube with two patent lumens and an occlusion balloon at the distal end that may be used to maintain the patient's airway. One lumen acts as an ET tube and the other acts as an esophageal tube, venting the stomach and facilitating gastric decompression.

The tube may be inserted blindly, usually in cardiac arrest situations, and may be used by those not trained in ET intubation or in cases in which ET intubation attempts have failed. If utilized properly, insertion in either the esophagus or trachea provides satisfactory oxygenation. In addition, if a spontaneously breathing patient has a tracheal placement, he can still breathe through multiple small holes in the unused lumen. The tube also allows gastric contents to be suctioned immediately upon insertion.

Equipment

- ETC
- 50-ml syringe for air insertion into proximal balloon
- 15-ml syringe to insert distal balloon
- Stethoscope to auscultate for proper position
- Suction device
- Bag-valve mask
- Oropharyngeal or nasal pharyngeal airway
- O_2 source
- Water-soluble lubricant
- Placement confirmation devices (CO_2 detector, pulse oximeter)

Procedure

To prepare to use the ETC, you should first:

- Determine cuff integrity according to the manufacturer's directions.
- Lubricate as necessary with water-soluble lubricant.
- Check that all necessary components and accessories are at hand.
- Reconfirm your original assessment.
- Inspect the upper airway and remove any visible obstruction.
  To insert the ETC:
- Position the patient's head in a neutral position.
- Insert with the ETC curvature in the same direction as the natural curvature of the pharynx.
- Grasp the tongue and lower jaw between your index finger and thumb and lift upward.
- Insert the ETC gently but firmly until the black rings on the tube are positioned between the patient's teeth.
- Place the proximal cuff between the base of the tongue and the hard palate.
- Apply cricoid pressure (Sellick maneuver) while the neck is extended to facilitate tracheal placement.
- If the tube doesn't insert easily, withdraw and retry. A maximum of three 30-second attempts with hyperventilation between each attempt is allowed.
- Inflate the large proximal balloon to stop ventilatory gases from exiting through the pharynx to the mouth or nose; inflate the pharyngeal cuff as per the manufacturer's instructions, usually with 100 to 140 cc of air, and the distal cuff with 15 to 20 cc of air.
- Ventilate through the primary tube.
  Confirm the placement of the tracheal portion of the tube by auscultating for breath sounds and assess its esophageal portion by auscultating

---

Key points

Understanding the esophageal-tracheal combitube

- A plastic tube with two patent lumens (one acts as an endotracheal [ET] tube, the other as an esophageal tube) and an occlusion balloon at the distal end
- May be inserted blindly, usually in cardiac arrest situations
- May be used by those not trained in ET intubation or in cases in which ET intubation attempts have failed
- Insertion in either the esophagus or trachea provides satisfactory oxygenation
- Allows gastric contents to be suctioned immediately upon insertion

over the stomach. The ETC is correctly placed in the esophagus when air is blown into the esophageal tube and breath sounds are present bilaterally and epigastric sounds are absent. The ETC is correctly placed in the trachea when breath sounds are absent and epigastric sounds are present and the printed ring is at the level of the teeth.

If lung inflation doesn't occur, attach the O_2 source to the other lumen and initiate ventilation. Hyperventilate for a minimum of 30 seconds. Then use the other tube to remove gastric fluid or gas with the catheter provided in the airway kit or with a gastric tube. Ventilate through the secondary tube. Reassess placement by auscultation and, if confirmed, continue to ventilate.

If both breath and epigastric sounds are absent:
- Immediately deflate both cuffs.
- Slightly withdraw the tube, and then reinflate the cuffs.
- Ventilate and reassess for placement.

If breath and epigastric sounds are still absent:
- Immediately deflate the cuffs and extubate.
- Suction as necessary.
- Insert an oropharyngeal or nasopharyngeal airway.
- Hyperventilate.
- Assess for placement by using the end-tidal CO_2 detector.
- Continue ongoing respiratory assessment and treatment.
- Deflate the balloon of the lumen not in use.

Special considerations
- Doesn't control an airway or provide ventilation as well as ET intubation
- Only used as a temporary measure
- Contraindicated in any person shorter than 5' (1.5 m) and in those with active gag reflex, esophageal disease, or caustic substance ingestion
- Esophageal tears possible due to tube insertion or increased pressure distal to the placed tube during cardiopulmonary resuscitation (CPR)

Laryngeal mask airway

The LMA is a silicone rubber device that combines tracheal intubation and the use of a face mask. It's used to maintain an airway until absolute airway management can be attained.

The LMA has a shaft ranging from 5.25 to 12 mm in internal diameter (i.d.) attached at a 30-degree angle to a distal elliptical spoon-shaped mask with an inflatable rim resembling a miniature face mask. The shaft is marked with a longitudinal black line along the posterior aspect; five sizes are available.

The LMA is useful for situations in which intubation attempts have failed, bag-valve mask ventilation is unsuccessful, and the patient needs immediate airway management. It's simple to use and insert, but studies are still needed on the device's effectiveness in managing a difficult or traumatic airway.

Equipment needed

- LMA of appropriate size
- Stethoscope to auscultate for proper position
- Suction device
- Bag-valve mask
- Oropharyngeal or nasal pharyngeal airway
- O_2 source
- Water-soluble lubricant
- Placement confirmation devices (CO_2 detector, pulse oximeter)

Procedure

Before beginning the procedure:

- Assess the cuff for defects.
- Observe standard precautions.
- Assess the patient for gag reflex.
- Place the patient in the sniffing position.
- Perform the jaw-thrust maneuver.

   To insert the airway:

- Press the distal tip of the lubricated, deflated LMA cuff against the hard palate using your index finger to guide the tube over the back of the tongue (avoid lubricating the anterior surface of the mask, because the lubricant may be aspirated).
- Gently advance the tube until resistance is felt as the upper esophageal sphincter is engaged.
- Inflate the cuff (without holding the tube) with the appropriate amount of air.

   The tube will move outward about $5/8''$ (1.5 cm) and the cuff will position itself around the laryngeal inlet, resulting in a slight movement of the thyroid and cricoid cartilage. The longitudinal black line on the shaft of the tube should lie in the midline against the upper lip (deviation may result in misplacement of the cuff and partial airway obstruction).

   Confirm placement using auscultation and an end-tidal CO_2 detector. When correctly positioned, the tip of the LMA cuff lies at the base of the hypopharynx against the upper esophageal sphincter, the sides lie in the pyriform fossae, and the upper border of the mask lies at the base of the tongue, pushing it forward. If the LMA is correctly placed, ventilate the patient and assess the LMA's effect. If aspiration occurs, leave the LMA in place, tilt the person's head down, and suction through the LMA.

Special considerations

■ Contraindicated if a risk of aspiration exists

■ Doesn't guarantee an airway with a mask

■ Can only be used on a patient with an empty stomach

■ Likelihood of aspiration if vomiting occurs after insertion

■ Possible increase in difficulty of placement from cricoid pressure

■ Increased intragastric pressure and possible contribution to gastric regurgitation from high inflation pressure

■ Can't be used if the mouth can't be opened more than 5/8" (1.5 cm)

■ Skill and training necessary for insertion

Nasopharyngeal airway

The nasopharyngeal airway (nasal tube) is a soft rubber uncuffed tube with a smooth curvature that's inserted through the nose into the oropharynx. When positioned properly, it creates a wide air channel and permits positive pressure ventilation through the trachea.

The nasopharyngeal airway is tolerated fairly well by a semiconscious or conscious patient with an intact gag reflex. It's easier to insert than an oral airway and is useful for maintaining an airway in an adult with seizures, trismus, or cervical spine injuries.

Equipment needed

■ Gloves

■ Appropriate size airway

■ Water-soluble lubricant

Procedure

Use a nasal tube of the largest diameter size that will fit the patient's nares. Determine the size by measuring from the tip of the nose to the tip of the earlobe. The typical sizes are:

■ small adult — 6.0 to 7.0 i.d. (26 Fr.)

■ medium adult — 7.0 to 8.0 i.d. (30 Fr.)

■ large adult — 8.0 to 9.0 i.d. (34 Fr.).

Then assess the nares for patency. The patient should be in a supine position and the airway should be properly positioned using the head-tilt, chin-lift maneuver.

Apply a water-soluble lubricant to the distal half of the tube. Then, gently insert the tube bevel-side toward the patient's septum. Rotate the tube slightly if resistance occurs, but don't force entry. Auscultate the lungs for clear and equal breath sounds after you've inserted the tube. Also be sure to have suction equipment available.

Special considerations
- Nasopharyngeal airway may stimulate laryngospasm, gag reflex (and vomiting), or esophageal insertion and gastric distention if tube too long or inserted too far
- Aspiration or improper placement may cause hypoxia (if occurs, check respiration and provide ventilatory assist as needed)
- May injure nasal mucosa and cause nosebleed
- Contraindicated when basilar skull fracture suspected

Oral airway

The oral airway (oropharyngeal airway) is a C-shaped tubular or channeled device made of firm plastic or flexible vinyl (to prevent occlusion by teeth). It's inserted between the tongue and the posterior wall of the pharynx to lift the base of the tongue off the hypopharynx and establish an open airway.

The oral airway is generally used:
- during bag-valve mask ventilation to facilitate lung oxygenation and minimize gastric distention
- as a bite block with ET intubation to prevent accidental occlusion of the tube by biting.

Equipment needed
- Suction and tonsillar (oral suction) catheter
- Appropriate size oropharyngeal airway:
- infant or child — size 1 or 2 (60 or 70 mm)
- small adult — size 3 (80 mm)
- medium adult — size 4 (90 mm)
- large adult — size 5 (100 mm)
- Tongue blade to move the tongue out of the way (preferred method for infants and children)

Procedure
Before you begin, place the patient in the supine position and, if needed, suction the oropharynx area. Measure for appropriate airway size (from the corner of the mouth to the tip of the earlobe or the bottom of angle of jaw).

To insert the airway:
- Turn the airway upside down and insert it into the mouth.
- Turn it 180 degrees into proper position as the end of the airway reaches about the middle of the tongue (half the curved part is in the mouth).

The flange should rest on the lips, and the end of the airway should be in place between the base of the tongue and the back of the throat. Auscultate for breath sounds during ventilation. Clear and equal breath sounds indicate proper ventilation.

Key points

Understanding the oral airway
- A C-shaped tubular or channeled device made of firm plastic or flexible vinyl
- Used during bag-valve mask ventilation to facilitate lung oxygenation and minimize gastric distention

Special considerations

■ Possible trauma to the oral mucosa, lips, tongue or teeth; displacement of tongue back into pharynx; and airway occlusion from incorrect insertion
■ Potential for palate injury from inserting upside down in elderly patients or children (use of tongue blade to pull tongue to the front and insert airway right side up into the pharynx necessary)
■ Can cause gagging and vomiting or stimulate laryngospasm, necessitating removal and maintenance of patent airway

Pharyngotracheal lumen airway

The PTLA is a double-lumen tube that's inserted blindly into the pharynx. It's designed to quickly establish an open airway in an unconscious patient and allow artificial ventilation. It's typically used to facilitate an airway when ET intubation isn't possible.

One tube serves as an ET tube with a 20- to 30-cc distal cuff, while the second tube is shorter and ends at the hypopharynx, allowing air and fluids to be removed from the stomach during resuscitation. An inflatable 150- to 200-cc low-pressure cuff blocks the esophagus so secretions can't enter the airway. The cuff provides an adequate mask seal that allows the user to provide single-handed ventilation, freeing the other hand.

Equipment needed

■ PTLA
■ Stethoscope for auscultation of proper position
■ Suction device
■ Bag-valve mask
■ Oropharyngeal or nasal pharyngeal airway
■ O_2 source
■ Water-soluble lubricant
■ Placement confirmation devices (CO_2 detector, pulse oximeter)

Procedure

To use the PTLA:
■ Use blind insertion to place the lubricated PTLA into the trachea or esophagus.
■ Inflate both cuffs (pharyngeal tube 150- to 200-cc; ET tube, 20- to 30-cc air).
■ When the tube is in position, instill air into the pharyngeal tube and observe for lung inflation.
■ Attach the bag-valve mask and ventilate the patient.
■ If the lungs inflate, attach the bag-valve mask to the ET tube and ventilate.
■ If the lungs don't inflate, deflate the pharyngeal balloon.

Special considerations
- Inconsistent inflation volume
- Potential for cuff damage by teeth during insertion

Transtracheal catheter ventilation

Transtracheal catheter ventilation, also known as needle cricothyrotomy, is an emergency procedure used to deliver O_2 when airway obstruction can't be cleared by other methods. During the procedure, a through-the-needle catheter is inserted through the cricothyroid membrane. After the catheter is inserted, intermittent jet ventilation is delivered through the catheter.

Equipment needed
- High-pressure O_2 source (50-psi wall source with flowmeter set on flush)
- Through-the-needle catheter
- 5- or 10-ml syringe
- 3 or 3.5 Fr. ET tube adapter
- Hand-operated release valve attached by high-pressure tubing to a pressure-regulating valve
- Relief valve connected to catheter by tubing
- Antiseptic solution
- Pharyngeal suction equipment

Procedure
To prepare the equipment and patient:
- Attach the syringe to the through-the-needle catheter.
- Place the patient in a supine position with his neck aligned in a neutral position.
- Locate the small depression below the thyroid cartilage and clean the area with the antiseptic solution.

   To insert the catheter:
- Puncture the cricothyroid membrane at a 45-degree downward angle and cannulate the trachea.
- Pull back on the syringe as you slowly advance the catheter to maintain negative pressure; when you enter the trachea, air will be aspirated into the syringe.
- Advance the catheter while removing the needle and syringe. (See *Catheter placement in the trachea,* page 36.)
- Attach the hub of the catheter to the tubing while stabilizing the catheter.
- Connect the O_2 source and adjust the flow rate to 15 L/minute.
- Open the release valve; O_2 will flow into the trachea to the lungs for about 2 full seconds.

Key points

Understanding transtracheal catheter ventilation
- Emergency procedure performed when other airway methods fail
- Through-the-needle catheter inserted through the cricothyroid membrane
- Intermittent jet ventilation delivered through the catheter

Catheter placement in the trachea

The transtracheal catheter supplies oxygen to the lungs throughout the respiratory cycle. Usually performed as an emergency procedure, the catheter is advanced into the trachea while the needle and syringe are removed.

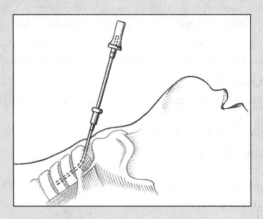

■ Close the valve when you note chest expansion (air then passively exits the glottis, mouth, and nose).
■ Adjust the O_2 flow to the minimum needed to produce chest expansion.
■ Observe the chest for deflation during exhalation.
■ Secure the tube.

The catheter hub can also be attached with a three-way stopcock to the narrow end of a 3 or 3.5 Fr. ET tube adapter. A bag-valve device is placed on the wider adapter end and the patient is manually ventilated with intermittent high-flow O_2 by occluding the open end of the Y connector for 1 second with 4 seconds between occlusions. (It can be used for up to 1 hour.)

Auscultate for bilateral breath sounds. If the chest doesn't passively deflate, suspect proximal airway obstruction and insert a second through-the-needle catheter through the cricothyroid membrane adjacent to the first.

Special considerations
■ Continuous observation required after catheter insertion for detection of dislodgment or kinking
■ Inability to suction airway through the catheter

■ Lack of adequate tidal volume in anyone over 33 lb (15 kg) when used with bag-valve or low-pressure, continuous-flow O_2 source
■ Risk of pneumothorax, hemorrhage, aspiration, and infection
■ Occurrence of oxygenation deficiency during prolonged insertion
■ Potential for mediastinal or subcutaneous emphysema from insertion trauma
■ Possible damage to thyroid cartilage resulting in voice changes, hoarseness, and difficulty pronouncing words

Ventilation devices

There are a number of devices and techniques used to ventilate the patient and help deliver O_2. They include the bag-valve device, barrier devices, automatic transport ventilators (ATVs), and manually triggered devices. When in place, these devices are used either to deliver room air or to deliver supplemental O_2.

Bag-valve device

A bag-valve device is an inflatable handheld resuscitation bag with a reservoir that can be directly attached to a face mask, ET tube, or tracheostomy tube.

The bag-valve device is used to provide manually delivered ventilation of room air or supplemental O_2 (if an O_2 source is available) by positive pressure to apneic patients or those with inadequate respirations.

When attached, the bag-valve device should fit tightly on the face, providing a good seal. If you use a device with an inflatable rim, it can be molded to facial contours.

Equipment needed
■ Oral or nasal airway, unless patient is intubated
■ Pharyngeal suctioning equipment
■ Bag-valve device with O_2 reservoir
■ Tubing to connect to O_2 source

Procedure
To prepare the patient and the device:
■ Suction the airway to ensure patency.
■ Insert an oral or nasal airway in an unconscious patient.
■ Connect tubing to the O_2 source and set the flow rate between 10 and 15 L/minute (this flow rate should yield from 90% to 100% O_2).
■ Attach the tubing to O_2 inlet of device.
■ Assess O_2 flow by placing the mask against your hand.

To attach the device to the patient:

■ Place the narrow end of the appropriate size mask over the patient's nose while lifting the patient's mandible with the fingers of both hands (the patient's mouth should be open under the mask, and the tip of the patient's chin should be at the rounded end of the mask).

■ If the patient is intubated, attach the adapter to the ET tube (see *How to apply a bag-valve device*).

■ Squeeze the bag and observe for the rise and fall of the chest.

Special considerations

■ Inadequate ventilation due to improper mask seal or improper bag squeezes

■ Potential for gastric distention that can trigger vomiting and aspiration or pneumothorax with too hard or too rapid bag squeezing

■ Potential for eye injury caused by direct pressure on the eyes with too large a mask

Barrier devices

A barrier device serves as a physical barrier between the patient and the rescuer; it's typically used with CPR in such areas as the workplace. Two categories of barrier devices are available: face shields and pocket face mask (also called mouth-to-mask) devices.

Face shield

A face shield contains a clear plastic or silicone portion that prevents contact between the rescuer and the patient. The shield is placed over the mouth and nose with the center opening placed over the patient's mouth. The face shield remains in place during ventilations and chest compressions.

Equipment needed

■ Face shield

Procedure

To use the device:

■ Establish a patent airway.

■ Place the shield with the center opening over the mouth and nose.

■ Slowly blow a sufficient volume of air into the center opening to make the patient's chest rise.

Special considerations

■ Difficult to ventilate adequately with this device

■ Necessary to obtain a supplemental O_2 source as soon as possible to prevent hypoxemia

How to apply a bag-valve device

Here's a step-by-step guide to applying a bag-valve device to the patient.

Cover the bridge
Place the mask over the patient's face so that the apex of the triangle covers the bridge of his nose and the base lies between his lower lip and chin.

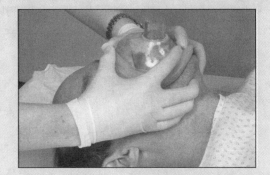

Keep the mouth open
Make sure that the patient's mouth remains open underneath the mask. Attach the bag to the mask and to the tubing leading to the oxygen source.

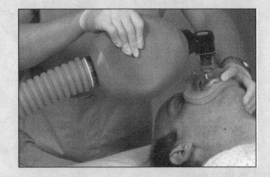

If the patient has a tube
If the patient has a tracheostomy tube or endotracheal tube in place, detach the mask from the bag and attach the handheld resuscitation bag directly to the tube.

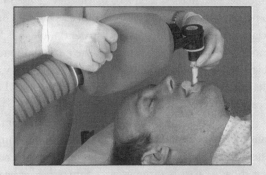

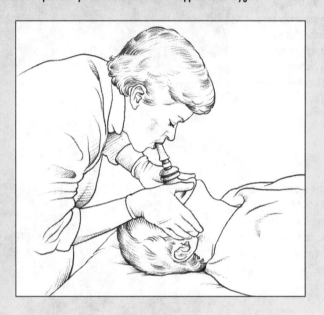

Pocket face mask

Portable and easy to use, a pocket face mask allows you to deliver a breath through a one-way valve while directing the patient's exhaled air away from you. Some devices contain an oxygen administration port that permits administration of supplemental oxygen.

Pocket face mask

A pocket face mask is a type of barrier device used to deliver enriched O_2 to patients with spontaneous ineffective respiration or to those requiring artificial ventilation. It's made of transparent, moldable plastic that allows visualization so that vomiting can be detected. Its components include an inflatable cushion, an O_2 port, a low-resistance one-way valve, and a disposable filter that prevents contact between the rescuer and the patient's secretions. (See *Pocket face mask*.)

The mask delivers 16% O_2 concentration from exhaled air. A higher concentration can be provided by connecting the mask to an O_2 source. The standard adult size can be used for infants by reversing the mask so that the nose part is at the infant's chin. Child sizes may also be used for an infant.

Equipment needed
- Pocket face mask
- Supplemental O_2 (optional)

Key points

Understanding the pocket face mask
- Used to deliver enriched O_2 to patients with spontaneous ineffective respiration or to those requiring artificial ventilation
- Delivers 16% O_2 concentration from exhaled air

Procedure

To prepare the mask and patient:

■ Establish a patent airway in the patient.

■ Snap the mask's filter firmly in place; the dome should be popped out.

■ Attach the one-way valve to the mask port, directing the exhalation port away from the narrow end.

    To attach the mask:

■ Position the mask on the patient's face to form a tight seal, with the narrow end at the bridge of the patient's nose and the rounded end between his lower lip and chin.

■ Apply pressure to both sides of the mask with the thumb sides of the hands.

■ Use the index, ring, and middle fingers to lift the mandible while maintaining head tilt.

■ Blow a sufficient volume slowly into the opening of the mask to make the chest rise.

■ Remove your mouth, allowing exhalation to occur.

■ Apply O_2 source at flow rate of 10 L/minute for 50% O_2 concentration as soon as possible.

Special considerations

■ Inadequate ventilation if mask isn't sealed tightly to face

■ Supplemental O_2 source necessary as soon as possible to prevent hypoxemia

Automatic transport ventilators

ATVs provide supplemental O_2 at a constant inspiratory flow rate for an extended period of time. The basic forms are time-cycled, volume-cycled, flow-cycled, and pressure-cycled:

■ Time-cycled devices stop delivery when a preset time for inspiration expires. The timing mechanism can be run by O_2 or electricity and the length of inspiration is set by the equipment operator.

■ Volume-cycled devices deliver a preset amount of O_2 and then stop.

■ Pressure-cycled devices stop when a preset airway pressure is met during the inspiratory phase.

■ Flow-cycled devices stop when the inspiratory flow rate drops to a preset critical level.

    Advantages for these devices include a controlled source of O_2 for the patient and freedom for the practitioner to perform other treatment measures.

Key points

Using automatic transport ventilators

■ Provide supplemental O_2 at a constant flow rate for an extended period of time

■ Control source of O_2

■ Free the practitioner to perform other treatment measures

Equipment needed
- ATV
- O_2 source
- Suction equipment

Procedure
To prepare the device:
- Check that the device is functioning properly.
- Use a bag-valve mask to assist ventilation until the equipment is ready (keep handy in the event that the O_2 supply is diminished).
- Have suction equipment ready.
  To attach the device:
- Turn on the unit and, if necessary, set the tidal volume (12 to 15 ml/kg is the guideline) and rate (8 to 12 breaths/minute).
- Set the peak inspiratory pressure at 60 cm H_2O pressure (should have the ability to increase to 80 cm).
- Attach the device to the proper airway adjunct.
- Observe the patient's respirations for adequate chest expansion (the tidal volume knob can be adjusted for more or less expansion).

  Assess for effectiveness using pulse oximetry or arterial blood gas analysis.

Special considerations
- Reliable O_2 and electrical source necessary
- Can't be used in children younger than age 5
- Potential for stopped ventilation if patient fights the equipment, causing increased airway resistance
- Potential for increased intrathoracic pressure and may cause hypotension by decreasing the blood flow to the heart
- Possible increased airway pressure causing barotrauma to the airway
- Gastric distension if the patient isn't intubated
- Respiratory alkalosis with delivery of too much O_2
- Bag-valve device should be kept nearby

Manually triggered devices

Manually triggered devices, such as the demand valve and Elder demand valve, are O_2-powered breathing devices that deliver positive-pressure ventilation by use of a manual control button. The devices are lightweight, portable, and easy to use.

These devices deliver O_2 under pressure to inflate the lungs and ventilate patients in respiratory arrest or with diminished breathing capacity.

Although they've been used in prehospital care for more than 25 years, they currently aren't recommended for use because of the high incidence of massive gastric inflation and barotrauma. Further studies are needed to compare their efficacy with that of bag-valve devices and ATVs.

Supplemental O$_2$ administration

In a respiratory emergency, supplemental O$_2$ administration reduces the patient's ventilatory effort. In a cardiac emergency, O$_2$ therapy helps meet the increased myocardial workload as the heart tries to compensate for hypoxemia. It's particularly important for a patient with compromised myocardium (as in cases of myocardial infarction or arrhythmia). Supplemental O$_2$ administration devices include nasal cannula, nonrebreather masks, simple masks, and Venturi masks.

Nasal cannula

A nasal cannula is the most frequently used low-flow O$_2$ delivery system for a spontaneously breathing patient who doesn't need precise concentrations. It's comfortable, easy to use, and composed of flexible plastic tubing with two nasal prongs (about ⅝″ long) and an adjustable elastic strap.

A nasal cannula provides 24% to 44% humidified O$_2$ concentration with 1 to 6 L/minute flow rates for patients with no or minimal respiratory distress. Every 1 L/minute increase equals a 4% O$_2$ concentration increase.

Equipment needed
- Nasal cannula
- O$_2$ source

Procedure
Assess the patient for nasal airway patency. Then:
- Attach the cannula tubing to the humidified O$_2$ source.
- Set the flow rate to the desired flow.
- Check the flow by holding the cannula against your hand.
- Place the cannula tubing behind the patient's ears and under his chin.
- Slide the adjuster to secure the tubing in position; if an elastic strap is present, slip it over the patient's head and secure it.

Special considerations
- Contraindicated for the patient with a nasal obstruction
- Can lead to variable O$_2$ concentration due to breathing pattern
- Flow rates greater than 6 L/minute dry mucous membranes and require a humidity source; may cause headaches
- Easily dislodged

Nonrebreather mask

This illustration shows the components of the nonrebreather mask.

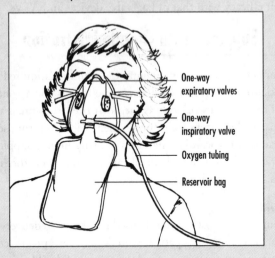

One-way expiratory valves

One-way inspiratory valve

Oxygen tubing

Reservoir bag

Nonrebreather mask

The nonrebreather mask is a face mask with an O_2 reservoir. It provides O_2 concentrations (60% to 90%) to spontaneously breathing patients with intact gag reflexes. On inhalation, the one-way inspiratory valve opens, directing O_2 from a reservoir bag into the mask. On exhalation, gas exits the mask through the one-way expiratory valves and enters the atmosphere. The patient breathes air only from the bag. (See *Nonrebreather mask.*)

Procedure

To prepare the mask:
- Attach tubing to the O_2 source and adjust to the desired O_2 flow rate, which should be 12 to 15 L/minute.
- Choose a face mask size that fits from the bridge of the nose to the tip of the chin.
- Inflate the reservoir bag by occluding the outlet to the mask.
    To attach the mask:
- Mold the metal nose piece to conform to the bridge of the nose.
- Place the elastic strap over the patient's head and adjust the strap so that the mask fits comfortably and securely over the chin, cheeks, and nose; this prevents intake of room air, which will dilute O_2 concentration.

Key points

Understanding the nonrebreather mask

- Is a face mask with an O_2 reservoir
- Provides O_2 concentrations (60% to 90%)
- Directs O_2 from the reservoir bag into the mask via a one-way inspiratory valve
- Has one-way expiratory valves that direct gas out into the atmosphere

- Adjust the O_2 flow so the reservoir bag remains two-thirds inflated during inspiration and expiration, never completely collapsing.
- Don't allow the reservoir bag to kink.

Special considerations

- Varying O_2 concentration depending on the manufacturer's design, patient's respiratory pattern, O_2 flow rate, proper fit of the mask, and removal of the one-way valve from side exhalation ports
- Possible rebreathing of accumulated CO_2 due to an inhalation valve malfunction or kink in the bag
- Can be uncomfortable and hot
- Must be removed for the patient to eat, talk, or expectorate
- Increased risk of aspiration

Simple mask

A simple face mask, also called a basic face mask, is a low-flow system that allows O_2 to enter through a bottom port and exit through side holes. The face mask is capable of delivering 40% to 60% humidified O_2 concentrations to patients with adequate spontaneous respiration for short periods of time. Air is exhaled through holes in the side of the mask.

The face mask comes in various standard sizes for the adult and pediatric face with an adjustable strap to assist with proper fit.

Equipment needed

- Face mask
- O_2 tubing
- O_2 source

Procedure

To prepare the mask:

- Attach tubing to the O_2 source and adjust to the desired flow rate (ideal flow rate is 8 to 10 L/minute with a minimum of 5 L/minute).
- Choose a face mask size that fits from the bridge of nose to the tip of the chin.
    To attach the mask:
- Mold the metal nose piece to conform to the bridge of the nose.
- Place the elastic strap over the patient's head and adjust the strap so that the mask fits comfortably and securely over the chin, cheeks, and nose; this prevents the intake of room air that will dilute O_2 concentration.
- Pad with gauze to promote an airtight seal if the seal can't be secure due to facial contour.

Key points

Understanding the simple mask

- Low-flow system that allows O_2 to enter through a bottom port and exit through side holes
- Capable of delivering 40% to 60% humidified O_2 concentrations

Venturi mask

This illustration shows the components of the Venturi mask.

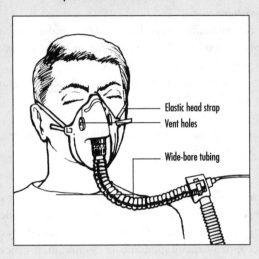

- Elastic head strap
- Vent holes
- Wide-bore tubing

Special considerations
■ Potential for improper fitting due to generic standard sizes, which can cause dilution of the O_2 concentration delivered
■ Potential for air to enter and dilute the O_2 concentration delivered if improperly placed
■ Varying delivered O_2 concentration depending on the flow rate and the patient's respirations
■ Covering the mouth or nose may make the patient feel like he's suffocating
■ Removal necessary to allow the patient to eat, drink, or expectorate
■ Increased risk of aspiration

Venturi mask

The Venturi mask is a face mask designed to mix room air with O_2. It allows varying percentages of O_2 to be administered at a constant concentration of 24% to 50%, regardless of the patient's respiratory rate. (See *Venturi mask*.)

The Venturi mask increases the spontaneous breathing efficiency of patients with chronic lung disease and does so without drying mucous mem-

Key points

Understanding the Venturi mask

■ Designed to mix room air with O_2
■ Allows varying percentages of O_2 to be administered at a constant concentration of 24% to 50%, regardless of the patient's respiratory rate

branes. A wide-bore flexible tube attaches between the adapters and the mask, allowing inhaled O_2 and room air to mix. The mask has a perforated cuff that allows exhaled air to flow into the atmosphere. Adapters can change the size of the orifice and O_2 flow.

Equipment needed
- Venturi mask
- Color-coded adapter
- Flexible tubing
- O_2 source

Procedure
To prepare the mask:
- Attach the appropriate color-coded adapter to the flexible tube, and then attach the O_2 source.
- Turn the O_2 flowmeter to the prescribed rate, initially 24% O_2 concentration at 3 L/minute flow.
- Check that flow is occurring.
    To attach the mask:
- Position the mask on the patient's face, adjusting the elastic strap as necessary.
- Add a humidification hood, if indicated, to protect the air entrapment ports and provide humidified oxygenation.

Special considerations
- Maintain a good seal for proper delivery of O_2 concentration
- Altered O_2 delivery concentration if intake ports obstructed
- Removal necessary to allow patient to eat, drink, or expectorate

Test your knowledge

Take the following quiz to test your knowledge of airway management.

1. Without oxygen, irreversible brain damage occurs within:

A. 45 seconds.
B. 5 minutes.
C. 10 minutes.
D. 20 minutes.

Correct answer: B

Irreversible brain damage occurs within 5 minutes without oxygenation. Brain cell death occurs within 10 minutes.

2. Which is the preferred method for opening the airway of an unconscious patient who may have suffered a neck injury?

    A. Head-tilt, chin-lift
    B. Chin-lift
    C. Jaw-thrust, chin-lift
    D. Jaw-thrust

Correct answer: D

The jaw-thrust maneuver is the preferred method for opening an airway in an unconscious patient, especially if a neck injury is suspected.

3. After performing endotracheal (ET) intubation, you auscultate the patient's chest. You find that breath sounds aren't audible. Based on this finding, you've most likely:

    A. intubated the esophagus.
    B. intubated the left mainstem bronchus.
    C. intubated the right mainstem bronchus.
    D. wedged the tube against the carina.

Correct answer: A

If breath sounds aren't audible after ET intubation, you've most likely intubated the patient's esophagus. Remove the tube and oxygenate the patient with 100% oxygen for 1 minute and then reattempt ET intubation.

4. The preferred tidal volume when delivering bag-valve device ventilation is:

    A. 5 to 10 ml/kg.
    B. 7 to 10 ml/kg.
    C. 10 to 15 ml/kg.
    D. 15 to 20 ml/kg.

Correct answer: C

A tidal volume of 10 to 15 ml/kg with the bag-valve device will adequately inflate the average person's lungs.

5. A bag-valve device without a reservoir has an oxygen (O_2) delivery concentration of 50%. With a reservoir, the O_2 concentration increases to:

    A. 65%.
    B. 75%.
    C. 85%.
    D. just under 100%.

Correct answer: D

O$_2$ concentration increases from 50% without a reservoir to nearly 100% with a reservoir. For that reason, a bag-valve device should include a reservoir.

6. When using a laryngoscope and straight blade for intubation, place the tip of the blade:

A. under the tongue.
B. under the epiglottis.
C. into the vallecula.
D. through the vocal cords.

Correct answer: B

The tip of the straight blade is inserted under the epiglottis to elevate it anteriorly and expose the glottic opening. The curved blade is inserted into the vallecula.

7. The most common cause of airway obstruction is:

A. food.
B. the patient's tongue.
C. small toys.
D. false teeth.

Correct answer: B

The tongue is the most common cause of airway obstruction. As the neck muscles of a person relax, the tongue may slide into the airway causing an obstruction. If the person is unconscious, the tongue loses muscle tone and muscles of the lower jaw relax, allowing the tongue to remain in an obstructed position.

8. Cricoid pressure is used to:

A. prevent vomiting.
B. displace the trachea posteriorly.
C. compress the trachea.
D. displace the tongue.

Correct answer: B

Cricoid pressure technique involves applying pressure to the cricoid cartilage in order to displace the trachea posteriorly. This prevents gastric inflation, thereby reducing the risk of vomiting and aspiration.

9. For proper assessment of breathing, the victim should be:

A. lying on the left side.
B. lying on the right side.
C. in a supine position.
D. in a prone position.

Correct answer: C

For effective assessment of breathing, the victim must be in a supine position and on a flat surface.

10. A potential complication of using the bag-valve device may be:

A. facial injury.
B. ventricular fibrillation.
C. dry mucous membranes.
D. pneumothorax.

Correct answer: D

Squeezing the bag-valve device too hard or too rapidly may cause a pneumo-thorax.

Cardiac arrhythmia recognition

Contraction of the heart, prompted by the heart's conduction system, causes blood to move throughout the body. When there's a disturbance in conduction—called a cardiac arrhythmia—blood flow is interrupted and the entire body may be placed in jeopardy. Therefore, early recognition and treatment of cardiac arrhythmias is essential.

This chapter briefly discusses normal cardiac conduction and explains how to apply cardiac rhythm monitoring devices. It then lists life-threatening cardiac arrhythmias and describes their characteristics so that you can identify them quickly and correctly.

Cardiac conduction

The cardiovascular system contains pacemaker cells, specialized cells that enable the heart to generate a precise rhythm. These cells have three unique characteristics:

- automaticity—the ability to generate an electrical impulse automatically
- conductivity—the ability to pass the impulse to the next cell
- contractility—the ability to shorten the fibers in the heart when receiving the impulse.

Cardiac conduction begins in the sinoatrial (SA) node and proceeds to the other elements of the cardiac conduction system. (See *Cardiac conduction system,* page 52.)

Sinoatrial node

The SA node, located on the endocardial surface of the right atrium near the superior vena cava, is the heart's normal pacemaker. Under normal conditions, the SA node generates an impulse 60 to 100 times per minute. The SA node's firing spreads an impulse throughout the right and left atria, resulting in atrial contraction.

Atrioventricular node

The atrioventricular (AV) node, situated low in the septal wall of the right atrium, slows the impulse conduction between the atria and ventricles. This "resistor" node provides time for the contracting atria to fill the ventricles with blood before the lower chambers contract.

Key points

Cardiac conduction
- SA node—normal pacemaker
- AV node—impulse conduction
- AV node will generate impulse if SA node fails.
- Ventricles will generate impulse if SA and AV nodes fail.

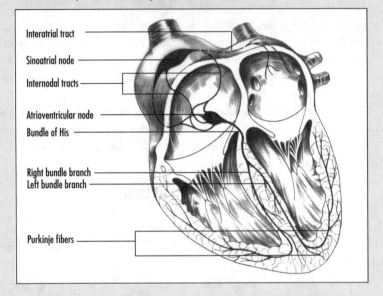

Cardiac conduction system

Each electrical impulse travels from the sinoatrial node through the internodal and interatrial tracts, producing atrial contraction. The impulse slows momentarily as it passes through the atrioventricular junction to the bundle of His. Then, it descends the left and right bundle branches and reaches the Purkinje fibers, stimulating ventricular contraction.

Interatrial tract
Sinoatrial node
Internodal tracts
Atrioventricular node
Bundle of His
Right bundle branch
Left bundle branch
Purkinje fibers

From the AV node to the myocardium

From the AV node, the impulse travels to the bundle of His (modified muscle fibers), branching off to right and left bundles. Then the impulse travels to the Purkinje fibers, the distal portions of the left and right bundle branches. These fibers fan across the surface of the ventricles from the endocardium to the myocardium. As the impulse spreads, it signals the blood-filled ventricles to contract.

Safety mechanisms

The conduction system has two built-in safety mechanisms. If the SA node fails to fire, the AV node will generate an impulse 40 to 60 times per minute. If the SA node and AV node both fail, the ventricles can generate their own impulse 20 to 40 times per minute.

Abnormal impulses

Abnormal impulse conduction occurs from disturbances in automaticity, conduction, or both.

Automaticity can increase or decrease. Tachycardia, for instance, commonly is caused by an increase in the automaticity of pacemaker cells below the SA node. Likewise, a decrease in the automaticity of cells in the SA node can cause the development of bradycardia or an escape rhythm.

Conduction may occur too quickly, as in Wolff-Parkinson-White (WPW) syndrome, or too slowly, as in AV block. An example of a combined automaticity and conduction disturbance is atrial tachycardia with a 4:1 block.

Monitoring and interpreting cardiac rhythms

An electrocardiogram (ECG) is used to monitor the precise sequence of electrical events occurring in the cardiac cycle. There are two types of ECG recordings, the 12-lead and the single lead, commonly known as a rhythm strip. Using an ECG, you can observe an ECG complex, the electrical events occurring in one cardiac cycle. An ECG complex consists of five waveforms, labeled with the letters P, Q, R, S, and T. The middle three letters — Q, R, and S — are referred to as a unit, the QRS complex. (See *ECG waveform components,* page 54.)

Identifying cardiac arrhythmias is typically done by recognizing their effects on the ECG waveform. However, ECG interpretation doesn't replace the need for keen assessment skills. Always remember that ECG findings should correlate with the patient's physical condition.

Applying monitoring devices

An ECG monitor is a tool that provides continuous information about the heart's electrical activity. Electrodes applied to the patient's chest pick up the heart's electrical activity for display on the monitor.

Commonly monitored leads include three bipolar leads — I, II, and III — and MCL_1 and MCL_6, which are modified versions of the leads V_1 and V_6.

To ensure accurate lead monitoring, you must apply the electrodes correctly. A three-, four-, or five-electrode system may be used for cardiac monitoring. First, prepare the skin by briskly rubbing each site until the skin reddens. Clip any dense hair present at each site. Remove the backing from the electrodes and apply one electrode to each prepared site by pressing it against the patient's skin. Then attach leadwires or cable connections by clipping or snapping them to the electrode. Turn on the monitor. Select the lead you wish to view following the monitor's instructions. (See *Using a five-leadwire system,* page 55.)

Interpreting rhythm strips: The eight-step method

You can learn to analyze and interpret ECGs systematically and correctly by following an eight-step method. Begin by scanning the entire strip and identifying the waveform components. Then follow these steps.

ECG waveform components

An electrocardiogram (ECG) waveform has three basic components: the P wave, the QRS complex, and the T wave. These elements can be further divided into the PR interval, J point, ST segment, U wave, and QT interval.

P wave and PR interval

The P wave represents atrial depolarization. The PR interval represents the time it takes an impulse to travel from the atria through the atrioventricular nodes and the bundle of His. The PR interval measures from the beginning of the P wave to the beginning of the QRS complex.

QRS complex

The QRS complex represents ventricular depolarization—the time it takes for the impulse to travel through the bundle branches to the Purkinje fibers.

The Q wave appears as the first negative deflection in the QRS complex; the R wave, as the first positive deflection. The S wave appears as the second negative deflection or the first negative deflection after the R wave.

J point and ST segment

Marking the end of the QRS complex, the J point also indicates the beginning of the ST segment. The ST segment represents part of ventricular repolarization.

T wave and U wave

Usually following the same deflection pattern as the P wave, the T wave represents ventricular repolarization. The U wave follows the T wave but, because it signifies a problem, it isn't seen in most patients.

QT interval

The QT interval represents ventricular depolarization and repolarization. It extends from the beginning of the QRS complex to the end of the T wave.

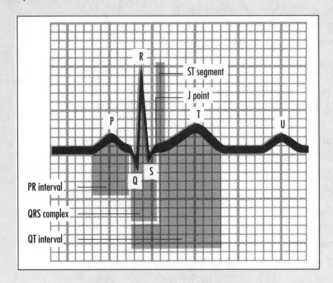

Step 1: Determine the rhythm.

To determine the heart's atrial and ventricular rhythms, use either the paper-and-pencil method or the calipers method. (See *Methods of determining rhythm*, page 56.) Then ask yourself, "Does the rhythm appear to be regular or irregular?"

Using a five-leadwire system

This illustration shows the correct placement of leadwires for a five-leadwire system. The chest electrode shown is located in the V, position, but you can place it in any of the chest-lead positions.

The electrodes are typically color-coded as follows:
- white — right arm (RA)
- black — left arm (LA)
- green — right leg (RL)
- red — left leg (LL)
- brown — chest (C).

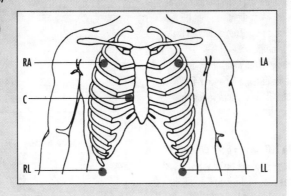

Step 2: Determine the rate.

Next, calculate the heart's atrial and ventricular rates, using the times ten method, the 1,500 method, or the sequence method. (See *Calculating the heart rate*, page 57.)

Determine if the rate is within normal limits (60 to 100 beats/minute). Then determine if the atrial (P-P interval) rate and ventricular (R-R interval) rate are continually the same measurement. Then determine if they're associated with each other.

Step 3: Evaluate the P wave.

Look at the rhythm strip and ask these questions:
- Are P waves present?
- Do the P waves have a normal shape (usually upright and rounded)?
- Are the P waves similar in size and shape?
- Do all of the P waves point in the same direction? Are they all upright, inverted, or diphasic?
- Is there a one-to-one relationship between P waves and QRS complexes?
- Is the distance between each P wave and its QRS complex the same?

Step 4: Determine the duration of the PR interval.

When you've determined the duration of the PR interval (normal duration is 0.12 to 0.20 second), determine if the PR interval is constant.

Methods of determining rhythm

To determine the heart's atrial and ventricular rhythms, use either the paper-and-pencil method or the calipers method.

Paper-and-pencil method

To use the paper-and-pencil method, place the electrocardiogram (ECG) strip on a flat surface; then position the straight edge of a piece of paper along the strip's baseline. Now move the paper up slightly so that the edge is near the peaks of the P waves. With a pencil, make dots on the paper at the first two P waves—the P-P interval.

Now move the paper across the strip from left to right, lining up the two dots with succeeding P-P intervals. If the distance for each P-P interval is the same, the atrial rhythm is regular. If the distance varies, the rhythm is irregular.

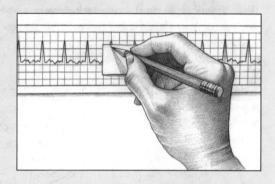

Calipers method

To use the calipers method, begin with the ECG strip on a flat surface. Place one point of the ECG calipers on the peak of the first P wave. Adjust the caliper legs so the other point is on the peak of the next P wave; this distance is the P-P interval. Now move the calipers, placing the first point on the peak of the second P wave. Note whether the other point is on the peak of the third P wave. Check the succeeding P-P intervals in this manner. If all the intervals are the same, the atrial rhythm is regular. If the intervals vary, the rhythm is irregular.

Using the same method, measure the R-R intervals of consecutive QRS complexes to determine whether the ventricular rhythm is regular or irregular.

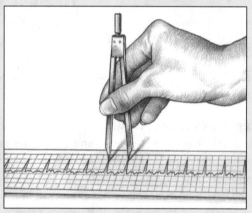

Step 5: Determine the duration of the QRS complex.

Look at the rhythm strip again and ask these questions:
- Are all the QRS complexes the same size and shape?
- What's the duration of the QRS complex? (Normal duration is 0.06 to 0.10 second.)
- Are all the QRS complexes the same distance from the T waves that follow them?
- Do all the QRS complexes point in the same direction?
- Are there any QRS complexes that appear to be different from the others on the strip? (If so, measure and describe each one individually.)

Step 6: Evaluate the T wave.

Examine the strip once more and ask these questions:
- Are T waves present?
- Do all the T waves have the same size and shape?

Calculating the heart rate

You can use one of three methods — the times ten method; the 1,500 method; or the sequence method — to determine atrial and ventricular heart rates from an electrocardiogram waveform.

Times ten method

The simplest, quickest, and most common technique, the times ten method is particularly useful if the patient's heart rhythm is irregular. Begin by obtaining a 6-second strip. Then count the number of P waves (to determine atrial rate) or R waves (to determine ventricular rate). Multiply by 10.

1,500 method

Use the 1,500 method only if the patient's heart rhythm is regular. First, identify two consecutive P waves on the rhythm strip. Next, select identical points in each wave and count the number of small squares between the points. Then divide 1,500 by the number of small squares counted (because 1,500 small squares equal 1 minute) to get the atrial rate. To calculate the ventricular rate, use the same procedure but with two consecutive R waves instead of P waves.

Sequence method

The sequence method gives you an estimated heart rate. First, find a P wave that peaks on a heavy black line. Assign the following numbers to the next six heavy black lines: 300, 150, 100, 75, 60, and 50, respectively.

   Then find the next P wave peak and estimate the atrial rate based on the number assigned to the nearest heavy black line. Estimate the ventricular rate following the same procedure but use the R wave instead of the P wave.

- Could a P wave be hidden in a T wave?
- Do the T waves point in the same direction as the QRS complexes?

Step 7: Determine the duration of the QT interval.

Note whether the duration of the QT interval falls within normal limits (0.36 to 0.44 second or 9 to 11 small squares).

Step 8: Evaluate any other components.

Finally, observe any other components on the ECG strip, including ectopic or aberrantly conducted beats and other abnormalities. Check the ST segment for any abnormalities, and look for a U wave. Note your findings.

Recognizing normal sinus rhythm

Before you can recognize an arrhythmia, you first need to be able to recognize normal sinus rhythm. Normal sinus rhythm records an impulse that starts in the sinus node and progresses to the ventricles through a normal conduction pathway — from the sinus node to the atria and AV node, through the bundle of His, to the bundle branches, and on to the Purkinje

Key points

Normal sinus rhythm
- Atrial and ventricular rhythms regular
- Atrial and ventricular rates 60 to 100 beats/minute
- PR interval 0.12 to 0.20 second
- QRS complex 0.06 to 0.10 second
- T wave upright and rounded
- QT interval 0.36 to 0.44 second

fibers. Normal sinus rhythm is the standard against which all other rhythms are compared.

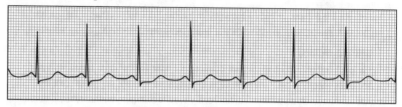

Interpretation

Rhythm. Atrial and ventricular rhythms are regular.

Rate. Atrial and ventricular rates are 60 to 100 beats/minute.

P wave. Normally shaped (upright and rounded). All P waves are similar in size and shape. There's a P wave for every QRS complex.

PR interval. Within normal limits (0.12 to 0.20 second).

QRS complex. Within normal limits (0.06 to 0.10 second).

T wave. Normally shaped (upright and rounded).

QT interval. Within normal limits (0.36 to 0.44 second).

Recognizing narrow complex tachycardias

Narrow complex tachycardias are arrhythmias that involve an accelerated heart rate and a narrow QRS complex. They include sinus tachycardia, atrial fibrillation, atrial flutter, atrial tachycardia, multifocal atrial tachycardia, WPW syndrome, and junctional tachycardia.

Sinus tachycardia

Sinus tachycardia is an acceleration of the firing of the SA node beyond its normal discharge rate, resulting in a heart rate of 100 to 160 beats/minute. Rates greater than 160 beats/minute may indicate ectopic focus. Persistent sinus tachycardia, especially with acute myocardial infarction (MI) may lead to ischemia and myocardial damage by raising oxygen requirements.

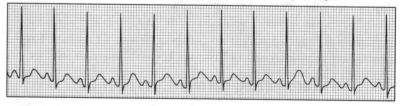

Interpretation

Rhythm. Atrial and ventricular rhythms are regular.

Rate. Atrial and ventricular rates are greater than 100 beats/minute (usually between 100 and 160 beats/minute).

Key points

Sinus tachycardia
- Atrial and ventricular rhythms regular
- Atrial and ventricular rates greater than 100 beats/minute
- PR interval normal
- QRS complex normal

Treatment
- Correction of underlying cause

P wave. Normal size and configuration. P wave precedes each QRS complex.

PR interval. Within normal limits and constant.

QRS complex. Normal duration and configuration.

T wave. Normal size and configuration.

QT interval. Within normal limits but commonly shortened.

Possible causes

- Caffeine, nicotine, and alcohol ingestion
- Digoxin toxicity
- Hypothyroidism and hyperthyroidism
- Normal cardiac response to demand for increased oxygen during exercise, fever, stress, pain, and dehydration
- Any other occurrence that decreases vagal tone and increases sympathetic tone
- May develop as a normal part of the inflammatory response after an MI (In acute MI, it may be one of the first signs of heart failure, cardiogenic shock, pulmonary embolism, or infarct extension.)
- Treatment with adrenergics, anticholinergics, and antiarrhythmics

Signs and symptoms

- Usually asymptomatic
- Rapid, regular pulse greater than 100 beats/minute
- Palpitations or angina caused by increased myocardial oxygen consumption and reduced coronary blood flow

Treatment

- Treatment aims to correct the underlying cause.
- If the patient is symptomatic, propranolol may be given.

Atrial fibrillation

Atrial fibrillation, sometimes called A-fib, is defined as chaotic, asynchronous, electrical activity in atrial tissue. It stems from the firing of a number of impulses in reentry pathways. Like atrial flutter, atrial fibrillation results in a loss of atrial kick. The ectopic impulses may fire at a rate of 400 to 600 times/minute, causing the atria to quiver instead of contract.

The ventricles respond only to those impulses that make it through the AV node. On an ECG, atrial activity is no longer represented by P waves but by erratic baseline waves called fibrillatory waves or f waves. This rhythm may be either sustained or paroxysmal (occurring in bursts). It can be proceeded by or the result of premature atrial contractions (PACs).

Key points

Atrial fibrillation
- Atrial and ventricular rhythms grossly irregular
- Atrial rate exceeds 400 beats/minute; ventricular rate 40 to 250 beats/minute
- P wave absent

Treatment
- Synchronized cardioversion (100 to 200 joules initially), if unstable
- Esmolol I.V. and calcium channel blockers, such as diltiazem and verapamil
- In patients with impaired heart function, either digoxin, diltiazem, or amiodarone

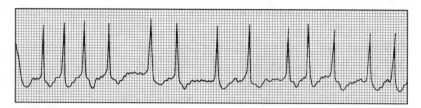

Interpretation

Rhythm. Atrial and ventricular rhythms are grossly irregular.

Rate. The atrial rate (almost indiscernible) usually exceeds 400 beats/minute. The ventricular rate usually varies from 40 to 250 beats/minute.

P wave. Absent. Erratic baseline f waves appear instead. Those chaotic f waves represent atrial tetanization from rapid atrial depolarizations.

PR interval. Indiscernible.

QT interval. Unmeasurable.

Other. The patient may develop an atrial rhythm that frequently varies between a fibrillatory line and flutter waves. This is called atrial fib-flutter.

Possible causes

- Rheumatic heart disease, valvular disorders (especially mitral stenosis), hypertension, MI, coronary artery disease (CAD), heart failure, cardiomyopathy, and pericarditis
- Thyrotoxicosis
- Chronic obstructive pulmonary disease (COPD)
- Drugs such as digoxin
- Cardiac surgery
- Increased sympathetic activity from exercise (occasionally)

Signs and symptoms

- Irregular pulse rhythm with a normal or rapid rate; peripheral pulse often slower than apical pulse
- Signs and symptoms of decreased cardiac output (if ventricular rate is rapid)

Treatment

- If the patient is hemodynamically unstable, synchronized cardioversion (100 to 200 joules initially) should be administered immediately.
- In patients with otherwise normal heart function, administer esmolol I.V. and a calcium channel blocker, such as diltiazem or verapamil, to control ventricular rate.
- In patients with impaired heart function (heart failure or ejection fraction less than 40%), use either digoxin, diltiazem, or amiodarone to control the ventricular rate.

Atrial flutter

Atrial flutter is a supraventricular tachycardia (SVT) characterized by an atrial rate of 250 to 400 beats/minute, though it's generally around 300 beats/minute. Originating in a single atrial focus, this rhythm results from reentry and, possibly, increased automaticity. The significance of atrial flutter depends on the extent to which the ventricular rate is accelerated. The faster this rate, the more dangerous the arrhythmia. Even a small rise in the rate can cause angina, syncope, hypotension, heart failure, and pulmonary edema.

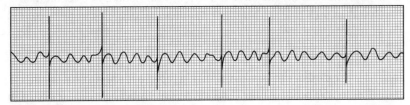

Interpretation

Rhythm. Atrial rhythm is regular. Ventricular rhythm depends on the AV conduction pattern; it's often regular, although cycles may alternate. An irregular pattern may herald atrial fibrillation or indicate a block.

Rate. Atrial rate is 250 to 400 beats/minute. Ventricular rate depends on the degree of AV block; usually it's 60 to 100 beats/minute, but it may accelerate to 125 to 150 beats/minute.

P wave. Saw-toothed or picket fence appearance.

PR interval. Unmeasurable.

QRS complex. Duration is usually within normal limits, but the complex may be widened if flutter waves are buried within.

T wave. Not identifiable.

QT interval. Unmeasurable.

Other. Atrial fib-flutter, a rhythm that frequently varies between a fibrillatory line and flutter waves, may appear.

Possible causes

■ Acute or chronic cardiac disorder, mitral or tricuspid valve disorder, cor pulmonale, and cardiac inflammation such as pericarditis
■ Transient complication of MI
■ Digoxin toxicity
■ Hyperthyroidism
■ Alcoholism
■ Cardiac surgery

Signs and symptoms

■ None or palpitations

■ Cardiac, cerebral, and peripheral vascular effects (if ventricular filling and coronary artery blood flow are compromised)

Treatment

■ If the patient is hemodynamically unstable, synchronized cardioversion (100 to 200 joules initially) should be administered immediately.

■ In patients with otherwise normal heart function, administer esmolol I.V. and a calcium channel blocker, such as diltiazem or verapamil, to control ventricular rate.

■ In patients with impaired heart function (heart failure or ejection fraction less than 40%), use either digoxin, diltiazem, or amiodarone to control the ventricular rate.

Atrial tachycardia

In atrial tachycardia, the atrial rhythm is ectopic, and the atrial rate ranges from 150 to 250 beats/minute. This arrhythmia is benign when it occurs in a healthy person; however, it can be dangerous when it occurs in a patient with an existing cardiac disorder.

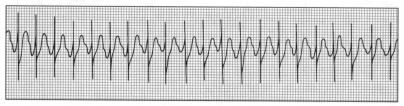

Interpretation

Rhythm. Atrial and ventricular rhythms are regular.

Rate. The atrial rate is characterized by three or more successive ectopic atrial beats at a rate of 150 to 250 beats/minute. The rate rarely exceeds 250 beats/minute. The ventricular rate depends on the AV conduction ratio.

P wave. Usually positive, the P wave may be aberrant, invisible, or hidden in the previous T wave. If visible, it precedes each QRS complex.

PR interval. May be unmeasurable if the P wave can't be distinguished from the preceding T wave.

QRS complex. Duration and configuration are usually normal.

T wave. Usually distinguishable but may be distorted by the P wave.

QT interval. Usually within normal limits but may be shorter because of the rapid rate.

Possible causes

■ Digoxin toxicity (the most common cause)

■ Primary cardiac disorders, such as MI, cardiomyopathy, pericarditis, valvular heart disease, and WPW syndrome

■ Secondary cardiac problems, such as hyperthyroidism, cor pulmonale, and systemic hypertension
■ COPD
■ In healthy persons: physical or psychological stress, hypoxia, hypokalemia, excessive use of caffeine or other stimulants, and use of marijuana

Signs and symptoms
■ Rapid apical or peripheral pulse rates
■ Signs and symptoms of decreased cardiac output, such as hypotension, syncope, and blurred vision

Treatment
■ Attempt vagal stimulation.
■ Administer adenosine.

Multifocal atrial tachycardia
Multifocal atrial tachycardia results from an extremely rapid firing of multifocal ectopic sites. Very rare in healthy individuals, this arrhythmia is usually found in acutely ill patients with pulmonary disease or elevated atrial pressures.

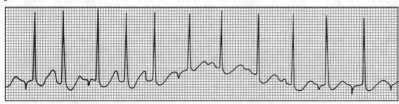

Interpretation
Rhythm. Atrial and ventricular rhythms are irregular.
Rate. Atrial and ventricular rates range from 100 to 250 beats/minute.
P wave. Configuration varies, usually with at least three unique P waves.
PR interval. Varies.
QRS complex. Duration and configuration are usually normal but may become aberrant if the arrhythmia persists.
T wave. Usually distorted.
QT interval. May be indiscernible.

Possible causes
■ Atrial distention from elevated pulmonary pressure, usually seen in patients with COPD

Signs and symptoms
■ Palpitations
■ Rapid apical or peripheral pulse rates

Key points

Multifocal atrial tachycardia
■ Atrial and ventricular rhythms irregular
■ Atrial and ventricular rates 100 to 250 beats/minute
■ Varying P wave configuration
■ Varying PR interval

Treatment
■ Calcium channel blocker (verapamil or diltiazem) or beta-adrenergic blocker along with digoxin
■ In a patient with impaired left ventricular function: diltiazem, amiodarone, and digoxin

■ Signs and symptoms of decreased cardiac output, such as blurred vision, syncope, and hypotension

Treatment

■ First, distinguish multifocal atrial tachycardia from atrial fibrillation because both may cause an irregularly irregular rhythm.

■ In the patient with an otherwise healthy heart, administer a calcium channel blocker (verapamil or diltiazem) or beta-adrenergic blocker as well as digoxin to control the ventricular rate.

■ In the patient with impaired left ventricular function, administer either diltiazem, amiodarone, or digoxin.

Wolff-Parkinson-White syndrome

WPW syndrome occurs when an anomalous atrial bypass tract (bundle of Kent) develops outside the AV junction, connecting the atria and the ventricles. This pathway can conduct impulses either to the ventricles or to the atria. With retrograde conduction, reentry can arise, resulting in a re-entrant tachycardia. Usually WPW syndrome is considered insignificant if tachycardia doesn't occur or if the patient has no associated cardiac disease. When tachycardia does occur in WPW syndrome, decreased cardiac output may develop.

Most likely congenital in origin, WPW syndrome occurs predominantly in young children and in adults ages 20 to 35.

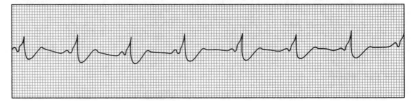

Interpretation

Rhythm. Atrial and ventricular rhythms are regular.

Rate. Atrial and ventricular rates are within normal limits, except when SVT occurs.

P wave. Normal in size and configuration.

PR interval. Short (less than 0.12 second).

QRS complex. Duration greater than 0.10 second. Beginning of the QRS complex may be slurred, producing a delta wave, the hallmark of WPW.

ST segment. Usually normal but may go in a direction opposite the QRS complex.

QT interval. Usually within normal limits.

T wave. Usually normal but may be deflected in a direction opposite the QRS complex.

Key points

Wolff-Parkinson-White (WPW) syndrome

■ Delta wave (the hallmark of WPW)

■ Atrial and ventricular rhythms regular

■ Atrial and ventricular rates within normal limits, except when SVT occurs

■ PR interval less than 0.12 second

■ QRS complex greater than 0.10 second

Treatment

■ Adenosine I.V.

■ Esmolol I.V.

Other. The delta wave is the hallmark of WPW syndrome. The syndrome may develop abrupt episodes of premature SVT, atrial fibrillation, and atrial flutter with a rate as fast as 300 beats/minute.

Possible causes
■ Most likely congenital in origin

Signs and symptoms
■ Usually none
■ If tachyarrhythmias develop with a high ventricular response: palpitations, possible syncope, sudden-onset chest pain, and shortness of breath

Treatment
■ Administer adenosine I.V.
■ Administer esmolol I.V.

Junctional tachycardia

Junctional tachycardia, considered an SVT, is three or more premature junctional contractions occurring in a row. This happens when an irritable focus from the AV junction has enhanced automaticity and overrides the SA node to function as the heart's pacemaker. The atria are depolarized by means of retrograde conduction, and conduction through the ventricles is normal. Usually the rate measures between 100 and 200 beats/minute.

The significance of this arrhythmia depends on the rate, the underlying cause, and the severity of the accompanying cardiac disease. At higher ventricular rates, junctional tachycardia may compromise cardiac output by affecting ventricular filling.

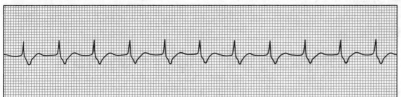

Interpretation
Rhythm. Atrial and ventricular rhythms are usually regular. The atrial rhythm may be difficult to determine if the P wave is absent or hidden in the QRS complex or preceding T wave.
Rate. Atrial and ventricular rates exceed 100 beats/minute (usually between 100 and 200 beats/minute). Atrial rate may be difficult to determine if the P wave is absent or hidden in the QRS complex or if it precedes the T wave.
P wave. Usually inverted. It may occur before or after the QRS complex, be hidden in the QRS complex, or be absent.

Key points

Junctional tachycardia
■ Atrial and ventricular rhythms usually regular
■ Atrial and ventricular rates usually between 100 and 200 beats/minute
■ P wave usually inverted, hidden, or absent
■ If P wave precedes the QRS complex, PR interval less than 0.12 second; otherwise unmeasurable

Treatment
■ Discontinuation of digoxin therapy
■ I.V. amiodarone, beta-adrenergic blockers, or calcium channel blockers

PR interval. If the P wave precedes the QRS complex, the PR interval is shortened (less than 0.12 second); otherwise, the PR interval can't be measured.

QRS complex. Duration within normal limits; configuration is usually normal.

T wave. Usually normal configuration but may be abnormal if the P wave is hidden in the T wave. Fast rate may make T wave indiscernible.

QT interval. Usually within normal limits.

Possible causes

- Digoxin toxicity (most common cause)
- Cardiomyopathy
- Enhanced automaticity
- Hypoxia
- Inferior wall MI and ischemia
- Myocarditis
- Vagal stimulation
- Valve replacement surgery

Signs and symptoms

- Pulse rate greater than 100 beats/minute
- Usually asymptomatic if the patient can compensate
- Possibly signs and symptoms of decreased cardiac output if compensation is poor

Treatment

- Discontinue digoxin therapy.
- Administer I.V. amiodarone, beta-adrenergic blockers, or calcium channel blockers.

Recognizing wide complex tachycardias

Wide complex tachycardias are arrhythmias that involve an accelerated heart rate and a wide QRS complex. They include premature ventricular contractions (PVCs), monomorphic ventricular tachycardia, polymorphic ventricular tachycardia, torsades de pointes, and ventricular fibrillation.

Premature ventricular contractions

PVCs are ectopic beats originating low in the ventricles that occur earlier than one would normally expect. PVCs may occur singly, in pairs, or in threes; in many cases they're followed by a compensatory pause. PVCs that occur every other beat are known as bigeminy; those that occur every third beat are known as trigeminy. PVCs may be uniform, arising from the same ectopic focus, or they may be multiform, arising from different ventricular

---

Key points

Premature ventricular contractions (PVCs)

- Atrial and ventricular rhythms irregular; underlying rhythm possibly regular
- P wave usually absent in the ectopic beat but may appear after the QRS complex
- PR interval unmeasurable, except in the underlying rhythm
- QRS complex duration greater than 0.12 second with bizarre configuration
- Compensatory pause possible after T wave

Treatment

- Correction of electrolyte imbalance
- Procainamide, amiodarone, or sotalol, if symptomatic

When PVCs spell danger

Here are some examples of patterns of dangerous premature ventricular contractions (PVCs).

Paired PVCs

Two PVCs in a row are called a pair, or couplet (see highlighted areas). A pair can produce ventricular tachycardia because the second contraction usually meets refractory tissue. A salvo—three or more PVCs in a row—is considered a run of ventricular tachycardia.

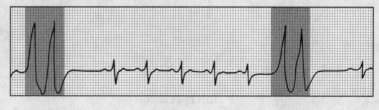

Multiform PVCs

PVCs that look different from one another arise from different sites or from the same site with abnormal conduction (see highlighted areas). Multiform PVCs may indicate severe heart disease or digoxin toxicity.

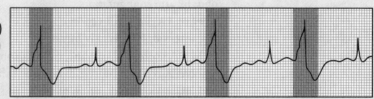

Bigeminy and trigeminy

PVCs that occur every other beat (bigeminy) or every third beat (trigeminy) can result in ventricular tachycardia or ventricular fibrillation (see highlighted areas).

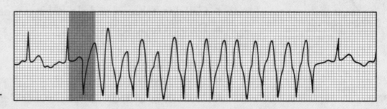

R-on-T phenomenon

In R-on-T phenomenon, the PVC occurs so early that it falls on the T wave of the preceding beat (see highlighted areas). Because the cells haven't fully repolarized, ventricular tachycardia or ventricular fibrillation can result.

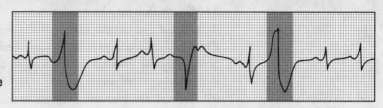

sites or from one site with changing patterns of conduction. (See *When PVCs spell danger*.)

The significance of this arrhythmia depends on how well the ventricle functions and how long the arrhythmia lasts. Cardiac output will diminish because of insufficient ventricular filling time.

Generally, PVCs are more serious if they occur in a patient with heart disease. In an ischemic or damaged heart, PVCs will more likely develop into ventricular tachycardia, flutter, or fibrillation.

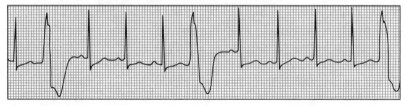

Interpretation

Rhythm. Atrial and ventricular rhythms are irregular during PVCs; the underlying rhythm may be regular.

Rate. Atrial and ventricular rates reflect underlying rhythm.

P wave. Usually absent in the ectopic beat but, with retrograde conduction to the atria, the P wave may appear after the QRS complex. Usually normal if present in underlying rhythm.

PR interval. Unmeasurable, except in the underlying rhythm.

QRS complex. Occurs earlier than expected; duration exceeds 0.12 second; bizarre configuration.

T wave. Occurs in direction opposite QRS complex.

QT interval. Not usually measured.

Other. A horizontal baseline, called a compensatory pause, may follow the T wave. A compensatory pause exists if the P-P interval encompassing the PVC has twice the duration of a normal sinus beat's P-P interval.

Possible causes

- Caffeine, tobacco, and alcohol ingestion
- Digoxin toxicity
- Exercise
- Hypocalcemia
- Hypokalemia
- Myocardial irritation by pacemaker electrodes or pulmonary artery catheter
- Myocardial ischemia and infarction
- Sympathomimetic drugs (such as epinephrine and isoproterenol)
- Proarrhythmic effect of antiarrhythmic agents

Signs and symptoms

- Possibly asymptomatic
- A longer-than-normal pause immediately after the premature beat
- Signs of decreased cardiac output if PVCs are frequent
- Palpitations

Treatment

■ Treatment is required only when PVCs are frequent or the patient has intolerable symptoms.
■ Administer oxygen.
■ Correct electrolyte imbalances.
■ Administer procainamide, amiodarone, or sotalol. Lidocaine may be administered as a second-choice drug.

Monomorphic ventricular tachycardia

Monomorphic ventricular tachycardia is the most common form of ventricular tachycardia. In this life-threatening arrhythmia, all of the QRS complexes are of the same morphology, indicating that they originate from the same location in the ventricles. Three or more PVCs occur in succession, at a rate of more than 100 beats/minute. The arrhythmia may be paroxysmal or sustained.

Because atrial and ventricular activity are dissociated and ventricular filling time is short, cardiac output may drop sharply. Monomorphic ventricular tachycardia may lead to ventricular fibrillation.

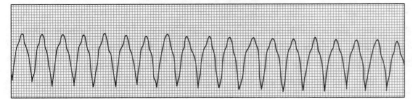

Interpretation

Rhythm. Atrial rhythm is unmeasurable. Ventricular rhythm is usually regular but may be slightly irregular.
Rate. Atrial rate is unmeasurable. Ventricular rate is usually rapid (100 to 250 beats/minute).
P wave. Usually absent. May be obscured by and is dissociated from the QRS complex. Retrograde and upright P waves may be present.
PR interval. Unmeasurable.
QRS complex. Duration greater than 0.12 second; bizarre appearance, usually with increased amplitude.
T wave. Occurs in opposite direction of QRS complex.
QT interval. Unmeasurable.

Possible causes

■ Usually caused by myocardial irritability and a circuit reentry, precipitated by a PVC or PAC that occurs in the vulnerable period of ventricular repolarization (R-on-T phenomenon)
■ Acute MI

- Cardiomyopathy
- CAD
- Drug toxicity
- Electrolyte imbalance
- Heart failure
- Mitral valve prolapse
- Pulmonary embolism
- Rheumatic heart disease

Signs and symptoms

- Possibly palpitations, dizziness, chest pain, and shortness of breath (if the patient is conscious)
- Signs and symptoms of low cardiac output
- Loss of consciousness and hemodynamic collapse

Treatment

- If the patient is stable and has otherwise normal cardiac function, administer procainamide or sotalol. If you're unable to administer procainamide or sotalol, administer amiodarone or lidocaine.
- If the patient is stable but has impaired left ventricular function, such as an ejection fraction less than 40% or heart failure, administer amiodarone or lidocaine, and then administer synchronized cardioversion.
- If the patient is unstable, prepare for immediate cardioversion. If pulseless ventricular tachycardia persists, administer epinephrine or vasopressin. Then resume attempts at defibrillation and consider other antiarrhythmics such as amiodarone.

Polymorphic ventricular tachycardia

Polymorphic ventricular tachycardia is a form of ventricular tachycardia in which the QRS complex morphology is unstable and continually varies because the site of origin changes throughout the ventricle. Polymorphic ventricular tachycardia is associated with a poorer prognosis than monomorphic ventricular tachycardia.

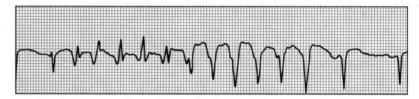

Interpretation

Rhythm. Atrial rhythm is unmeasurable. Ventricular rhythm is irregular.

Rate. Atrial rate is unmeasurable. Ventricular rate is usually rapid (100 to 250 beats/minute).

P wave. Absent.

PR interval. Unmeasurable.

QRS complex. Duration varies but is greater than 0.12 second; bizarre appearance; some may have increased amplitude.

T wave. Abnormal morphology.

QT interval. Within normal limits when the patient is in sinus rhythm.

Possible causes
- Acute MI
- CAD

Signs and symptoms
- Possibly palpitations, dizziness, chest pain, and shortness of breath (if the patient is conscious)
- Signs and symptoms of low cardiac output
- Loss of consciousness and hemodynamic collapse

Treatment
- Administer nitrates to treat ischemia, if present.
- Administer one of the following agents: beta-adrenergic blocker, lidocaine, amiodarone, procainamide, or sotalol.
- If cardiac function is impaired, administer amiodarone and then administer synchronized cardioversion.
- If the patient is unstable, prepare for defibrillation. If pulseless ventricular tachycardia persists, administer epinephrine or vasopressin. Then resume attempts at defibrillation and consider other antiarrhythmics such as amiodarone.

Torsades de pointes
A life-threatening arrhythmia, torsades de pointes is a polymorphic ventricular tachycardia characterized by prolonged QT interval and QRS polarity that seem to spiral around the isoelectric line. Any condition that causes a prolonged QT interval can also cause torsades de pointes.

Although the sinus rhythm sometimes resumes spontaneously, torsades de pointes usually degenerates to ventricular fibrillation.

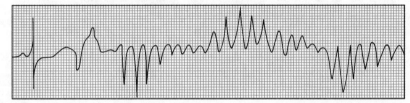

Key points

Torsades de pointes
- Atrial rhythm undetermined; ventricular rhythm regular or irregular
- Atrial rate undetermined; ventricular rate 150 to 250 beats/minute
- P wave unidentifiable
- PR interval absent
- QRS complex usually wide with a phasic variation in its electrical polarity
- ST segment indiscernible
- QT interval prolonged while patient is in sinus rhythm

Treatment
- Correction of any electrolyte imbalance
- Magnesium, isoproterenol, phenytoin, lidocaine
- Discontinuation of causative drug
- Defibrillation

Interpretation

Rhythm. Atrial rhythm can't be determined. Ventricular rhythm is regular or irregular.

Rate. Atrial rate can't be determined. Ventricular rate is 150 to 250 beats/minute.

P wave. Not identifiable because it's buried in the QRS complex.

PR interval. Not applicable because P wave can't be identified.

QRS complex. Usually wide with a phasic variation in its electrical polarity, shown by complexes that point downward for several beats and then turn upward for several beats and vice versa.

ST segment. Not discernible.

QT interval. Prolonged (indicating delayed ventricular repolarization) while the patient is in sinus rhythm.

Other. May be paroxysmal, starting and stopping suddenly.

Possible causes

- AV block
- Drug toxicity (particularly sotalol, quinidine, procainamide, and related antiarrhythmics such as disopyramide)
- Electrolyte imbalance (hypokalemia, hypocalcemia, and hypomagnesemia)
- Hereditary Q-T prolongation syndrome
- Myocardial ischemia
- Psychotropic drugs (phenothiazines and tricyclic antidepressants)
- SA disease that results in profound bradycardia

Signs and symptoms

- Possibly, palpitations, dizziness, chest pain, and shortness of breath if the patient is conscious
- Rapidly occurring signs or symptoms of low cardiac output, such as hypotension and altered consciousness
- If rapid and prolonged torsades de pointes, loss of consciousness, pulse, and respirations

Treatment

- If the patient is stable, correct the electrolyte imbalance, if present. Administer one of the following agents: magnesium, isoproterenol, phenytoin, or lidocaine. Overdrive pacing may be necessary.
- If torsades de pointes is being caused by a specific drug, discontinue the drug.

■ If torsades de pointes persists, administer defibrillation. Then administer epinephrine or vasopressin. Resume attempts at defibrillation and consider other antiarrhythmics such as amiodarone.

Ventricular fibrillation

Commonly called V-fib, ventricular fibrillation is a chaotic pattern of electrical activity in the ventricles in which electrical impulses arise from many different foci. It produces no effective muscular contraction and no cardiac output. If fibrillation continues, it eventually leads to ventricular asystole. Ventricular fibrillation is responsible for most sudden cardiac deaths in people outside of a hospital.

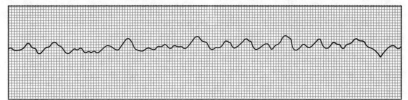

Interpretation

Rhythm. Atrial rhythm is unmeasurable. Ventricular rhythm has no pattern or regularity.

Rate. Atrial and ventricular rates are unmeasurable.

P wave. Absent.

PR interval. Unmeasurable.

QRS complex. Duration unmeasurable.

T wave. Unmeasurable.

QT interval. Unmeasurable.

Other. Coarse fibrillation indicates more electrical activity in the ventricles than fine fibrillation, and it's easier to convert. The f waves become finer as acidosis and hypoxemia develop.

Possible causes

■ Myocardial ischemia
■ Acute MI
■ Untreated ventricular tachycardia
■ Underlying heart disease
■ Acid-base imbalance
■ Electric shock
■ Severe hypothermia
■ Electrolyte imbalances, such as hypokalemia, hyperkalemia, and hypercalcemia

Signs and symptoms

- Absent pulse, heart sounds, and blood pressure
- Dilated pupils
- Loss of consciousness
- Rapid development of cyanosis
- Seizures (occasional)

Treatment

- Perform cardiopulmonary resuscitation (CPR). Administer defibrillation up to three times; first using 200 joules, then 200 to 300 joules, followed by 360 joules, if necessary.
- Next, continue CPR and administer vasopressin. If vasopressin is used first and is ineffective, follow with epinephrine.
- Resume attempts at defibrillation using 360 joules.
- Consider antiarrhythmics, such as amiodarone or lidocaine. If the patient is hypomagnesemic, administer magnesium. Administer procainamide if intermittent ventricular tachycardia or ventricular fibrillation recur.
- Continue attempts at defibrillation, if necessary.

Recognizing atrioventricular blocks

AV blocks result from interruption in the conduction of impulses between the atria and the ventricles. They can be partial, total, or involve only a delay of conduction. Blocks can occur at the AV node, bundle of His, or bundle branches. The clinical effect depends on how many impulses are completely blocked, how slow the ventricular rate is, and how the block affects the heart. Blocks with slow rates can decrease cardiac output. AV blocks are classified as first-degree, second-degree, or third-degree.

First-degree AV block

First-degree AV block occurs when impulses from the atria are consistently delayed during conduction through the AV node. It can be temporary and is the least dangerous of the AV blocks; however, it can progress to a more severe block.

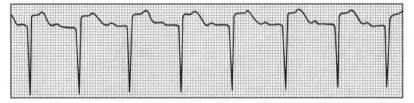

Interpretation

Rhythm. Atrial and ventricular rhythms are regular.

Rate. Atrial and ventricular rates are the same and within normal limits.

P wave. Normal size and configuration.

PR interval. Prolonged (exceeding 0.20 second) but constant. A PR interval of 0.21 to 0.24 second indicates slight first-degree AV block; a PR interval 0.25 to 0.29 second, a moderate first-degree AV block; a PR interval of 0.30 second or longer, a severe first-degree AV block. Usually the PR interval doesn't last longer than 0.35 second; however, in rare instances it may last up to 0.88 second. (If you see an exceptionally long PR interval, look for hidden P waves; these may indicate second-degree AV block.)

QRS complex. Duration usually remains within normal limits if the conduction delay occurs in the AV node. If the QRS duration exceeds 0.12 second, the conduction delay may be in the His-Purkinje fibers.

T wave. Normal size and configuration unless the QRS complex is prolonged.

QT interval. Usually within normal limits.

Possible causes

■ Drug toxicity; especially from digoxin, a beta-adrenergic blocker such as propranolol, a calcium channel blocker such as verapamil, or an antiarrhythmic, such as quinidine or procainamide

■ Chronic degenerative disease of the conduction system and inferior wall MI

■ Hypokalemia and hyperkalemia

■ Hypothermia

■ Hypothyroidism

Signs and symptoms

■ Usually none (however, the patient's peripheral pulse rate will be normal or slow with a regular rhythm)

■ Possibly signs and symptoms of decreased cardiac output, such as hypotension, syncope, and blurred vision, if the patient has a slow rate

Treatment

■ Treatment aims to correct the underlying cause.

■ Monitor carefully for worsening heart block, especially if severe myocardial damage is present.

Second-degree AV block (type I)

In type I (Wenckebach or Mobitz I) second-degree AV block, diseased tissues in the AV node delay conduction of impulses to the ventricles. As a re-

Key points

Second-degree AV block (type I)

■ Atrial rhythm regular; ventricular rhythm irregular

■ Atrial rate exceeds the ventricular rate

■ PR interval progressively longer with each cycle until a P wave appears without a QRS complex; the cycle then repeats

■ QRS complex periodically absent

■ T wave deflection may be opposite that of the QRS complex

Treatment

■ Correction of underlying cause

sult, each successive impulse arrives increasingly earlier in the refractory period. After several beats, an impulse arrives during the absolute refractory period when the tissue can't conduct it. The next impulse arrives during the relative refractory period and is conducted normally. The cycle is then repeated.

Type I second-degree AV block is usually transient. An asymptomatic patient has a good prognosis; however, the block may progress to a more serious type.

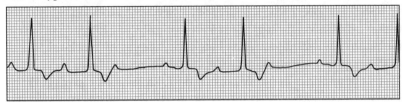

Interpretation

Rhythm. Atrial rhythm is regular, whereas ventricular rhythm is irregular. The R-R interval shortens progressively until a P wave appears without a QRS complex. The cycle then repeats.

Rate. The atrial rate exceeds the ventricular rate, but both usually remain within normal limits.

P wave. Normal size and configuration.

PR interval. Progressively, but typically only slightly, longer with each cycle until a P wave appears without a QRS complex. The PR interval after the nonconducted beat is shorter than the interval preceding it.

QRS complex. Duration usually remains within normal limits because the block commonly lies above the bundle of His. The complex is absent periodically.

T wave. Normal size and configuration, but its deflection may be opposite that of the QRS complex.

QT interval. Usually within normal limits.

Other. Usually distinguished by group beating; referred to as footprints of Wenckebach.

Possible causes

■ CAD

■ Inferior wall MI

■ Rheumatic fever

■ Digoxin toxicity and use of beta-adrenergic blockers, calcium channel blockers, quinidine, and procainamide

Signs and symptoms

■ Usually none

- Possibly a first heart sound that becomes progressively softer with intermittent pauses
- Hypotension and syncope (if ventricular rate is low)

Treatment
- For most patients, treatment addresses the underlying cause, thereby correcting heart block.

Second-degree AV block (type II)
Produced by a conduction disturbance in the His-Purkinje fibers, a type II (Mobitz II) second-degree AV block causes an intermittent conduction delay or block. On the ECG, you won't see any warning before a beat is dropped, as you do with type I second-degree AV block. In type II second-degree AV block, the PR and R-R intervals remain constant before the dropped beat. The arrhythmia frequently progresses to third-degree or complete heart block.

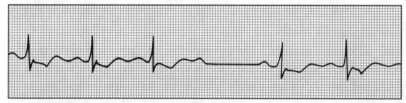

Interpretation
Rhythm. The atrial rhythm is regular, but the ventricular rhythm can be regular or irregular. Pauses correspond to the dropped beat. If the block is intermittent, the rhythm is often irregular. If the block stays constant (for example, 2:1 or 3:1), the rhythm is regular.

Rate. The atrial rate is usually within normal limits. The ventricular rate, slower than the atrial rate, may be within normal limits.

P wave. Normal size and configuration, but some P waves aren't followed by a QRS complex. The R-R interval containing such a nonconducted P wave equals two normal R-R intervals.

PR interval. Within normal limits or prolonged but always constant for the conducted beats. The PR interval following a nonconducted beat may be shortened.

QRS complex. Duration is within normal limits if the block occurs at the bundle of His; prolonged if it occurs below the bundle of His. The complex is absent periodically.

T wave. Usually normal size and configuration.

QT interval. Usually within normal limits.

Other. The PR and R-R intervals don't vary before a dropped beat, so no warning occurs.

Key points

Second-degree AV block (type II)
- Atrial rhythm regular; ventricular rhythm often irregular; pauses correspond to the dropped beat
- Ventricular rate possibly slower than atrial rate
- P wave normal size and configuration; R-R interval containing a nonconducted P wave equals two normal R-R intervals
- PR interval possibly prolonged, constant for the conducted beats, and shortened following a nonconducted beat
- QRS complex periodically absent

Treatment
- None if patient is asymptomatic
- With symptomatic bradycardia, administration of atropine and transcutaneous pacemaker

Possible causes

- Acute anterior-wall MI
- Degenerative changes in the conduction system
- Severe CAD
- Acute myocarditis

Signs and symptoms

- Normal or slow peripheral pulse rate
- Possible signs and symptoms of decreased cardiac output (if pulse rate is slow)

Treatment

- Usually, no immediate treatment is needed if the patient is asymptomatic.
- If symptomatic bradycardia is present, administer atropine and apply a transcutaneous pacemaker. Administer a dopamine infusion if patient is hypotensive. If hypotension is severe, administer an epinephrine infusion.

Third-degree AV block

When all supraventricular impulses are prevented from reaching the ventricles, the patient has third-degree AV block, also known as complete heart block. Just how significant the block is depends on the patient's response to any decline in ventricular rate and on the stability of the escape rhythm. Junctional escape rhythms are typically stable and may produce adequate cardiac output. Ventricular escape rhythms, however, are slower and less stable and pose the risk for intermittent or permanent ventricular standstill.

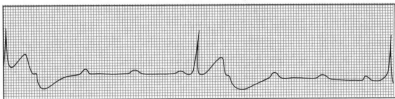

Interpretation

Rhythm. Atrial and ventricular rhythms are regular.

Rate. Atrial rate, which is usually within normal limits, exceeds ventricular rate. A ventricular escape rhythm ranges from 25 to 40 beats/minute. A junctional escape rhythm usually ranges from 40 to 60 beats/minute.

P wave. Normal size and configuration.

PR interval. Not applicable or measurable because the atria and ventricles beat independently (AV dissociation).

QRS complex. Configuration depends on where the ventricular beat originates. A high AV junctional pacemaker produces a narrow QRS complex; a ventricular pacemaker produces a wide, bizarre QRS complex.

Key points

Third-degree AV block

- Atrial rate within normal limits but exceeds ventricular rate; ventricular escape rhythm from 25 to 40 beats/minute; junctional escape rhythm from 40 to 60 beats/minute
- PR interval varies; the atria and ventricles beat independently
- QRS complex configuration related to origin of the ventricular beat

Treatment

- No treatment
- Administration of atropine and application of transcutaneous pacemaker, if patient is unstable

T wave. Normal size and configuration unless the QRS complex originates in the ventricle.

QT interval. May or may not be within normal limits.

Possible causes

- Severe digoxin toxicity, beta-adrenergic blockers, or calcium channel blockers
- Anterior- or inferior-wall MI
- Cardiac catheterization
- Myocarditis caused by Lyme disease
- Cardiac surgery
- Congenital heart defect

Signs and symptoms

- Slow peripheral pulse rate, usually less than 40 beats/minute, but a regular rhythm
- Possibly signs and symptoms of decreased cardiac output if the patient has a slow peripheral pulse rate
- Possibly no symptoms if the block results from a congenital abnormality

Treatment

- If the patient has adequate cardiac output, he may not need treatment.
- If symptomatic bradycardia is present, administer atropine and apply a transcutaneous pacemaker. Administer a dopamine infusion if patient is hypotensive. If hypotension is severe, administer an epinephrine infusion.

Recognizing other arrhythmias

Other common arrhythmias include sinus bradycardia, PACs, pulseless electrical activity (PEA), and asystole.

Sinus bradycardia

In sinus bradycardia, the sinus rate is below 60 beats/minute, and all impulses come from the SA node. This arrhythmia's significance depends on the symptoms and underlying cause. Sinus bradycardia is the most common arrhythmia seen in patients who have suffered an MI, regardless of its location.

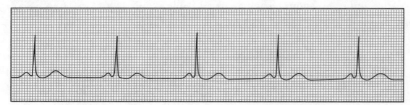

Interpretation

Rhythm. Atrial and ventricular rhythms are regular.

Rate. Atrial and ventricular rates are less than 60 beats/minute.

P wave. Normal size and configuration. P wave precedes each QRS complex.

PR interval. Within normal limits and constant.

QRS complex. Normal duration and configuration.

T wave. Normal size and configuration.

QT interval. Within normal limits but may be prolonged.

Possible causes

- Hyperkalemia
- Increased intracranial pressure
- Increased vagal tone that accompanies straining at stool, vomiting, intubation, mechanical ventilation, sick sinus syndrome, hypothyroidism, and hard physical exertion
- Possible result of inferior MI involving the right coronary artery, which supplies blood to the SA node
- Treatment with beta-adrenergic blockers, sympatholytic drugs, digoxin, morphine, or meperidine

Signs and symptoms

- Heart rate less than 60 beats/minute
- Fatigue, light-headedness, syncope, and palpitations
- Chest pain and premature beats (if heart disease exists and coronary blood flow is decreased)

Treatment

- Administer oxygen.
- Administer atropine. Use cautiously in patients with acute myocardial ischemia or MI — may cause excessive increases in heart rate, worsening ischemia, or increasing the zone of infarction.
- Initiate transcutaneous pacing, if available.
- Administer dopamine infusion if hypotension is present.
- Isoproterenol infusion titrated according to the patient's heart rate and rhythm; use only when atropine and dopamine have failed and transcutaneous and transvenous pacing aren't available.
- If symptoms are severe, add epinephrine infusion.

Premature atrial contractions

Originating outside the SA node, PACs usually arise from an irritable focus in the atria that supercedes the SA node as pacemaker for one or more beats. PACs can occur in groups of two in a row or every other beat (bigeminy). They're often followed by a pause as the SA node is reset. Ventricular conduction is normal.

PACs may precipitate a more serious arrhythmia, such as atrial flutter and atrial fibrillation in patients with heart disease. If PACs occur with an acute MI, they may signal heart failure or an electrolyte imbalance.

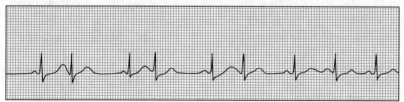

Interpretation

Rhythm. Atrial and ventricular rhythms are irregular as a result of the PACs, but the underlying rhythm may be regular.

Rate. Atrial and ventricular rates vary with the underlying rhythm.

P wave. Premature and abnormally shaped; possibly lost in the previous T wave.

PR interval. Usually within normal limits, but may be shortened or slightly prolonged for the ectopic beat, depending on the origin of the ectopic focus.

QRS complex. Duration and configuration are usually normal. If no QRS complex follows the P wave, a nonconducted PAC has occurred. With nonconducted PACs, the P wave is seen in a distorted T wave.

T wave. Usually has a normal configuration. However, if the P wave is hidden in the T wave, the T wave may be distorted.

QT interval. Usually within normal limits.

Other. A PAC is usually followed by a pause, which may be noncompensatory, compensatory, or longer than compensatory. Most commonly, the pause is noncompensatory. PACs may also be blocked, with only an early P wave present. The most common cause of a pause is a blocked PAC.

Possible causes

- Acute respiratory failure
- Heart failure
- Drugs that prolong the SA node's absolute refractory period, such as digoxin, quinidine, and procainamide
- Excessive use of caffeine, tobacco, and alcohol
- Ischemic heart disease
- Stress, fatigue, and overeating

Signs and symptoms

- Irregular pulse
- Palpitations

Key points

Premature atrial contractions

- Atrial and ventricular rhythms irregular; underlying rhythm possibly regular
- Atrial and ventricular rates varying with the underlying rhythm
- P wave premature and abnormally shaped; possibly lost in the previous T wave
- PR interval possibly shortened or slightly prolonged for the ectopic beat
- If the P wave is hidden in the T wave, distorted T wave

Treatment

- No treatment necessary

Treatment

- Typically, no treatment is necessary.
- Eliminate known causes, such as caffeine, tobacco, and alcohol.

Pulseless electrical activity

In PEA, formerly known as electromechanical dissociation, isolated electrical activity occurs sporadically without any evidence of effective myocardial contraction. PEA is commonly caused by a clinical condition that can be reversed when identified quickly and treated appropriately.

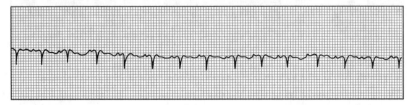

Interpretation

Rhythm. Atrial and ventricular rhythms are the same as the underlying rhythm. They eventually become irregular as the rate slows.

Rate. Atrial rate reflects the underlying rhythm. Ventricular rate also reflects the underlying rhythm but gradually decreases.

P wave. Same as the underlying rhythm but gradually flattens and disappears.

PR interval. Same as the underlying rhythm but eventually disappears as the P wave disappears.

QRS complex. Same as the underlying rhythm but eventually becomes progressively wider.

T wave. Same as the underlying rhythm but eventually becomes indiscernible.

QT interval. Same as the underlying rhythm but eventually becomes indiscernible.

Other. Typically within several minutes, a flat line tracing occurs indicating asystole.

Possible causes

- Failure in the calcium transport mechanism
- Extensive myocardial damage, such as rupture of the left ventricular wall and massive MI
- Tension pneumothorax, cardiac tamponade, hypovolemia from severe hemorrhage, hypoxemia, acidosis, pulmonary embolus, hypothermia, drug overdose, hyperkalemia, and advanced left-sided heart failure

Signs and symptoms

- Apnea and sudden loss of consciousness
- No blood pressure and pulse

Treatment

- Begin CPR immediately.
- Identify the cause of PEA and treat accordingly. The patient may need volume infusion for hypovolemia from hemorrhage; pericardiocentesis for cardiac tamponade; needle decompression or chest tube insertion for tension pneumothorax; surgery or thrombolytic therapy for massive pulmonary embolism; and ventilation for hypoxemia.
- Administer epinephrine.
- Administer sodium bicarbonate for preexisting hyperkalemia, preexisting acidosis, or tricyclic antidepressant overdose; to alkalinize urine in aspirin or other drug overdose; or if arrest period is prolonged.
- If the PEA rate is slow, administer atropine.

Asystole

Asystole refers to the total absence of ventricular activity. Some activity may be evident in the atria, but atrial impulses aren't conducted to the ventricles. Without ventricular electrical activity, ventricular contraction doesn't occur. As a result, no cardiac output or perfusion occurs. It's important to distinguish asystole from ventricular fibrillation, which may mimic this arrhythmia. In addition, make sure that all ECG leads are placed properly; otherwise, the resulting waveform may also resemble asystole. Asystole is associated with a low rate of survival. The only hope lies in identifying and reversing the underlying cause. As an ACLS provider, you'll need to focus on whether you should begin resuscitation and when you should stop if you initiate it.

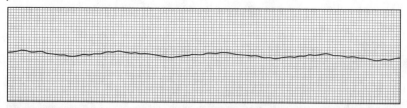

Interpretation

Rhythm. Atrial rhythm is (usually) indiscernible. No ventricular rhythm is present.
Rate. Atrial rate is (usually) indiscernible. No ventricular rate is present.
P wave. May or may not be present.

Key points

Asystole
- Atrial rhythm indiscernible (usually); ventricular rhythm absent
- Atrial rate indiscernible (usually); ventricular rate absent
- P wave possibly present
- PR interval unmeasurable
- QRS complex absent or occasional escape beats
- T wave absent
- Waveform almost a flat line

Treatment
- Cardiopulmonary resuscitation
- Confirmation that patient is in asystole by verifying the rhythm in another lead and checking lead and cable connections
- Consideration of transcutaneous pacing
- Administration of epinephrine and atropine

PR interval. Unmeasurable.

QRS complex. Absent or occasional escape beats.

T wave. Absent.

QT interval. Unmeasurable.

Other. Waveform is almost a flat line.

Possible causes

■ Severe metabolic deficit

■ Acute respiratory failure

■ Extensive myocardial damage, possibly from myocardial ischemia or MI, and ruptured ventricular aneurysm

Signs and symptoms

■ Loss of consciousness

■ Absence of peripheral pulses, blood pressure, or respirations

Treatment

■ Begin CPR.

■ Confirm that the patient is in asystole by verifying the rhythm in another lead, along with checking lead and cable connections.

■ Administer sodium bicarbonate for tricyclic antidepressant overdose, prolonged arrest period, and hypercarbic acidosis or to alkalinize the urine in overdoses.

■ Consider transcutaneous pacing.

■ Administer epinephrine.

■ Administer atropine.

■ If asystole persists, consider stopping resuscitation.

Test your knowledge

Take the following quiz to test your knowledge of normal and abnormal cardiac rhythms.

1. Identify the characteristics and interpret the rhythm strip below.

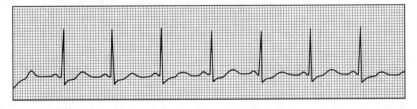

Rhythm _____

Rate _____

P wave _____

PR interval _____

QRS complex _____

T wave _____

QT interval _____

Interpretation _____

Answers to test strip:

Rhythm: Both atrial and ventricular rhythms regular

Rate: Atrial and ventricular rates both 79 beats/minute

P wave: Normal size and configuration

PR interval: 0.12 second

QRS complex: 0.08 second; normal size and configuration

T wave: Normal configuration

QT interval: 0.44 second

Other: None

Interpretation: Normal sinus rhythm

2. A patient with symptomatic sinus bradycardia at a rate of 40 beats/minute typically experiences:

    A. high blood pressure.

    B. chest pain and dyspnea.

    C. facial flushing and ataxia.

    D. no perceptible symptoms.

Correct answer: B

A patient with symptomatic bradycardia suffers from low cardiac output, which may produce chest pain and dyspnea. The patient may also have crackles, an S_3 heart sound, and a sudden onset of confusion.

3. Persistent tachycardia in a patient who has had a myocardial infarction (MI) may signal:

    A. chronic sick sinus syndrome.

    B. pulmonary embolism or stroke.

    C. impending heart failure or cardiogenic shock.

    D. respiratory failure.

Correct answer: C

Sinus tachycardia occurs in about 30% of patients after acute MI. It's considered a poor prognostic sign because it may be associated with massive heart damage, including heart failure and cardiogenic shock.

4. In a junctional tachycardia, the P wave can occur:

    A. within the T wave.
    B. on top of the preceding Q wave.
    C. before, during, or after the QRS complex.
    D. only at a normal interval.

Correct answer: C

In all junctional arrhythmias, the P wave is inverted and may appear before, during, or after the QRS complex.

5. In the strip below, the atrial and ventricular rhythms are regular at 47 beats/minute, the P wave is inverted, the PR interval is 0.08 second, the QRS complex is 0.06 second, the T wave is normal, and the QT interval is 0.42 second. You would interpret this rhythm as:

    A. wandering pacemaker.
    B. junctional tachycardia.
    C. junctional escape rhythm.
    D. pulseless electrical activity.

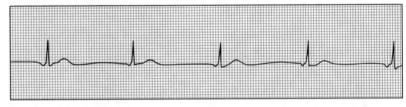

Correct answer: C

This strip shows junctional escape rhythm: rhythm is regular, rate is from 40 to 60 beats/minute, P wave is inverted, QRS complex is less than 0.12 second, and T wave and QT intervals are normal.

6. Premature ventricular contractions (PVCs) are most dangerous if they:

    A. are multiformed and increase in frequency.
    B. appear wide and bizarre.
    C. occur after the T wave.
    D. occur every third beat.

Correct answer: A

PVCs that have different shapes and increase in frequency may signal severe heart disease or digoxin toxicity and can progress to a lethal arrhythmia.

7. In the strip that follows, the ventricular rhythm is irregular, ventricular rate is 130 beats/minute, P wave is absent, PR interval and QT interval

aren't measurable, QRS complex is wide and bizarre with varying duration, and T wave is opposite the QRS complex. You would interpret this
rhythm as:

   A. ventricular fibrillation.
   B. ventricular tachycardia.
   C. idioventricular rhythm.
   D. sinus bradycardia.

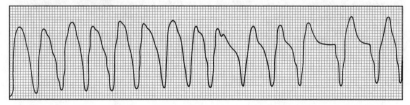

Correct answer: B

*This strip shows ventricular tachycardia: the rhythm is irregular, rate is from 100
to 200 beats/minute, P wave is absent, PR and QT intervals are unmeasurable,
QRS complex is wide and bizarre, and T wave is opposite the QRS complex.*

8. Torsades de pointes differs from monomorphic tachycardia in which of
the following ways?

   A. QRS complexes may vary from upward to downward.
   B. It may be life-threatening.
   C. It may degenerate to ventricular fibrillation.
   D. It may be caused by an electrolyte imbalance.

Correct answer: A

*Torsades de pointes is a polymorphic ventricular tachycardia characterized by
prolonged QT intervals and QRS polarity that seem to spiral around the isoelectric line, causing complexes that point upward and then downward.*

9. The term *pulseless electrical activity (PEA)* refers to a condition in which
there's:

   A. asystole on a monitor or rhythm strip.
   B. an extremely slow heart rate but no pulse.
   C. electrical activity in the heart but no actual contraction.
   D. contractions occurring without electrical activity occurring in the
   heart.

Correct answer: C

*PEA is electrical activity without mechanical contraction. The patient is in car-
diac arrest, with no blood pressure or pulse.*

10. Immediate treatment of ventricular defibrillation includes:

    A. epinephrine, defibrillation, and vasopressin.
    B. defibrillation (up to three times), atropine, and lidocaine.
    C. epinephrine, defibrillation (up to three times), and atropine.
    D. defibrillation (up to three times), epinephrine, and defibrillation.

Correct answer: D

Immediately administer defibrillation up to three times: 200 joules, then 200 to 300 joules, then 360 joules (if necessary). Then administer epinephrine or vasopressin. Resume attempts at defibrillation using 360 joules.

CHAPTER FIVE

Cardiovascular pharmacology

Cardiovascular pharmacologic therapy is an essential component of ACLS, although it's important to remember that drugs alone can't replace effective oxygenation and circulation. This chapter describes drugs commonly used in ACLS, with indications and dosages for adults. It also covers the most common drug interactions encountered in ACLS practice.

Here are some important general points to remember about medication administration.

■ Geriatric populations usually require smaller dosages than those given here. In addition, pediatric dosages are typically based on weight (such as those provided on resuscitation tapes) and aren't given here. If the adult patient you're treating has organ impairment (especially kidney or liver), you may need to reduce the dosage because metabolism and excretion of the drug may be altered significantly.

■ Remember that a patient may be taking over-the-counter (OTC) medications, illegal drugs, or herbal remedies or may be consuming food or beverages (alcohol, for example) that interact with the medication. Also, be aware that the patient may have known or unknown drug allergies; any medication has the potential to cause an anaphylactic reaction or hypersensitivity.

■ After administration of a medication, you should continually monitor the patient for the drug's effects, including adverse reactions. Monitoring the patient includes continual cardiac monitoring; assessing vital signs before, during, and after the administration of the medication; and any additional assessment as indicated by the drug's use (such as cardiac output measurement for medications that affect cardiac output).

Adrenergics

Adrenergics have various bodily effects, but generally serve as cardiac stimulants. They're typically used in ACLS to restore heart rate, rhythm, and blood pressure during resuscitation of the patient.

Epinephrine
Epinephrine is an adrenergic used as a bronchodilator, vasopressor, and cardiac stimulant. It's indicated for treatment of cardiac arrest (ventricular fibrillation [VF], pulseless ventricular tachycardia [VT], asystole, and pulseless

electrical activity [PEA]), symptomatic bradycardia (after atropine, dopamine, and transcutaneous pacing), severe hypotension, and severe allergic reactions (when combined with large fluid volumes, corticosteroids, or antihistamines).

Action

Epinephrine acts directly by stimulating alpha- and beta-adrenergic receptors in the sympathetic nervous system. Its main therapeutic effects include relaxation of bronchial smooth muscle, cardiac stimulation, and dilation of skeletal muscle vasculature. Epinephrine relaxes bronchial smooth muscle by stimulating beta$_2$-adrenergic receptors, and constricts bronchial arterioles by stimulating alpha-adrenergic receptors, resulting in relief of bronchospasm, reduced congestion and edema, and increased tidal volume and vital capacity. By inhibiting histamine release, it may reverse bronchiolar constriction, vasodilation, and edema.

As a cardiac stimulant, epinephrine produces positive chronotropic and inotropic effects by action on beta$_1$-receptors in the heart, increasing cardiac output, myocardial oxygen consumption, and force of contraction and decreasing cardiac efficiency. Vasodilation results from its effect on beta$_2$-receptors; vasoconstriction results from alpha-adrenergic effects.

Dosage

■ Administer 1 mg (10 ml of 1:10,000 solution) I.V. every 3 to 5 minutes during resuscitation; follow each dose with 20-ml I.V. flush; doses up to 0.2 mg/kg may be used if 1 mg dose fails
■ For continuous infusion, add 1 mg dose (1 ml of 1:1,000 solution) to 250 ml normal saline solution (NSS) or dextrose 5% in water (D$_5$W); initial dose is 1 mcg/minute and increased to 3 to 4 mcg/minute
■ May be given down the endotracheal tube (if placement is confirmed) by administering 2 to 2.5 mg diluted in 10 ml NSS; follow with several positive pressure ventilations
■ For profound bradycardia or hypotension, add 1 mg of 1:1,000 solution to 500 ml NSS and infuse at 1 mcg/minute and titrate to the desired hemodynamic response (2 to 10 mcg/minute)

Special considerations

■ If administered with alpha blockers, vasoconstriction and hypertensive effects may be counteracted.
■ If the patient is taking antidiabetics, the effect of the drug may also be decreased; dosage adjustments may be necessary and serum glucose levels should also be monitored.
■ Antihistamines and tricyclic antidepressants (TCAs) may potentiate drug's adverse cardiac effects; avoid concomitant use.

- Beta-adrenergic blockers can antagonize drug's cardiac and bronchodilating effects.
- Cardiac glycosides may sensitize the myocardium to drug's effects, causing arrhythmias.
- Intracardiac administration requires external cardiac massage to move drug into coronary circulation.

Isoproterenol

Isoproterenol (Isuprel) is an adrenergic used as a cardiac stimulant and as a temporary measure for treatment of symptomatic bradycardia if an external pacemaker isn't available. It's also used in torsades de pointes that doesn't respond to magnesium sulfate, for temporary control of bradycardia in heart transplant patients, and in counteracting poisoning from beta-adrenergic blockers.

Action

Isoproterenol acts on beta$_1$-adrenergic receptors in the heart, producing a positive chronotropic and inotropic effect. It usually increases cardiac output. In patients with atrioventricular (AV) block, isoproterenol shortens conduction time and the refractory period of the AV node and increases the rate and strength of ventricular contraction.

Dosage

- 1 mg dose mixed in 500 ml D$_5$W and infused at 2 to 10 mcg/minute and titrated to adequate heart rate
- In torsades de pointes, titrate until VT is suppressed

Special considerations

- Drug is contraindicated in patients with tachycardia caused by digoxin intoxication, preexisting arrhythmias (other than those that may respond to treatment with isoproterenol), and angina pectoris.
- Beta-adrenergic blockers antagonize drug's effects; there's an increased chance of arrhythmias when it's used with cardiac glycosides, potassium-depleting drugs, and other drugs that affect cardiac rhythm.
- Epinephrine and other adrenergics can cause additive reactions; drugs may be used together if at least 4 hours elapse between administration of the two drugs.
- Remember that the drug doesn't replace administration of blood, plasma, fluids, or electrolytes in patients with blood volume depletion.
- Prescription for the I.V. infusion rate should include specific guidelines for regulating flow or terminating infusion in relation to heart rate, premature beats, electrocardiogram (ECG) changes, precordial distress, blood pressure, and urine flow.

Key points

Isoproterenol
- Cardiac stimulant that produces positive chronotropic and inotropic effects
- Indications: symptomatic bradycardia, torsades de pointes, to counteract beta-adrenergic blockers
- Continuous infusion: 2 to 10 mcg/minute and titrated to adequate response

Key points

Norepinephrine
- Primarily produces vasoconstriction and cardiac stimulation
- Indications: severe cardiogenic shock, significant hypotension, ischemic heart disease, and shock
- Continuous infusion: 0.5 to 1.0 mcg/minute titrated to desired blood pressure (to maximum rate of 30 mcg/minute)

- Because of danger of arrhythmias, rate of infusion is usually decreased or temporarily stopped if heart rate exceeds 110 beats/minute. Use with infusion pump.

Norepinephrine

Norepinephrine (Levophed) is an adrenergic indicated in severe cardiogenic shock and significant hypotension (systolic blood pressure less than 70 mm Hg) with low total peripheral resistance. It's the medication of last resort for management of ischemic heart disease and shock.

Action

Norepinephrine stimulates alpha- and $beta_1$-receptors within the sympathetic nervous system. It primarily produces vasoconstriction and cardiac stimulation.

Dosage

- 4 mg dose mixed in 250 ml of D_5W or dextrose 5% in NSS (D_5NSS) and titrated to effect; 0.5 to 1.0 mcg/minute I.V. usually titrated to improve blood pressure (up to 30 mcg/minute may be administered)
- Higher dose may be required to achieve adequate perfusion with poison-induced hypotension

Special considerations

- Bradycardia, severe hypertension, and arrhythmias can occur.
- Alpha blockers may antagonize this drug's effects; avoid concomitant use.
- Don't use this drug with monoamine oxidase (MAO) inhibitors, methyldopa, and TCAs; severe hypertension can occur.
- Administering norepinephrine isn't a substitute for blood or fluid replacement therapy. If volume deficit exists, replace fluid before administering vasopressors.
- Monitor extremities for color and temperature.
- Use a central venous catheter or large vein to minimize risk of extravasation. Phentolamine (Regitine) 5 to 10 mg in 10 to 15 ml NSS is used to infiltrate the area to minimize tissue necrosis if extravasation occurs.

Dobutamine hydrochloride

Dobutamine (Dobutrex) is an adrenergic, $beta_1$ agonist. It's indicated to increase cardiac output in cardiac decompensation situations with systolic blood pressure of 70 to 100 mm Hg and no accompanying signs of shock.

Action

Dobutamine works by selectively stimulating $beta_1$-adrenergic receptors to increase myocardial contractility and stroke volume. This results in increased cardiac output (a positive inotropic effect). At therapeutic doses, drug decreases peripheral resistance (afterload), reduces ventricular filling pressure (preload), and may facilitate AV node conduction. Systolic blood pressure and pulse pressure may remain unchanged or may be increased from increased cardiac output.

Dosage

■ Administer at 2 to 20 mcg/kg/minute I.V., titrated so that cardiac rate isn't greater than 10% of baseline

Special considerations

■ Avoid dobutamine administration when systolic blood pressure is less than 100 mm Hg and signs of shock exist. Before drug therapy, correct hypovolemia with appropriate plasma volume expanders.

■ Drug may cause tachycardia, fluctuations in blood pressure, headache, and nausea.

■ Dobutamine must be administered by I.V. infusion using an infusion pump or other device to control flow rate. Hemodynamic monitoring is also necessary to monitor its effect.

■ Drug is contraindicated in suspected or known poisoning or drug-induced shock.

■ When drug is used with beta-adrenergic blockers, increased peripheral resistance and predominance of alpha-adrenergic effects may occur.

■ When used with TCAs, drug may potentiate pressor response — monitor patient closely.

■ This drug is also incompatible with alkaline solutions (sodium bicarbonate).

Dopamine hydrochloride

Dopamine (Intropin) is an adrenergic; it's also classified as a vasopressor. Dopamine is indicated as a secondary drug (after atropine) for symptomatic bradycardia. It's also used for hypotension (systolic blood pressure greater than or equal to 70 to 100 mm Hg) accompanied by signs and symptoms of shock.

Action

Dopamine stimulates dopaminergic, beta-adrenergic, and alpha-adrenergic receptors of the sympathetic nervous system. It has a direct stimulating effect on beta$_1$-receptors (in I.V. doses of 2 to 10 mcg/kg/minute) and little or no effect on beta$_2$-receptors.

Dopamine's effects are dose-dependent. In I.V. doses of 0.5 to 2 mcg/kg/minute, it acts on dopaminergic receptors (dopaminergic response), causing vasodilation in the renal, mesenteric, coronary, and intracerebral vascular beds. Low to moderate doses result in cardiac stimulation (positive inotropic effects). In I.V. doses above 10 mcg/kg/minute, it stimulates alpha-receptors resulting in increased peripheral resistance and renal vasoconstriction.

Dosage

- Low dose: 1 to 4 mcg/kg/minute I.V. infusion
- Cardiac dose: 5 to 10 mcg/kg/minute I.V. infusion
- Vasopressor dose: 10 to 20 mcg/kg/minute I.V. infusion

Special considerations

- Dopamine is contraindicated in uncorrected tachyarrhythmias, pheochromocytoma, or VF.
- Administer drug into large vein to prevent possibility of extravasation (central venous access is recommended).
- Adjust dose to meet individual needs of patient and to achieve desired response. Reduce dose as soon as hemodynamic condition is stabilized. Severe hypotension may result with abrupt withdrawal; taper gradually.
- Don't mix other drugs in dopamine solutions.
- Hypovolemia should be corrected with appropriate plasma volume expanders before starting dopamine therapy.
- Beta-adrenergic blockers antagonize cardiac effects of dopamine.
- Use with phenytoin may cause hypotension and bradycardia.

Vasopressin

Vasopressin (antidiuretic hormone, or ADH) is a posterior pituitary hormone indicated as an alternative vasopressor to epinephrine in the treatment of adult shock-refractory VF. It may also provide hemodynamic support in vasodilatory shock by maintaining coronary perfusion pressure.

Action

Vasopressin acts at the renal tubular level to increase cyclic adenosine monophosphate (cAMP), which in turn increases water permeability at the renal tubule and collecting duct. This results in increased urine osmolality and decreased urine flow rate. Vasopressin also directly stimulates vasoconstriction of capillaries and small arterioles.

Dosage

- Cardiac arrest: 40 U I.V. push as a one-time dose

Special considerations

- Drug may provoke cardiac ischemia and angina.
- Because of the risk of necrosis and gangrene, use extreme caution to avoid extravasation with this drug.

Analgesics

Analgesics are used in ACLS primarily to help alleviate cardiac pain and to promote relaxation. Morphine sulfate is the most common analgesic recommended for these actions.

Morphine sulfate

Morphine sulfate is an opioid used as a narcotic analgesic. It's a schedule II controlled substance indicated for chest pain that doesn't respond to nitrates. Morphine sulfate is also given to patients with acute pulmonary edema (if blood pressure is adequate).

Action

Morphine sulfate is an opium alkaloid. It's thought to work through the opiate receptors, altering the patient's perception of pain. The drug also has a central depressant effect on respiration and on the cough reflex center.

Dosage

■ Give 2 to 4 mg I.V. over 1 to 5 minutes; repeat every 5 to 30 minutes and titrate to effect

Special considerations

■ Drug may compromise respirations and should be used with caution in patients with compromised respiratory state or acute pulmonary edema.
■ Drug can cause hypotension in volume-depleted patients.
■ If needed, reverse morphine's effects with naloxone (Narcan) 0.4 to 2 mg I.V.
■ Central nervous system (CNS) depressants can potentiate drug's respiratory and CNS depression, sedation, and hypotensive effects.
■ Adverse reactions include hypotension, bradycardia, shock, cardiac arrest, tachycardia, and hypertension; respiratory depression, apnea, and respiratory arrest can also occur with morphine.
■ Rapid morphine I.V. administration may result in overdose because of the delay in maximum CNS effect (30 minutes).

Nitrates

Nitrates are used to prevent or relieve angina. (See *How antianginal agents relieve angina,* page 96.) The most commonly used nitrate is nitroglycerin.

Nitroglycerin

Nitroglycerin (Nitro-Bid I.V., Tridil) functions as an antianginal and vasodilator. It's indicated in suspected ischemic pain in the initial 24 to 48

How antianginal agents relieve angina

Angina occurs when the coronary arteries, the heart's primary source of oxygen, supply insufficient oxygen to the myocardium. This increases the heart's workload, which in turn increases heart rate, preload (blood volume in ventricles at end of diastole), afterload (pressure in arteries leading from ventricles), and force of myocardial contractility. The antianginal agents (nitrates, beta-adrenergic blockers, and calcium channel blockers) relieve angina by decreasing one or more of these four factors. This diagram summarizes how antianginal agents affect the cardiovascular system.

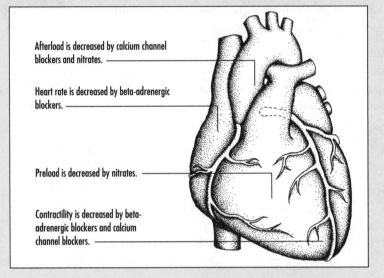

Afterload is decreased by calcium channel blockers and nitrates.

Heart rate is decreased by beta-adrenergic blockers.

Preload is decreased by nitrates.

Contractility is decreased by beta-adrenergic blockers and calcium channel blockers.

hours in patients with acute myocardial infarction (MI) and heart failure, large anterior wall infarction, persistent or recurrent ischemia, hypertension, recurrent angina, persistent pulmonary congestion, and hypertensive urgency with acute coronary syndrome.

Action

Nitroglycerin relaxes vascular smooth muscle of both the venous and arterial beds, resulting in decreased myocardial oxygen consumption. It dilates coronary vessels, leading to redistribution of blood flow to ischemic tissue.

Because peripheral vasodilation decreases venous return to the heart (preload), nitroglycerin also helps to treat pulmonary edema and heart failure. Arterial vasodilation decreases arterial impedance (afterload), thereby decreasing left ventricular work and aiding the failing heart.

Dosage

■ I.V. bolus: 12.5 to 25 mcg; infusion of 10 to 20 mcg/minute increased by 5 to 10 mcg/minute every 5 to 10 minutes until the desired hemodynamic or clinical response occurs

- Sublingual route: 1 tablet (0.3 to 0.4 mg) and repeat every 5 minutes
- Aerosol spray: 0.5 to 1.0 second at 5-minute intervals (provides 0.4 mg per dose)

Special considerations

- In I.V. form, drug is contraindicated in patients with cardiac tamponade, restrictive cardiomyopathy, or constrictive pericarditis.
- Also, use drug cautiously in patients with hypotension or volume depletion.
- Nitroglycerin's administration as I.V. infusion requires special nonabsorbent tubing supplied by the manufacturer because regular plastic tubing may absorb up to 80% of drug. Infusion should be prepared in a glass bottle or container.
- Toxicity of drug may cause hypotension, persistent throbbing headache, palpitations, flushing of the skin, nausea and vomiting, bradycardia, heart block, tissue hypoxia, metabolic acidosis, and circulatory collapse. Circulatory collapse or asphyxia may cause death.

Beta-adrenergic blockers

Beta-adrenergic blockers are a group of medications indicated for suspected MI and unstable angina in the absence of complications. They're effective antianginal agents that can reduce incidence of VF and are used as adjunctive agents with fibrinolytic therapy because they may reduce nonfatal reinfarction and recurrent ischemia. Beta-adrenergic blockers are also used for conversion to normal sinus rhythm or to slow ventricular response (or both) in supraventricular tachyarrhythmias (SVTs), such as paroxysmal SVT (PSVT), atrial fibrillation, or atrial flutter.

Beta-adrenergic blockers are considered second-line agents after adenosine, diltiazem, or digoxin. They've been known to reduce myocardial ischemia and damage in acute MI patients with elevated heart rate, blood pressure, or both. They're also used for emergency antihypertensive therapy for hemorrhagic and acute ischemic stroke.

Beta-adrenergic blockers may reduce blood pressure by adrenergic receptor blockade, thereby decreasing cardiac output by decreasing the sympathetic outflow from the CNS and by suppressing renin release. (See *Major effects of beta-adrenergic blockers,* page 98.)

Beta-adrenergic blockers help treat chronic stable angina by decreasing myocardial contractility and heart rate (negative inotropic and chronotropic effect), thus reducing myocardial oxygen consumption. The mechanism of action in patients with MI is unknown. However, the drug does reduce frequency of premature ventricular contractions (PVCs), chest pain, and

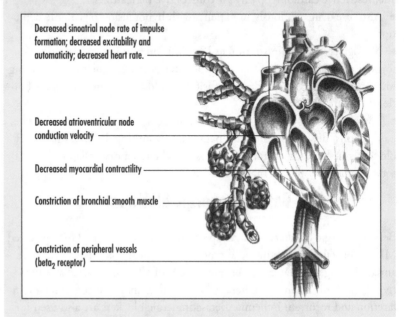

Major effects of beta-adrenergic blockers

Beta-adrenergic blockers block the action of endogenous catecholamines and other sympathomimetic agents at beta-receptor sites, thus counteracting the stimulating effects of those agents. This illustration depicts the effects of beta-adrenergic blockers on the pulmonary and cardiovascular systems.

Decreased sinoatrial node rate of impulse formation; decreased excitability and automaticity; decreased heart rate.

Decreased atrioventricular node conduction velocity

Decreased myocardial contractility

Constriction of bronchial smooth muscle

Constriction of peripheral vessels (beta$_2$ receptor)

enzyme elevation. (For precautions that apply to all beta-adrenergic blockers, see *General precautions for beta-adrenergic blockers*.)

Atenolol

Atenolol (Tenormin) is a beta-adrenergic blocker used as an antihypertensive and antianginal agent. It has been shown to reduce the incidence of VF in post-MI patients who didn't receive fibrinolytic agents.

Action
(See "Beta-adrenergic blockers," page 97.)

Dosage
- Give 5 mg I.V. over 5 minutes; then another 5 mg I.V. 10 minutes later
- If tolerated well in 10 minutes, give 50 mg by mouth; then continue with 50 mg by mouth twice per day

Special considerations
- Alpha-adrenergic drugs (such as those found in OTC cold remedies), indomethacin, and nonsteroidal anti-inflammatory agents (NSAIDs), may

General precautions for beta-adrenergic blockers

Observe these general precautions when administering beta-adrenergic blockers.

■ Severe hypotension can occur if I.V. beta-adrenergic agents are administered with I.V. calcium channel blocking agents (such as verapamil or diltiazem).

■ When administering beta-adrenergic blockers with other antihypertensive medications (such as labetalol), increased hypotension may occur.

■ Avoid using these drugs in patients with bronchospastic diseases, cardiac failure, or severe abnormalities in conduction.

■ Myocardial depression may occur as a reaction to drugs.

■ Beta-adrenergic blockers are contraindicated in the presence of a heart rate less than 60 beats per minute, systolic blood pressure less than 100 mm Hg, severe left-sided heart failure, hypoperfusion, or second- or third-degree atrioventricular block.

■ Beta-adrenergic blockers may require altered dosage requirements in stable diabetic patients.

■ Signs and symptoms of overdose to these drugs include severe hypotension, bradycardia, heart failure, and bronchospasm. Treat bradycardia with atropine (0.25 to 1 mg); if no response, administer isoproterenol cautiously. Treat cardiac failure with cardiac glycosides and diuretics and hypotension with glucagon or vasopressors; epinephrine is preferred. Treat bronchospasm with isoproterenol and aminophylline.

cause the antihypertensive effects of atenolol to be antagonized. Use together er cautiously. See *General precautions for beta-adrenergic blockers.*

Esmolol hydrochloride

Esmolol (Brevibloc) is a class II antiarrhythmic and ultra-short-acting selective beta-adrenergic blocker. It decreases heart rate, contractility, and blood pressure. It's recommended for the acute treatment of PSVT, rate control in non-preexcited atrial fibrillation (AF) or atrial flutter, ectopic atrial tachycardia, and polymorphic VT due to torsades de pointes.

Action

See "Beta-adrenergic blockers," page 97.

Dosage

■ Give 0.5 mg/kg I.V. over one minute, followed by continuous infusion of 50 mcg/kg/minute with a maximum infusion of 300 mcg/kg/minute
■ Titrate to maintain effect
■ Half-life is 2 to 9 minutes

Special considerations

■ This drug may increase serum digoxin levels by 10% to 20%.
■ Morphine may increase esmolol blood levels.
■ When used with reserpine and other catecholamine-depleting drugs, drug may cause additive bradycardia and hypotension.

Key points

Esmolol hydrochloride
■ Ultra-short-acting selective beta-adrenergic blocker that decreases heart rate, contractility, and blood pressure
■ Indications: SVT, atrial fibrillation or flutter, noncompensatory sinus tachycardia
■ 0.5 mg/kg I.V. over one minute, followed by continuous infusion of 50 mcg/kg/minute with a maximum of 300 mcg/kg/minute; titrate to maintain effect

■ Esmolol solutions are incompatible with diazepam, furosemide, sodium bicarbonate, and thiopental sodium.

■ Up to 50% of all patients treated with esmolol develop hypotension; this can be reversed within 30 minutes by decreasing the dose or, if needed, by stopping the infusion.

■ Drug is recommended only for short-term use, no longer than 48 hours.

■ When the patient's heart rate becomes stable, esmolol is replaced by alternative (longer-acting) antiarrhythmics, such as propranolol, digoxin, or verapamil.

■ Use an infusion control device with esmolol; dilute to a maximum level of 10 mg/ml before infusion.

Labetalol hydrochloride

Labetalol (Normodyne) is a beta-adrenergic blocker used as an antihypertensive.

Action

See "Beta-adrenergic blockers," page 97.

Dosage

■ Give 20 mg I.V. push over 1 to 2 minutes; repeat injections of 40 to 80 mg every 10 minutes to a maximum dose of 300 mg I.V.

■ As an alternative, give initial dose as a bolus, then start labetalol infusion at initial rate of 2 mg/minute until satisfactory response is obtained; usual cumulative dose is 50 to 200 mg

Special considerations

■ This drug may cause ventricular arrhythmias, orthostatic hypotension, and bronchospasm.

■ Labetalol masks common signs and symptoms of shock.

Metoprolol tartrate

Metoprolol (Lopressor) is a beta-adrenergic blocker is used as an antihypertensive and in adjunctive treatment of acute MI to reduce the incidence of VF.

Action

See "Beta-adrenergic blockers," page 97.

Dosage

■ Give 5 mg slowly I.V. at 5-minute intervals for a total of 15 mg

■ Following I.V. dose, give 50 mg by mouth twice per day for 24 hours; then increase to 100 mg twice per day

Special considerations

■ When used to treat hypertension or angina, drug is contraindicated in sinus bradycardia, heart block greater than first-degree, cardiogenic shock, or overt cardiac failure.

■ When used to treat MI, metoprolol is contraindicated in patients with heart rate less than 45 beats/minute, second- or third-degree heart block, PR interval of 0.24 second or longer with first-degree heart block, systolic blood pressure less than 100 mm Hg, or moderate-to-severe cardiac failure.

■ Adrenergics increase drug's beta-adrenergic effects; use together cautiously.

Propranolol hydrochloride

Propranolol hydrochloride (Inderal) is a beta-adrenergic blocker used as an antihypertensive, antianginal, and antiarrhythmic and in adjunctive therapy of MI to reduce the incidence of VF.

Action

See "Beta-adrenergic blockers," page 97.

Dosage

■ Give 0.1 mg/kg by slow I.V. push, divided into three equal doses at 2- to 3-minute intervals, not to exceed 1 mg/minute

Special considerations

■ Drug is contraindicated in patients with bronchial asthma, sinus bradycardia and heart block greater than first-degree, cardiogenic shock, and heart failure (unless failure is caused by a tachycardia that can be treated with propranolol).

■ When used with atropine, TCAs, or other drugs with anticholinergic effects, possible antagonized propranolol-induced bradycardia may occur.

■ Given with epinephrine, propranolol may lead to severe vasoconstriction; monitor blood pressure and observe patient carefully.

■ Drug's use with NSAIDs may result in possible antagonized hypotensive effects.

■ Sympathomimetics (such as isoproterenol, MAO inhibitors) may result in antagonized beta-adrenergic stimulating effects of this drug; monitor patient closely.

■ Reactions to drug include bradycardia, hypotension, heart failure, intermittent claudication, and intensification of AV block.

■ Never administer propranolol as an adjunct in treatment of pheochromocytoma, unless the patient has been pretreated with alpha blockers.

General precautions for calcium channel blockers

Adverse reactions to calcium channel blockers include hypotension, arrhythmias, and heart failure. Follow these general precautions when administering calcium channel blockers.

■ Don't use these drugs for wide complex tachycardias of uncertain origin, or for poison- or drug-induced tachycardia.

■ Avoid use in patients with Wolff-Parkinson-White syndrome plus rapid atrial fibrillation or flutter, in patients with sick sinus syndrome, or in patients with atrioventricular block without a pacemaker.

■ Avoid use in patients receiving oral beta-adrenergic blockers.

■ Don't use I.V. doses with I.V. beta-adrenergic blockers (severe hypotension may result).

Calcium channel blockers

Calcium channel blockers are used to prevent angina that doesn't respond to other antianginal agents. (See *General precautions for calcium channel blockers.*)

Calcium channel blockers work by decreasing myocardial oxygen demand, decreasing the force of myocardial contractibility, and decreasing afterload. They also increase the oxygen supply to the myocardium by dilating the coronary arteries. (See *How calcium channel blockers work.*)

Diltiazem hydrochloride

Diltiazem (Cardizem) is a calcium channel blocker used as an antianginal. It's indicated to control ventricular rate in atrial fibrillation and atrial flutter. Diltiazem is also used in converting reentrant arrhythmias that require AV nodal conduction for their continuation. It's used after adenosine to convert PSVT to sinus rhythm.

Action

Diltiazem works by dilating systemic arteries. This dilation decreases total peripheral resistance and afterload, slightly reduces blood pressure, and increases cardiac index when the drug is given in high doses (over 200 mg). The afterload reduction and the resulting decrease in myocardial oxygen consumption account for diltiazem's effectiveness in controlling chronic stable angina.

Diltiazem also decreases myocardial oxygen demand and cardiac work by reducing heart rate, relieving coronary artery spasm (through coronary artery vasodilation), and dilating peripheral vessels. These effects serve to relieve ischemia and pain.

In patients with Prinzmetal's angina, diltiazem inhibits coronary artery spasm, increasing myocardial oxygen delivery.

Key points

Diltiazem hydrochloride

■ Dilates systemic arteries, controls ventricular rate, converts antianginal rhythm

■ Indications: vasospasmic angina, hypertension, atrial fibrillation, atrial flutter, and PSVT

■ 0.25 mg/kg I.V. over 2 minutes; may be repeated in 15 minutes at 0.35 mg/kg over 2 minutes

■ Maintenance infusion: 5 to 15 mg/hour, titrated to heart rate

How calcium channel blockers work

Calcium channel blockers prevent calcium transport across the cell membrane. This causes the cardiac muscle and the smooth muscle of the coronary arteries to contract less forcefully.

Under normal conditions, a protein complex prevents muscle contraction by keeping actin and myosin (the contractile proteins) apart. Actin and myosin must interact for a muscle to contract. When the muscle cell is stimulated, calcium ions enter the cell. This influx of calcium releases more calcium from the sarcoplasmic reticulum inside the muscle cell.

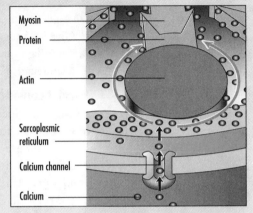

When enough calcium is released, it binds with the protein complex. The actin and myosin then can interact and the muscle contracts.

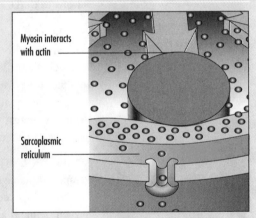

Calcium channel blockers prevent calcium from entering the cell, thereby preventing calcium release from the sarcoplasmic reticulum.

Although all the calcium channel blockers exert this effect on cardiac muscle, one compound may prove to be more effective for a specific heart condition than another. In general, however, calcium channel blockers can:
- reduce electrical excitation and mechanical contraction of the heart
- relieve excruciating anginal pain caused by spasms of coronary arteries
- allow more rest for damaged tissue
- reduce peripheral arterial resistance and myocardial oxygen demand.

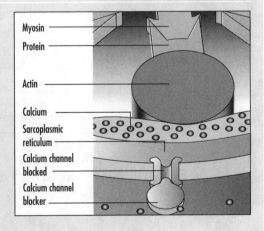

By impeding the slow inward influx of calcium at the AV node, diltiazem decreases conduction velocity and increases refractory period, thereby decreasing the impulses transmitted to the ventricles in atrial fibrillation or flutter. The end result is a decreased ventricular rate.

Dosage
- Give 0.25 mg/kg I.V. over 2 minutes; may be repeated in 15 minutes at 0.35 mg/kg over 2 minutes
- Maintenance infusion: 5 to 15 mg/hour, titrated to heart rate

Special considerations
- Drug may increase serum levels of digoxin.
- Furosemide forms precipitate when mixed with diltiazem injection. Don't administer together.
- Sublingual nitroglycerin may be administered concomitantly with diltiazem, as needed, if patient has acute angina symptoms.
- Heart block, asystole, and hypotension are the most serious overdose reactions to diltiazem and need immediate attention.

Verapamil hydrochloride
Verapamil hydrochloride (Calan, Isoptin) is a calcium channel blocker with antianginal, antihypertensive, and antiarrhythmic effects. It's indicated as an alternative drug (after adenosine) to terminate PSVT with narrow QRS complex, adequate blood pressure, and preserved left ventricular function. Verapamil controls ventricular response with atrial fibrillation, flutter, or multifocal atrial tachycardia.

Action
Verapamil manages unstable and chronic stable angina by reducing afterload, thereby decreasing oxygen consumption. It also decreases myocardial oxygen demand and cardiac workload by exerting a negative inotropic effect: reducing heart rate, relieving coronary artery spasm (via coronary artery vasodilation), and dilating peripheral vessels.

Verapamil reduces blood pressure mainly by dilating peripheral vessels. Its negative inotropic effect blocks reflex mechanisms that lead to increased blood pressure.

The drug's primary effect is on the AV node; slowed conduction reduces the ventricular rate in atrial tachyarrhythmias and blocks reentry paths in paroxysmal supraventricular arrhythmias.

Dosage
- Give 2.5 to 5 mg I.V. bolus over 2 minutes with a second dose of 5 to 10 mg, if needed, in 15 to 30 minutes to a maximum dose of 20 mg

Special considerations

■ Drug is contraindicated in patients with severe left ventricular dysfunction, cardiogenic shock, second- or third-degree AV block (except in presence of functioning pacemaker), atrial flutter or fibrillation and accessory bypass tract syndrome, severe heart failure (unless secondary to verapamil therapy), and severe hypotension.

■ I.V. verapamil is contraindicated in patients receiving I.V. beta-adrenergic blockers and in those with VT or other wide-complex tachycardia.

■ Drug's use with antihypertensives and drugs that attenuate alpha-adrenergic response may result in hypotension. When used with disopyramide, the combination may result in combined negative inotropic effects.

■ Verapamil's use with flecainide may add to negative inotropic effect and prolong AV conduction. Digoxin doses may be reduced by half with concurrent use of verapamil. Stop disopyramide 48 hours before starting verapamil therapy and don't reinstitute until 24 hours after verapamil has been stopped.

■ Use reduced doses with severely compromised cardiac function and with those patients receiving beta-adrenergic blockers.

■ Heart block, asystole, and hypotension are verapamil's most serious adverse reactions and require immediate attention

■ In elderly patients, administer I.V. doses over at least 3 minutes to minimize risk of adverse reactions.

Antiarrhythmic agents

Antiarrhythmic agents are used to treat abnormal electrical activity of the heart. There are seven classes: I, IA, IB, IC, II, III, and IV. (See *Classes of antiarrhythmics,* page 106.) In general, antiarrhythmic agents are used to treat, suppress, or prevent three major mechanisms of arrhythmias: increased automaticity, decreased conductivity, and reentry. When used in combination, antiarrhythmic agents may have a more powerful effect.

Adenosine

Adenosine (Adenocard) is a naturally occurring nucleoside indicated to convert PSVT to sinus rhythm. It's also used in the treatment of PSVT associated with accessory bypass tracts (Wolff-Parkinson-White syndrome).

Action

Adenosine acts on the AV node to slow conduction and inhibit reentry pathways.

Key points

Adenosine
■ Acts on the AV node to slow conduction and inhibit reentry pathways
■ Indications: PSVT
■ 6 mg I.V. by rapid bolus injection (over 1 to 3 seconds)
■ 12 mg I.V. if arrhythmia isn't eliminated in 1 to 2 minutes (a third dose of 12 mg I.V. may be given if necessary)

Classes of antiarrhythmics

Here are the seven classes of antiarrhythmics.

Class I (moricizine hydrochloride)
- Stabilizes the myocardial membrane
- Used to manage life-threatening ventricular arrhythmias, such as sustained ventricular tachycardia
- Interactions include cimetidine and theophylline
- Most serious adverse reaction is appearance of new arrhythmias or the exacerbation of existing arrhythmias

Class IA (disopyramide phosphate and procainamide hydrochloride)
- Used to treat various atrial and ventricular arrhythmias; they alter the myocardial cell membrane and interfere with autonomic control of pacemaker cells
- Increase the conduction rate of the atrioventricular (AV) node
- May interact with other antiarrhythmics and anticholinergic drugs
- Can also produce arrhythmias

Class IB (lidocaine hydrochloride)
- Used to treat ventricular arrhythmias; decreases the action potential duration and the effective refractory period
- May interact with other antiarrhythmics
- May interact with propranolol
- Commonly cause central nervous system (CNS) disturbances, such as confusion and paresthesia, and upper GI distress

Class IC (flecainide acetate and propafenone hydrochloride)
- Used to treat certain types of severe, refractory ventricular arrhythmias
- Flecainide may also be used to prevent paroxysmal supraventricular tachycardia in patients without structural heart disease
- Act primarily by decreasing depolarization

- May interact with other antiarrhythmics and various other drugs
- Use is limited because they can cause new arrhythmias
- Other adverse reactions include CNS, GI, and cardiovascular disturbances

Class II (beta-adrenergic blockers, esmolol hydrochloride, and propranolol hydrochloride)
- Used to treat various atrial and ventricular arrhythmias
- Use is limited by multiple effects and their ability to cause breakthrough ectopy
- May interact with phenothiazines, antihypertensives, and anticholinergics
- Most common adverse reactions involve the cardiovascular system and usually occur when the drugs are initially given

Class III (amiodarone hydrochloride)
- Used to treat ventricular arrhythmias
- Exact mechanism unclear
- May interact with other antiarrhythmics, warfarin, and antihypertensives
- Adverse reactions vary widely and include pulmonary toxicity, corneal microdeposits, photosensitivity, and thyroid imbalance

Class IV (calcium channel blockers, verapamil, and diltiazem)
- Used to treat supraventricular arrhythmias with rapid ventricular response rates
- Act by increasing the effective refractory period of the AV node and slowing the conduction rate between the atria and ventricles
- May interact with many drugs
- May cause cardiovascular alterations, such as orthostatic hypotension and new arrhythmias

Dosage
- Give 6 mg I.V. by rapid bolus injection (over 1 to 3 seconds), followed by NSS bolus of 20 ml
- Administer 12 mg I.V. if arrhythmia isn't eliminated in 1 to 2 minutes
- Administer a third dose of 12 mg I.V., if necessary

Special considerations

■ Adenosine can interact with other medications. Use cautiously with carbamazepine because higher degrees of heart block may occur with concurrent use. Dipyridamole may potentiate effects of drug; smaller doses may be needed. Methylxanthines antagonize effects of adenosine.

■ Patients receiving theophylline may need higher doses or may not respond to adenosine therapy. Likewise, caffeine may antagonize effects of adenosine and higher doses may be needed, or the patient may not have any response at all.

■ Drug is contraindicated with second- or third-degree heart block unless an artificial pacemaker is present.

■ Adverse reactions include hypotension. Because half-life of adenosine is less than 10 seconds, adverse effects of overdose usually dissipate rapidly and are self-limiting.

Amiodarone hydrochloride

Amiodarone hydrochloride (Cordarone) is a ventricular and supraventricular antiarrhythmic used in recurrent VF, unstable VT, supraventricular arrhythmias, atrial fibrillation, angina, and hypertrophic cardiomyopathy.

Action

Amiodarone has mixed class IC and III antiarrhythmic effects, but is considered a class III drug. It increases the action potential duration (repolarization inhibition). With prolonged therapy, amiodarone slows conduction through the AV node and prolongs the refractory period. Its vasodilating effect decreases cardiac workload and myocardial oxygen consumption. It affects sodium, potassium, and calcium channels as well as alpha- and beta-adrenergic blocking properties.

Dosage

■ For cardiac arrest: give 300 mg I.V. push; repeat with 150 mg I.V. push in 3 to 5 minutes
■ Maximum cumulative dose: 2.2 g I.V./24 hours
■ For wide complex tachycardia (stable): give rapid infusion of 150 mg I.V. over first 10 minutes (15 mg/minute) and repeat every 10 minutes as needed; slow infusion of 360 mg I.V. over 6 hours (1 mg/minute) may be given as an alternative
■ Maintenance infusion: 540 mg I.V. over 18 hours (0.5 mg/minute)

Special considerations

■ Watch for hypersensitivity to drug. Don't use in patients with severe sinoatrial (SA) node disease resulting in preexisting bradycardia.

■ Unless an artificial pacemaker is present, drug is also contraindicated with second- or third-degree AV block and in those with syncope caused by bradycardia.

■ Concomitant use with beta-adrenergic blockers or calcium channel blockers may cause sinus bradycardia, sinus arrest, and AV block. Use together cautiously.

■ Drug's use with digoxin, flecainide, lidocaine, phenytoin, procainamide, quinidine, and theophylline may lead to increased serum levels of these drugs, resulting in enhanced effects. Use together cautiously. In addition, digoxin, quinidine, phenytoin, and procainamide doses should be decreased during amiodarone therapy to avoid toxicity.

■ Disopyramide, phenothiazines, quinidine, and TCAs in concurrent use with amiodarone may cause additive effects that lead to a prolonged QT interval, possibly resulting in torsades de pointes. Don't use together.

■ Adverse reactions to drug are more prevalent with high doses, but usually resolve within about 4 months after drug therapy stops.

■ Amiodarone I.V. infusions exceeding 2 hours must be administered in glass or polyolefin bottles containing D_5W.

■ Amiodarone can't be removed by dialysis.

■ Bradycardia, hypotension, arrhythmias, heart failure, heart block, or sinus arrest can occur with drug's use.

Atropine sulfate

Atropine sulfate is an antiarrhythmic indicated for symptomatic bradycardia and bradyarrhythmia (junctional or escape rhythm). It's also indicated after epinephrine or vasopressin for asystole or bradycardic PEA.

Action

Atropine is an anticholinergic (parasympatholytic) that blocks the effects of acetylcholine on the SA and AV nodes, thereby increasing SA and AV node conduction velocity. It also increases sinus node discharge rate and decreases the effective refractory period of the AV node. The result is an increased heart rate. (See *How atropine speeds heart rate*.)

Dosage

■ If asystole or PEA is present: 1 mg by I.V. push; repeat every 3 to 5 minutes to maximum of 0.03 to 0.04 mg/kg

■ To treat bradycardia: 0.5 to 1 mg I.V. every 3 to 5 minutes as needed, not to exceed total dose of 0.04 mg/kg; shorter dosing interval of 3 minutes and a higher dose (0.04 mg/kg) may be used in severe clinical condition

■ Endotracheal administration: dilute in 10-ml NSS

■ Effects on heart rate peak within 2 to 4 minutes after I.V. administration

How atropine speeds heart rate

When acetylcholine is released, the vagus nerve stimulates the sinoatrial (SA) and atrioventricular (AV) nodes, which inhibits electrical conduction. This slows the heart rate. The cholinergic blocker atropine competes with acetylcholine for binding with cholinergic receptors on SA and AV nodal cells. By blocking the effects of acetylcholine, atropine speeds the heart rate.

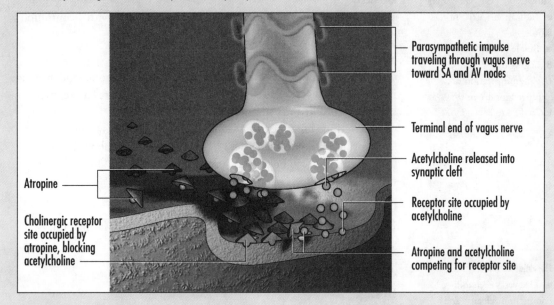

Parasympathetic impulse traveling through vagus nerve toward SA and AV nodes

Terminal end of vagus nerve

Acetylcholine released into synaptic cleft

Receptor site occupied by acetylcholine

Atropine and acetylcholine competing for receptor site

Atropine

Cholinergic receptor site occupied by atropine, blocking acetylcholine

Special considerations

■ With I.V. administration, drug may cause paradoxical initial bradycardia, which usually disappears within 2 minutes.

■ Use drug with caution in myocardial ischemia and hypoxia, because myocardial oxygen demand is increased with atropine.

■ Avoid atropine's use in hypothermic bradycardia.

■ Drug is ineffective for infranodal (type II) AV block and new third-degree block with wide QRS complex; paradoxical slowing may occur.

■ Other anticholinergics and drugs with anticholinergic effects produce additive effects; avoid concurrent use.

■ Signs of atropine overdose reflect excessive cardiovascular and CNS stimulation; treat with physostigmine administration.

■ Tachycardia may occur after higher doses of drug.

Disopyramide and disopyramide phosphate

Disopyramide (Rythmodan) and disopyramide phosphate (Norpace) are class IA antiarrhythmics indicated for treatment of VT and other ventricular arrhythmias believed to be life-threatening.

Key points

Disopyramide and disopyramide phosphate

■ Prolongs action potential

■ Indications: VT and other ventricular arrhythmias believed to be life-threatening

■ Administer 2 mg/kg I.V. over 10 minutes followed with a continuous infusion of 0.4 mg/kg/hour

Action

Disopyramide depolarizes phase 0 and prolongs action potential. It has membrane-stabilizing effects and also prolongs effective refractory period similar to procainamide.

Dosage

■ Administer 2 mg/kg I.V. over 10 minutes, followed with a continuous infusion of 0.4 mg/kg/hour

Special considerations

■ Infuse slowly, because these drugs have potent anticholinergic, negative inotropic, and hypotensive effects. They may cause heart failure, hypotension, heart block, and arrhythmias.

■ Discontinue use if heart block develops, QRS widens by greater than 25%, or if QT interval lengthens by greater than 25% above baseline.

■ NSS or D_5W can be used as compatible solutions to dilute disopyramide.

Dofetilide

Dofetilide is an antiarrhythmic indicated to treat atrial fibrillation.

Action

The precise action of dofetilide is unknown.

Dosage

■ Give I.V. single infusion of 8 mcg/kg over 30 minutes

■ I.V. administration not approved for use in the United States

Special considerations

■ Adverse reactions to drug include QT prolongation, which may be associated with torsades de pointes.

■ Patients with a history of heart failure may be more likely to have adverse reactions to drug.

■ Drug has limited use due to its required slow infusion.

Flecainide acetate

Flecainide (Tambocor) is a class IC antiarrhythmic indicated to treat ventricular arrhythmias and supraventricular arrhythmias in patients without coronary artery disease. It's also used to terminate atrial fibrillation, atrial flutter, ectopic atrial tachycardia, AV nodal reentrant tachycardia, and SVT associated with an accessory pathway.

Action

Flecainide decreases excitability, conduction velocity, and automaticity due to slowed atrial, AV node, His-Purkinje system, and intraventricular conduction. It causes a slight but significant prolongation of refractory periods in these tissues.

Dosage
- Infuse 2 mg/kg body weight at 10 mg/minute I.V.; mix only with D_5W
- I.V. administration not approved for use in United States

Special considerations
- Avoid use of drug in patients with impaired left ventricular function because of significant negative inotropic effects.
- Adverse reactions to drug include bradycardia, worsened arrhythmias, heart failure, cardiac arrest, hypotension, and neurologic symptoms (oral paresthesia and visual blurring).
- Drug may increase plasma digoxin levels by 15% to 25%.
- Flecainide's negative inotropic properties may be additive with disopyramide and verapamil. Propranolol and other beta-adrenergic blockers may cause increased toxicity to drug.
- Drug can alter endocardial-pacing thresholds in patients with pacemakers.
- Hypokalemia and hyperkalemia may alter the drug's effect.
- Because of the drug's long half-life, its full therapeutic effect may take 3 to 5 days; I.V. lidocaine may be administered concomitantly for the first several days.

Ibutilide fumarate
Ibutilide (Corvert) is a supraventricular antiarrhythmic used for conversion of atrial fibrillation or flutter.

Action
Ibutilide prolongs action potential in isolated cardiac myocytes and increases atrial and ventricular refractoriness, namely class III electrophysiologic effects.

Dosage
- Adults weighing 60 kg (132 lb) or more: give 1 mg I.V. over 10 minutes, diluted or undiluted; a second dose may be repeated after 10 minutes
- Adults weighing less than 60 kg: give 0.01 mg/kg I.V. over 10 minutes

Special considerations
- Drug may cause AV block, bradycardia, bundle-branch block, hypotension, nonsustained monomorphic and polymorphic VT, palpitations, prolonged QT segment, sustained polymorphic VT, tachycardia, and ventricular extrasystoles.
- Class Ia and class III antiarrhythmics can cause prolonged refractoriness when used with ibutilide; don't use within 4 hours after infusion. In addi-

---

Key points

Ibutilide fumarate
- Prolongs action potential in isolated cardiac myocytes and increases atrial and ventricular refractoriness, namely class III electrophysiologic effects
- Indications: atrial fibrillation or flutter
- Adults weighing 60 kg (132 lb) or more: give 1 mg I.V. over 10 minutes, diluted or undiluted; a second dose may be repeated after 10 minutes
- Adults weighing less than 60 kg: give 0.01 mg/kg I.V. over 10 minutes

tion, drugs that prolong the QT interval, phenothiazine, TCAs and tetra-cyclic antidepressants, and certain antihistamines, such as H_1-receptor antagonists, may cause arrhythmias when used with drug.

- Polymorphic VT, including torsades de pointes, develops in 2% to 5% of patients with ibutilide.
- Patients with atrial fibrillation that lasts more than 2 to 3 days must be adequately anticoagulated, generally for at least 2 weeks, before drug is administered.
- Monitor ECG continuously during drug administration and for at least 4 hours afterward or until QT returns to baseline.
- Drug can worsen ventricular arrhythmias. Make sure that a cardiac monitor, intracardiac pacing, a cardioverter or a defibrillator, and a drug for sustained VT is available.

Lidocaine

Lidocaine is a ventricular antiarrhythmic indicated for cardiac arrest from VF or VT, stable VT, wide-complex tachycardia of uncertain type, and wide-complex PSVT.

Action

As a class IB antiarrhythmic, lidocaine suppresses automaticity and shortens the effective refractory period and action potential duration of His-Purkinje fibers. It also suppresses spontaneous ventricular depolarization during diastole. The drug seems to act preferentially on diseased or ischemic myocardial tissue. By exerting its effects on the conduction system, it inhibits reentry mechanisms and halts ventricular arrhythmias.

Dosage

- A single dose of 1.5 mg/kg I.V. may suffice as treatment
- Endotracheal administration: 2 to 4 mg/kg
- Maintenance infusion: usually a simultaneous constant infusion of 1 to 4 mg/minute (30 to 50 mcg/kg/minute)
- In cardiac arrest: give 50 to 100 mg (1 to 1.5 mg/kg) I.V. dose initially; in refractory VF, may give additional 0.5 to 0.75 mg/kg I.V. push and repeat in 5 to 10 minutes; maximum dose 3 mg/kg
- In perfusing arrhythmia with stable VT, wide-complex tachycardia of uncertain type, or significant ectopy: 1 to 1.5 mg/kg I.V. push; repeat 0.5 to 0.75 mg/kg every 5 to 10 minutes with a maximum total dose of 3 mg/kg

Special considerations

- Drug is contraindicated in patients with hypersensitivity to amide-type local anesthetics, and in those with Stokes-Adams syndrome, Wolff-Parkinson-White syndrome, and severe degrees of SA, AV, or intraventricular block in absence of artificial pacemaker.

■ Beta-adrenergic blockers and cimetidine may cause lidocaine toxicity from reduced hepatic clearance. Other antiarrhythmics (such as phenytoin, procainamide, propranolol, and quinidine) may cause additive or antagonist effects and additive toxicity with drug.

■ Use infusion pump or microdrip system and timer to monitor lidocaine infusion precisely. Never exceed infusion rate of 4 mg/minute, if possible. A faster rate greatly increases risk of toxicity.

■ Therapeutic serum levels of drug range from 2 to 5 μg/ml.

■ Effects of lidocaine overdose include signs and symptoms of CNS toxicity, such as seizures or respiratory depression, and cardiovascular toxicity (as indicated by hypotension).

■ Watch for signs of excessive depression of cardiac conductivity (such as sinus node dysfunction, PR-interval prolongation, QRS-interval widening, and appearance or exacerbation of arrhythmias). If they occur, reduce dosage or stop drug.

Procainamide hydrochloride

Procainamide (Pronestyl) is a ventricular antiarrhythmic and supraventricular antiarrhythmic. It's indicated for a wide variety of arrhythmias and is also used for stable wide-complex tachycardias of unknown origin as well as for atrial fibrillation with rapid rate in Wolff-Parkinson-White syndrome.

Action

As a class IA antiarrhythmic, procainamide depresses phase 0 of the action potential. It's considered a myocardial depressant because it decreases myocardial excitability and conduction velocity and may depress myocardial contractility. Procainamide also possesses anticholinergic activity, which may modify direct myocardial effects.

In therapeutic doses, the drug reduces conduction velocity in the atria, ventricles, and His-Purkinje system. It controls atrial tachyarrhythmias by prolonging the effective refractory period and increasing the action potential duration in the atria, ventricles, and His-Purkinje system; the tissue remains refractory even after returning to resting membrane potential. Procainamide shortens the effective refractory period of the AV node. The drug's anticholinergic action also may increase AV node conductivity. Suppression of automaticity in the His-Purkinje system and ectopic pacemakers accounts for procainamide's effectiveness in treating ventricular premature beats.

At therapeutic doses, procainamide prolongs the PR and QT intervals. Procainamide exerts a peripheral vasodilatory effect; with I.V. administration, it may cause hypotension.

Key points

Procainamide hydrochloride

■ Depresses phase 0 of the action potential: decreases myocardial excitability and conduction velocity and may depress myocardial contractility; also possesses anticholinergic activity that may modify direct myocardial effects

■ Indications: wide variety of arrhythmias

■ For cardiac arrest and arrhythmia suppression: 20 mg/minute I.V. infusion with a maximum total dose of 17 mg/kg

■ Maintenance infusion: 1 to 4 mg/minute

Dosage

■ In cardiac arrest and for arryhthmia suppression: give 20 mg/minute I.V. infusion with a maximum total dose of 17 mg/kg
■ Maintenance infusion: 1 to 4 mg/minute

Special considerations

■ Drug is contraindicated in patients with hypersensitivity to procaine and related drugs; complete, second-, or third-degree heart block in the absence of an artificial pacemaker; myasthenia gravis; systemic lupus erythematosus; and atypical VT (torsades de pointes).
■ Drug's use with antihypertensives may cause additive hypotensive effects. Other antiarrhythmics may cause additive or antagonistic cardiac effects; possible additive toxic effects.
■ Infusion pump or microdrip system and timer should be used to monitor procainamide infusion precisely.
■ Drug toxicity may cause severe hypotension, widening QRS complex, junctional tachycardia, intraventricular conduction delay, VF, oliguria, and confusion.
■ Watch for prolonged QT and QRS intervals (50% or greater widening), heart block, or increased arrhythmias. When these ECG signs appear, stop drug and monitor patient closely.
■ Monitor therapeutic serum levels of procainamide: most patients are controlled at 4 to 8 μg/ml; may exhibit toxicity at levels greater than 16 μg/ml. Monitor levels of NAPA (procainamide's active metabolite) as well; some doctors feel that procainamide and NAPA levels should be 10 to 30 μg/ml.

Propafenone hydrochloride

Propafenone (Rythmol) is a sodium channel antagonist that functions as an antiarrhythmic. It's used for suppression of ventricular and supraventricular arrhythmias.

Action

Propafenone reduces the inward sodium current in myocardial cells and Purkinje fibers. It has weak beta-adrenergic blocking effects and slows the upstroke velocity of the action potential (phase 0 of the depolarization cycle). Propafenone slows conduction in the AV node, His-Purkinje system, and intraventricular conduction system, as well as prolonging the refractory period in the AV node.

Dosage

■ Infuse 1 to 2 mg/kg at 10 mg/minute slowly
■ I.V. administration not approved for use in the United States

Special considerations

■ Drug is contraindicated in patients with severe or uncontrolled heart failure; cardiogenic shock; SA, AV, or intraventricular disorders of impulse conduction in the absence of a pacemaker; bradycardia; marked hypotension; or electrolyte imbalance.

■ Propafenone causes dose-related increase in plasma digoxin levels. Quinidine competitively inhibits one of the metabolic pathways for propafenone, increasing its half-life; don't give together.

■ Adverse reactions to drug include atrial fibrillation, bradycardia, bundle branch block, angina, chest pain, edema, first-degree AV block, hypotension, increased QRS complex duration, intraventricular conduction delay, palpitations, heart failure, and proarrhythmic events (VT, PVCs, VF).

Sotalol

Sotalol (Betapace) is a beta-adrenergic blocker used as an antiarrhythmic; it's indicated for documented, life-threatening ventricular arrhythmias.

Action

Sotalol depresses sinus heart rate, slows AV conduction, increases AV nodal refractoriness, and prolongs the refractory period of atrial and ventricular muscle and AV accessory pathways in anterograde and retrograde directions. It also decreases cardiac output and lowers systolic and diastolic blood pressure.

Dosage

■ Administer 1.0 to 1.5 mg/kg, then infuse at a rate of 10 mg/minute
■ I.V. administration not approved for use in the United States

Special considerations

■ Drug should be avoided in patients with poor perfusion because of significant negative inotropic effects. It's contraindicated in patients with severe sinus node dysfunction, sinus bradycardia, second- and third-degree AV block in the absence of an artificial pacemaker, congenital or acquired long QT syndrome, cardiogenic shock, uncontrolled heart failure, or bronchial asthma.

■ Drug given with calcium channel antagonists may result in enhanced myocardial depression. In addition, use it cautiously with drugs that prolong QT interval (procainamide, amiodarone).

■ Drug may cause increased blood glucose levels and masked symptoms of hypoglycemia in diabetics.

■ The most common signs and symptoms of sotalol overdose are bradycardia, heart failure, hypotension, bronchospasm, and hypoglycemia. If overdose occurs, stop drug and observe patient closely.

Key points

Sotalol
■ Depresses sinus heart rate, slows AV conduction, increases AV nodal refractoriness, and prolongs the refractory period of atrial and ventricular muscle and AV accessory pathways in anterograde and retrograde directions
■ Indications: life-threatening ventricular arrhythmias
■ 1.0 to 1.5 mg/kg, then infuse at a rate of 10 mg/minute (I.V. administration not approved for use in the United States)

■ Patients given drug should be carefully observed until QT intervals are normalized.

Anticoagulants

Aspirin and heparin (and its derivatives) are used in cardiac patients for their anticoagulant properties. These medications, given prophylactically, have decreased the recurrence of MI.

Aspirin

Aspirin is a nonnarcotic analgesic with antipyretic, anti-inflammatory, and antiplatelet activity. It's indicated in all patients with acute coronary syndrome, especially reperfusion candidates, and in anyone with signs of ischemic pain (chest pain described as pressure, heavy weight, squeezing, or crushing).

Action

Aspirin produces analgesia by its effect on the hypothalamus (central action) and by blocking generation of pain impulses (peripheral action). The peripheral action may involve blocking of prostaglandin synthesis. As an anti-inflammatory, aspirin is believed to inhibit prostaglandin synthesis. At low doses, it appears to impede clotting by blocking prostaglandin synthetase action, preventing formation of platelet-aggregating substance thromboxane A_2. This interference with platelet activity is irreversible and can prolong bleeding time.

At high doses (1,000 mg), aspirin interferes with prostacyclin production, a potent vasoconstrictor and inhibitor of platelet aggregation, possibly negating its anticlotting properties.

Dosage

■ Give 160 to 325 mg by mouth (preferably chewable), or rectally if patient can't take orally, as soon as possible

Specific precautions

■ Drug is contraindicated in patients with bleeding disorders, those with NSAID-induced sensitivity reactions, and in children with chickenpox or flulike symptoms; use cautiously in patients with GI lesions, impaired renal function, hypoprothrombinemia, vitamin K deficiency, thrombotic thrombocytopenic purpura, or hepatic impairment.

■ Anticoagulants and thrombolytics may potentiate platelet-inhibiting effects of aspirin.

■ Other GI irritating drugs (such as antibiotics, corticosteroids, and other NSAIDs) may potentiate adverse GI effects of aspirin; use together with caution.

■ Enteric-coated products are absorbed slowly and aren't suitable for acute therapy.

Heparin

Heparin is an anticoagulant and is indicated as adjuvant therapy in acute MI. It's also indicated when fibrinolytics (such as alteplase) are administered.

Action

Heparin potentiates the effects of antithrombin, which inhibits conversion of fibrinogen to fibrin. It also inhibits the action of factors IX, X, XI, and XII. The drug inactivates fibrin-stabilizing factor, preventing formation of a stable fibrin clot.

Because heparin doesn't have fibrinolytic action, it can't dissolve existing clots.

Dosage

■ Give initial bolus of 60 IU/kg with a maximum bolus dose of 4,000 IU; then 12 IU/kg/hour I.V. infusion (maximum of 1,000 IU/hour for patients weighing more than 70 kg); infusion may be rounded to the nearest 50 IU
■ Adjust dosage to maintain activated partial thromboplastin time (aPTT) 1.5 to 2.0 times the control values for 48 hours or until angiography; for activated coagulation time, 2 to 3 times the control value
■ Target range for aPTT after the first 24 hours: between 50 and 70 seconds (may vary with the laboratory)
■ Follow facility policy for heparin protocol

Special considerations

■ Drug is incompatible with alteplase, amiodarone, diazepam, diltiazem, dobutamine, morphine sulfate, phenytoin sodium, quinidine gluconate, solutions with a phosphate buffer, sodium carbonate, or sodium oxalate.
■ Drug is contraindicated in those with hypersensitivity to heparin (except in life-threatening situations), severe thrombocytopenia (possible exacerbation), uncontrollable bleeding (except when caused by disseminated intravascular coagulation), and severe, uncontrolled hypertension.
■ Use drug extremely cautiously in patients with hemorrhaging (or at risk for it) and in those with GI conditions such as ulcerative colitis. Severe hemorrhage, acute thrombocytopenia, and new thrombus formation (white clot syndrome) can occur with drug.
■ Drug given with antihistamines and cardiac glycosides may cause diminished anticoagulant effect. Aspirin, dipyridamole, other NSAIDs, and indomethacin with drug may cause impaired platelet aggregation and possible increased risk of bleeding.

Key points

Heparin
■ Potentiates the effects of antithrombin, which inhibits conversion of fibrinogen to fibrin
■ Also inhibits the action of factors IX, X, XI, and XII; inactivates fibrin-stabilizing factor and prevents formation of a stable fibrin clot
■ Indications: adjuvant therapy in acute MI and fibrinolytic therapy
■ Initial bolus of 60 IU/kg with a maximum bolus dose of 4,000 IU, then 12 IU/kg/hour I.V. infusion (maximum of 1,000 IU/hour for patients weighing more than 70 kg); infusion may be rounded to the nearest 50 IU
■ Adjust dosage to maintain aPTT 1.5 to 2.0 times the control values for 48 hours or until angiography

When platelet counts fall

A platelet count at or below 100,000 contraindicates heparin. As an alternative to heparin, direct antithrombins may be used, which may provide the anticoagulant effect of heparin without decreasing platelet counts. These agents include:

■ desirudin (Revasc), administered at 0.1 mg/kg I.V. bolus and followed by infusion of 0.1 mg/kg/hour for 72 hours

■ lepirudin (Refludan), administered at 0.4 mg/kg I.V. bolus followed by infusion of 0.15 mg/kg/hour for 72 hours.

An alternative to I.V. dosing is a subcutaneous dose of dalteparin and enoxaparin at 1 mg/kg twice per day for 2 to 8 days, administered concurrently with aspirin.

■ If overdose occurs, give 1% solution of protamine sulfate by slow infusion. Don't infuse more than 50 mg in a 10-minute period. Hemodialysis doesn't remove the drug.

■ Monitor patient for bleeding, which may occur at any site and may be difficult to detect. Frequently monitor hematocrit and check stools for occult blood to detect asymptomatic bleeding. Regularly inspect venipuncture and wound sites and the skin for bleeding.

■ Frequently monitor platelet count and coagulation tests, such as prothrombin time, aPTT, and activated coagulation time. (See *When platelet counts fall.*)

Antidotes

Antidotes are used to reverse the effects of medications or situations in which the patient's life might be in danger. Among these are digoxin immune FAB, flumazenil, glucagon, and naloxone hydrochloride.

Digoxin immune FAB

Digoxin immune FAB (Digibind) is an antibody fragment that works as a cardiac glycoside antidote by preventing or reversing toxic effects of cardiac glycosides. It's indicated for potentially life-threatening digoxin toxicity (life-threatening arrhythmias, hyperkalemia with a plasma level greater than 5 mEq/L).

Action

With digoxin immune FAB, specific antigen-binding fragments bind with free digoxin intravascularly or in extracellular spaces, making them unavailable for binding at their sites of action.

Key points

Digoxin immune FAB

■ Prevents or reverses toxic effects of cardiac glycosides

■ Indications: life-threatening digoxin toxicity

■ Average dose: 400 mg — dosage based on ingested amount of serum level of digoxin

Dosage

■ Adults and children: dosage based on ingested amount or serum level of digoxin
■ I.V. dose given with average dose of 10 vials (400 mg); some individuals may require up to 20 vials (800 mg)
■ If cardiac arrest is imminent: may be given rapidly by direct I.V. injection into vein or I.V. line containing a free-flowing, compatible solution, using a 0.22-micron filter needle

Special considerations

■ Digoxin levels greater than 2.5 ng/ml may be toxic. Ingestion of more than 10 mg of digoxin (in adults) or 4 mg (in children) at one time may cause cardiac arrest; therefore, Digibind should be used.
■ Obtain serum digoxin levels 8 hours after last dose to ensure accuracy.
■ Closely monitor serum potassium level during and after administration of drug.

Flumazenil

Flumazenil (Romazicon) is a benzodiazepine antagonist. It's indicated to treat respiratory depression and sedative effects resulting from pure benzodiazepine overdose.

Action

Flumazenil competitively inhibits the actions of benzodiazepines on the gamma-aminobutyric acid–benzodiazepine receptor complex.

Dosage

■ Initially, give 0.2 mg I.V. over 15 seconds; if patient doesn't reach desired level of consciousness, administer 0.3 mg I.V. over 30 seconds; if still not responding adequately, give 0.5 mg I.V. over 30 seconds; repeat 0.5 mg doses at 1-minute intervals until a cumulative dose of 3 mg has been given

Special considerations

■ Don't give more than 5 mg of drug over 5 minutes initially. Sedation that persists after this dosage is unlikely to be caused by benzodiazepines. (See *When flumazenil is contraindicated,* page 120.)
■ If the patient becomes sedated again, drug dosage may be repeated after 20 minutes; however, no more than 1 mg should be given at any one time, and no more than 3 mg/hour.
■ Monitor patient closely for resedation after reversal of benzodiazepine effects, which may occur because the duration of action of flumazenil is shorter than that of all benzodiazepines. Duration of monitoring depends on the specific drug being reversed. Monitor closely after long-acting ben-

Key points

Flumazenil
■ Inhibits action of benzodiazapines
■ Indications: benzodiazepine overdose
■ 0.2 mg I.V., then 0.3 mg I.V. if desired response doesn't occur — may increase to 0.5 mg and repeat at 1-minute intervals

When flumazenil is contraindicated

Before receiving flumazenil, patients should have a secure airway and I.V. access. The patient should also be awakened gradually. In addition, flumazenil is contraindicated in patients who:
■ have been given a benzodiazepine for a potentially life-threatening condition (such as to control intracranial pressure or status epilepticus)
■ show signs of serious cyclic antidepressant overdose
■ are at risk for mixed overdose (especially in cases when seizures are likely to occur).
   Flumazenil should be given as a series of small injections, not as a single bolus dose, to control reversal of sedation to the desired endpoint and to minimize risk of adverse effects.
   Flumazenil should be used with caution in patients who:
■ are at high risk for developing seizures
■ are withdrawing from sedative-hypnotics
■ are displaying some signs of seizure activity (such as myoclonus)
■ may be at risk for unrecognized benzodiazepine dependence (such as those in the intensive care unit)
■ are experiencing alcohol or other drug dependencies because of increased risk of benzodiazepine tolerance
■ have a head injury.

zodiazepines such as diazepam, or after high doses of short-acting benzodiazepines such as midazolam.

Glucagon

Glucagon is an antihypoglycemic (reverses low blood glucose levels). It's indicated as adjuvant treatment of toxic effects of calcium channel blockers or beta-adrenergic blockers.

Action

Glucagon promotes hepatic glycogenolysis and gluconeogenesis, raising serum glucose levels. It also relaxes GI smooth muscle and produces a positive inotropic and chronotropic myocardial effect.

Dosage

■ Give 1 to 5 mg I.V. over 2 to 5 minutes

Special considerations

■ Drug is incompatible with sodium chloride solution and other solutions with a pH of 3 to 9.5 because it may cause precipitation.
■ Drug may cause vomiting and hypoglycemia.
■ If hypoglycemic patient doesn't respond to drug, give I.V. dextrose.
■ Drug may fail to relieve coma because of markedly depleted hepatic stores of glycogen or irreversible brain damage caused by prolonged hypoglycemia.

Key points

Glucagon
■ Promotes hepatic glycogenolysis and gluconeogenesis, raising serum glucose levels; also relaxes GI smooth muscle and produces a positive inotropic and chronotropic myocardial effect
■ Indications: adjuvant treatment of toxic effects of calcium channel blockers or beta-adrenergic blockers
■ 1 to 5 mg I.V. over 2 to 5 minutes

■ Drug has been used as a cardiac stimulant in managing toxicity resulting from use of beta-adrenergic blockers, quinidine, and TCAs.

Naloxone hydrochloride

Naloxone hydrochloride (Narcan) is an antidote used as a narcotic (opioid) antagonist. It's indicated for respiratory and neurologic depression due to opiate intoxication.

Action

In patients who have received an opioid agonist or other analgesic with narcotic-like effects, naloxone antagonizes most of the effects; especially respiratory depression, sedation, and hypotension. Because the duration of action is shorter than that of the opioid, effects may return. The precise mechanism of action is unknown, but is thought to involve competitive antagonism of more than one opiate receptor in the CNS.

Dosage

■ Give 0.4 mg I.V. repeated every 2 to 3 minutes; higher doses may be used for complete narcotic reversal; up to 10 mg can be administered over a short period (less than 10 minutes)

■ In suspected opiate-addicted patients, dosage should be titrated until ventilations are adequate; begin with 0.2 mg every 2 minutes for three doses, then 1.4 mg I.V. push

Special considerations

■ Drug given with cardiotoxic drugs may cause potential serious cardiovascular effects. Avoid using together.

■ Tachycardia, hypertension (with higher-than-recommended doses), hypotension, VF, and cardiac arrest can occur with drug.

■ Withdrawal symptoms can occur in narcotic-dependent patients with higher-than-recommended doses of drug.

■ Because naloxone's duration of activity is shorter than that of most narcotics, continued monitoring and repeated doses are usually necessary to manage acute narcotic overdose in a non-addicted patient.

■ Drug isn't effective in treating respiratory depression caused by non-opioid drugs.

■ Drug can be diluted in D_5W or NSS; use within 24 hours after mixing.

ACE inhibitors

Angiotensin-converting enzyme (ACE) inhibitors are used to reduce mortality and improve left ventricular function in post-acute MI patients. They prevent adverse left ventricular remodeling, delay progression of heart failure, and decrease sudden death and recurrent MI.

Key points

Naloxone hydrochloride
■ Precise mechanism of action is unknown, but is thought to involve competitive antagonism of more than one opiate receptor in the CNS
■ Indications: opiate intoxication
■ 0.4 mg I.V. repeated every 2 to 3 minutes; up to 10 mg can be administered over a short period (less than 10 minutes)

General precautions for ACE inhibitors

Observe these general precautions when administering angiotensin-converting enzyme (ACE) inhibitors.

■ ACE inhibitors are contraindicated in pregnancy as they may cause fetal injury or death; they are also contraindicated in angioedema.

■ These medications are usually started in first 24 hours after fibrinolytic therapy has been completed and blood pressure has stabilized.

■ Excessive hypotension can occur when these medications are used with diuretics or other antihypertensives.

■ Risk of hypoglycemia can occur in diabetics when therapy with these drugs is initiated.

■ These drugs may cause lithium toxicity and can also increase risk of hyperkalemia in patients taking potassium-sparing diuretics.

■ These drugs may cause angioedema.

■ Potassium-containing salt substitutes may cause hyperkalemia in patients taking ACE inhibitors.

■ Use these drugs with caution in patients with renal impairment.

ACE inhibitors are indicated in suspected MI and ST segment elevation in two or more precordial leads, in hypertension, and in heart failure (without hypotension) in patients not responding to digoxin or diuretics. It should also be used when there are clinical signs of acute MI with left ventricular dysfunction and left ventricular ejection fraction of greater than 40%.

ACE inhibitors reduce blood pressure by interrupting the renin-angiotensin-aldosterone cycle. They specifically prevent the conversion of angiotensin I to angiotensin II, a potent vasoconstrictor. Reduced formation of angiotensin II decreases peripheral arterial resistance, thus decreasing aldosterone secretion. This, in turn, decreases sodium and water retention and decreases blood pressure. It also decreases systemic vascular resistance (afterload) and pulmonary capillary wedge pressure (preload), thus increasing cardiac output in patients with heart failure. (See *General precautions for ACE inhibitors*.)

Captopril

Captopril (Capoten) is an ACE inhibitor used to treat hypertension and heart failure.

Action

See "ACE inhibitors," page 121.

Key points

Captopril

■ Interrupts the renin-angiotensin-aldosterone cycle, as well as decreases systemic vascular resistance

■ Indications: hypertension and heart failure

■ 6.25 mg P.O. initially as a single dose; advance to 25 mg t.i.d., and then to 50 mg t.i.d. as tolerated

Dosage

■ Give 6.25 mg by mouth initially as a single dose; advance to 25 mg three times per day, and then to 50 mg three times per day as tolerated

Special considerations

■ Drug may increase serum digoxin and lithium levels, leading to toxicity.
■ Aspirin and other NSAIDs may decrease drug's antihypertensive effect.
■ Several weeks of therapy may be required before beneficial effects of drug are seen.
■ Overdose of captopril is manifested primarily by severe hypotension.

Enalapril

Enalapril (Vasotec) is an ACE inhibitor used to treat hypertension and heart failure.

Action

See "ACE inhibitors," page 121.

Dosage

■ By mouth: Give 2.5 mg as a single dose initially, and then increase to 20 mg twice per day
■ I.V.: Give 1.25 mg initially over 5 minutes, then 1.25 to 5.0 mg every 6 hours
■ Give drug slowly in I.V. form over at least 5 minutes; may be diluted in 50 ml of compatible solution (such as D_5W, NSS for injection, D_5LR, D_5NSS for injection, or Isolyte E) and infused over 15 minutes

Special considerations

■ Be aware that patients with diabetes, impaired renal failure, or heart failure can develop hyperkalemia when given enalapril. Hyperkalemia can also develop in patients concurrently receiving drugs that increase serum potassium level.

Lisinopril

Lisinopril (Prinivil, Zestril) is an ACE inhibitor used to treat hypertension and heart failure, as well as to improve survival rate after acute MI.

Action

See "ACE inhibitors," page 121.

Dosage

■ For hypertension: 20 to 40 mg by mouth daily
■ For heart failure: 5 mg by mouth daily
■ For acute MI: 5 mg by mouth within first 24 hours of onset of symptoms, then 5 mg by mouth after 24 hours, then 10 mg given after 48 hours, then 10 mg daily for 6 weeks

Key points

Ramipril

■ Interrupts the renin-angiotensin-aldosterone cycle, and decreases systemic vascular resistance
■ Indications: hypertension and heart failure
■ 2.5 mg P.O. initially as a single dose, and increase to 5 mg P.O. b.i.d. as tolerated

Key points

Nitroprusside sodium

■ A potent vasodilator indicated for hypertensive crisis
■ Known to reduce afterload in heart failure, acute pulmonary edema, and acute mitral or aortic valve regurgitation
■ Acts directly on vascular smooth muscle, causing peripheral vasodilation
■ For hypertension, begin at 0.10 mcg/ kg/minute and titrate upward every 3 to 5 minutes to desired effect (up to 5.0 mcg/kg/minute)
■ Can cause cyanide toxicity; check serum thiocyanate levels every 72 hours; levels above 100 µg/ml are associated with cyanide toxicity, which can produce profound hypotension, metabolic acidosis, dyspnea, ataxia, and vomiting; if such symptoms occur, stop infusion and reevaluate therapy

Special considerations

■ Use cautiously in patients with impaired renal function because hyperkalemia may occur.

Ramipril

Ramipril (Altace) is an ACE inhibitor used to treat hypertension and heart failure.

Action

See "ACE inhibitors," page 121.

Dosage

■ Give 2.5 mg by mouth initially as a single dose, and increase to 5 mg by mouth twice per day as tolerated

Special considerations

■ Closely assess renal function during the first few weeks of therapy, especially in patients with severe heart failure or hypertension.

Vasodilating antihypertensive agents

Vasodilating antihypertensive agents include direct vasodilators (typically nitroprusside) and calcium channel blockers (typically verapamil hydrochloride). Direct vasodilators act on arteries, veins, or both and commonly produce adverse reactions related to reflex activation of the sympathetic nervous system. Calcium channel blockers produce arteriolar relaxation, which reduces the mechanical activity of vascular smooth muscle. These drugs usually are used as adjuncts in treating hypertension rather than as primary agents.

Nitroprusside is discussed here. For a discussion of verapamil hydrochloride, see page 104.

Nitroprusside sodium

Nitroprusside (Nipride) is a potent vasodilator indicated for hypertensive crisis. It's known to reduce afterload in heart failure, acute pulmonary edema, and acute mitral or aortic valve regurgitation.

Action

Nitroprusside acts directly on vascular smooth muscle, causing peripheral vasodilation.

Dosage

■ Titrate I.V. infusion to blood pressure; begin at 0.10 mcg/kg/minute and titrate upward every 3 to 5 minutes to desired effect (up to 5.0 mcg/kg/minute)

Special considerations
■ Drug's action occurs within 1 to 2 minutes.
■ Other antihypertensives may potentiate drug's effects.
■ Epinephrine given with drug causes increased blood pressure during therapy. Don't use together.
■ Prepare drug in solution using D_5W solution; because of light sensitivity, foil-wrap I.V. solution (but not tubing). Fresh solutions have faint brownish tint; discard after 24 hours.
■ Infuse drug with infusion pump. Drug is best run piggyback through a peripheral line with no other drugs; don't adjust rate of main I.V. line while drug is running because even small boluses can cause severe hypotension.
■ Drug can cause cyanide toxicity. Check serum thiocyanate levels every 72 hours; levels above 100 µg/ml are associated with cyanide toxicity, which can produce profound hypotension, metabolic acidosis, dyspnea, ataxia, and vomiting. If such symptoms occur, stop infusion and reevaluate therapy.

Diuretic agents

Diuretics are used to treat cardiac patients experiencing edema. Close monitoring of electrolyte levels and accurately assessing fluid balance (intake, output) is important when using diuretics.

Furosemide
Furosemide (Lasix), a loop diuretic, is an antihypertensive as well as a highly potent diuretic. It's indicated as adjunctive therapy of acute pulmonary edema in patients with systolic blood pressure greater than 90 to 100 mm Hg without signs and symptoms of shock. Furosemide is also used in hypertensive emergencies and in cases of increased intracranial pressure (ICP).

Action
Furosemide inhibits sodium and chloride reabsorption in the proximal part of the ascending loop of Henle, promoting excretion of sodium, water, chloride, and potassium. Its antihypertensive effect may result from renal and peripheral vasodilation, a temporary increase in glomerular filtration rate, and a decrease in peripheral vascular resistance.

Dosage
■ Give 0.5 to 1.0 mg/kg I.V. infusion over 1 to 2 minutes; if no response, increase to 2.0 mg/kg and give slowly over 1 to 2 minutes

Special considerations
■ Drug may decrease hypoglycemic effects in diabetic patients.

Key points

Furosemide
■ Inhibits sodium and chloride reabsorption in the proximal part of the ascending loop of Henle, promoting excretion of sodium, water, chloride, and potassium
■ Indications: acute pulmonary edema, hypertensive emergencies, increased ICP
■ Give 0.5 to 1.0 mg/kg I.V. infusion over 1 to 2 minutes; if no response, increase to 2.0 mg/kg and give slowly over 1 to 2 minutes

■ When given with antihypertensives, drug may increase risk of hypotension.

■ Cardiac glycosides and lithium may increase risk of drug's toxicity because of furosemide-induced hypokalemia; monitor patient for arrhythmias.

■ NSAIDs may inhibit diuretic response.

■ Give I.V. furosemide slowly, over 1 to 2 minutes. For I.V. infusion, dilute furosemide in D_5W, NSS, or LR, and use within 24 hours. If high-dose furosemide therapy is needed, administer as a controlled infusion not exceeding 4 mg/minute.

■ Signs and symptoms of overdose include profound electrolyte and volume depletion, which may precipitate circulatory collapse.

Mannitol

Mannitol (Osmitrol) is an osmotic diuretic indicated to reduce increased ICP and to prevent acute renal failure.

Action

Mannitol increases the osmotic pressure of glomerular filtrate. This inhibits tubular reabsorption of water and electrolytes, thus promoting diuresis and urinary elimination of certain drugs. Reduction of ICP occurs because the drug elevates plasma osmolality, enhancing flow of water into extracellular fluid.

Dosage

■ For increased intracranial pressure: give 1.5 to 2 g/kg as a 15% to 20% solution I.V. over 30 to 60 minutes

Special considerations

■ Drug is contraindicated in patients with severe pulmonary congestion, pulmonary edema, severe heart failure, severe dehydration, metabolic edema, progressive renal disease or dysfunction, or active intracranial bleeding except during craniotomy. Use with extreme caution in patients with compromised renal function; monitor vital signs (including central venous pressure) hourly as well as input and output, weight, renal function, and fluid balance.

■ Drug may enhance possibility of digoxin toxicity.

■ Drug should be administered I.V. via an in-line filter with great care to avoid extravasation.

■ Mannitol solutions commonly crystallize at low temperatures; place crystallized solutions in a hot water bath, shake vigorously to dissolve crystals, and cool to body temperature before use. Don't use solutions with undissolved crystals.

■ Monitor serum and urinary sodium and potassium levels daily with drug.

Key points

Mannitol
■ Increases the osmotic pressure of glomerular filtrate, enhancing flow of water into extracellular fluid
■ Indications: increased ICP, renal failure, drug intoxication
■ 1.5 to 2 g/kg I.V. over 30 to 60 minutes

Electrolytes and buffers

Electrolytes and buffering agents are used for electrolyte replacement therapy. Calcium chloride, magnesium sulfate, and sodium bicarbonate are the drugs most frequently used in ACLS.

Calcium chloride

Calcium chloride is a calcium supplement used for patients experiencing electrolyte imbalances. It's indicated for known or suspected hyperkalemia (as in renal failure) and in hypocalcemia. It serves as an antidote for calcium channel blocker overdose or beta-adrenergic blocker overdose. It may also be given prophylactically before I.V. calcium channel blockers to prevent hypotension.

Action

Calcium chloride is essential for maintaining the functional integrity of the nervous, muscular, and skeletal systems, as well as for maintaining cell membrane and capillary permeability.

Dosage

■ Give 2 to 4 mg/kg (usually 2 ml) slow I.V. push and repeat at 10-minute intervals as needed

Special considerations

■ Don't use drug routinely in cardiac arrhythmias.
■ Don't mix drug with sodium bicarbonate.
■ Drug may antagonize the therapeutic effects of calcium channel blockers such as verapamil. It also increases digoxin toxicity when used with digoxin; administer very cautiously, if at all, to patients receiving digoxin. In addition, calcium competes with magnesium, thus decreasing the amount of bioavailable magnesium, so use together cautiously.
■ Give calcium chloride I.V. only; don't use scalp vein in children as it may cause tissue necrosis. Give I.V. calcium slowly through small-bore needle into large vein. Severe necrosis and sloughing of tissue may occur after extravasation. Calcium gluconate is less irritating to veins and tissue than calcium chloride. Crash carts usually contain both gluconate and chloride. Be sure to specify form to be administered.
■ Hypercalcemia may result when large doses of drug are given to patients with chronic renal failure. Acute hypercalcemia syndrome is characterized by markedly elevated plasma calcium level, lethargy, weakness, nausea and vomiting, and coma; it may lead to sudden death.
■ Assess Chvostek's and Trousseau's signs periodically to check for tetany and monitor patient for symptoms of hypercalcemia (nausea, vomiting,

Key points

Calcium chloride
■ Essential for maintaining the functional integrity of the nervous, muscular, and skeletal systems, and for maintaining cell membrane and capillary permeability
■ Indications: hyperkalemia, hypocalcemia, calcium channel blocker overdose
■ Give 2 to 4 mg/kg slow I.V. push and repeat at 10-minute intervals as needed

headache, mental confusion, anorexia) with drug, and report them immediately.

Magnesium sulfate

Magnesium sulfate is a mineral and electrolyte indicated for use in cardiac arrest only when torsades de pointes is suspected or hypomagnesia is present. It's also indicated in refractory VF (after lidocaine), torsades de pointes with a pulse, and in life-threatening ventricular arrhythmias due to digoxin toxicity.

Action

Magnesium sulfate depresses the CNS and respiratory system. It acts peripherally, causing vasodilation; moderate doses result in flushing and sweating, while high doses may lead to hypotension.

Dosage

■ Administer drug by constant infusion pump, if available; maximum infusion rate is 150 mg/minute. Rapid drip causes feeling of heat. Level of magnesium sulfate for I.V. administration shouldn't exceed 20% at a rate no greater than 150 mg/minute (1.5 ml of a 10% concentration or equivalent). To calculate grams of magnesium in a percentage of solution: X% = X g/100 ml (for example, 25% = 25 g/100 ml = 250 mg/ml).
■ In cardiac arrest (for hypomagnesia or torsades de pointes): give 1 to 2 g (2 to 4 ml of 50% solution) diluted in 10 ml of D_5W I.V. push
■ In torsades de pointes without cardiac arrest: give loading dose of 1 to 2 g in 50 to 100 ml D_5W over 5 to 60 minutes I.V.; follow with 0.5 to 1.0 g/hour I.V. and titrate to control torsades de pointes
■ In acute MI: give loading dose of 1 to 2 g in 50 to 100 ml D_5W over 5 to 60 minutes I.V.; follow with 0.5 to 1.0 g/hour I.V. for up to 24 hours

Special considerations

■ When drug is given with cardiac glycosides, it may exacerbate arrhythmias.
■ Drug co-administered with I.V. calcium can cause changes in cardiac conduction in digitalized patients and may lead to heart block; avoid concomitant use.
■ In I.V. bolus form, drug must be injected slowly (to avoid respiratory or cardiac arrest); hypotension, circulatory collapse, depressed cardiac function, and respiratory paralysis can occur.
■ Signs and symptoms of magnesium overdose include a sharp drop in blood pressure and respiratory paralysis, ECG changes (increased PR, QRS, and QT intervals), heart block, and asystole. Treatment requires artificial ventilation and I.V. calcium salt to reverse respiratory depression and heart block.

Sodium bicarbonate

Sodium bicarbonate is an alkalinizing agent used as a systemic hydrogen ion buffer. (See *Indications for sodium bicarbonate.*)

Action

Sodium bicarbonate is an alkalinizing drug that dissociates to provide bicarbonate ion. Excess bicarbonate (bicarbonate not needed to buffer hydrogen ions) causes systemic alkalinization and, when excreted, urinary alkalinization as well.

Dosage

- Give 1 mEq/kg I.V. bolus and repeat half of this dose every 10 minutes (depending on blood gas values if rapidly available)
- Calculate based on bicarbonate concentration

Special considerations

- If monitoring blood gas results, be aware that an acute change in partial pressure of arterial carbon dioxide ($PaCO_2$) of 1 mm Hg is associated with an increase or decrease in pH of 0.008 U (relative to normal $PaCO_2$ of 40 mm Hg and normal pH of 7.4).
- Avoid extravasation of sodium I.V. solutions. Addition of calcium salts may cause precipitate; bicarbonate may inactivate catecholamines in solution (epinephrine, phenylephrine, and dopamine).
- Clinical signs of sodium overdose include depressed consciousness and obtundation from hypernatremia, tetany from hypocalcemia, arrhythmias from hypokalemia, and seizures from alkalosis. Correct fluid, electrolyte, and pH abnormalities. Monitor vital signs and fluid and electrolyte levels closely.

Key points

Sodium bicarbonate
- An alkalinizing agent used as a systemic hydrogen ion buffer
- Indications: hyperkalemia, preexisting acidosis, overdose, prolonged resuscitation
- Give 1 mEq/kg I.V. bolus and repeat half of this dose every 10 minutes (depending on blood gas values if rapidly available); calculate based on bicarbonate concentration

Contraindications and precautions for fibrinolytic agents

Contraindications for fibrinolytic agents include:
- active internal bleeding (except menses) within 21 days
- history of cerebrovascular, intracranial, or intraspinal event within 3 months (stroke, arteriovenous malformation, neoplasm, aneurysm, recent trauma, recent surgery)
- major surgery or serious trauma within 14 days
- aortic dissection
- severe, uncontrolled hypertension
- known bleeding disorders
- prolonged cardiopulmonary resuscitation with evidence of thoracic trauma
- lumbar puncture within 7 days
- recent arterial puncture at noncompressible site.
   Observe these special precautions when using fibrinolytic agents:
- during the first 24 hours of fibrinolytic therapy for ischemic stroke, don't administer aspirin or heparin
- initiate two peripheral I.V. lines, using one exclusively for fibrinolytic administration
- adjuvant therapy for acute myocardial infarction includes administration of 160 to 325 mg aspirin chewed as soon as possible, and heparin therapy initiated immediately and continued for 48 hours if alteplase or retavase is used
- monitor for adverse reactions, including cerebral hemorrhage; hypotension; arrhythmias; severe, spontaneous bleeding (cerebral, retroperitoneal, genitourinary, GI); and bleeding at puncture sites
- avoid I.M. injections, venipuncture, and arterial puncture during therapy; use pressure dressings or ice packs on recent puncture sites to prevent bleeding; if arterial puncture is needed, select a site on the arm and apply pressure for 30 minutes afterward.

Fibrinolytic agents

Fibrinolytic agents are thrombolytic enzymes that promote the enzyme plasmin, which in turn dissolves fibrin and fibrous strands that bind clots. They are indicated for acute MI in adults with:
- ST segment elevation (greater than or equal to 1 mm in two or more leads)
- evidence of new left bundle-branch block on ECG
- history and symptoms strongly suspicious of myocardial injury, such as bundle-branch block obscuring ST analysis
- an onset of acute MI symptoms of less than 12 hours.

Note that certain conditions contraindicate the use of fibrinolytic agents. (See *Contraindications and precautions for fibrinolytic agents.*)

Alteplase

Alteplase (recombinant alteplase [Activase] tissue plasminogen activator [tPA]) is a thrombolytic enzyme indicated for acute MI and acute ischemic stroke.

Action

Alteplase exerts thrombolytic action due to an enzyme that catalyzes the conversion of tissue plasminogen to plasmin in the presence of fibrin. This fibrin specificity produces local fibrinolysis in the area of recent clot formation, with limited systemic proteolysis. In patients with acute MI, this allows for reperfusion of ischemic cardiac muscle and improved left ventricular function with a decreased risk of heart failure.

Dosage

■ In acute MI for adults weighing over 67 kg: give 15 mg I.V. push, then administer 50 mg over 30 minutes; then 35 mg over 60 minutes
■ In acute MI for adults weighing less than 67 kg: give accelerated infusion over 1.5 hours; give 15 mg I.V. bolus initially, then administer 0.75 mg/kg I.V. over the next 30 minutes (not to exceed 50 mg), and 0.50 mg/kg over the next 60 minutes (not to exceed 35 mg); the total dose shouldn't exceed 100 mg
■ An alternative 3-hour infusion may be given; give 60 mg I.V. in the first hour with an initial 6 to 10 mg given as a bolus; then give 20 mg/hour for 2 additional hours
■ In acute ischemic stroke: infuse 0.9 mg/kg (maximum 90 mg) I.V. over 60 minutes; give 10% of the total dose as an initial I.V. bolus over 1 minute; give the remaining dose over the next 60 minutes

Special considerations

■ Drugs that antagonize platelet function (abciximab, aspirin, and dipyridamole) may increase risk of bleeding if given before, during, or after alteplase therapy; avoid concomitant use.
■ Expect to begin alteplase infusions as soon as possible after onset of MI symptoms.
■ Administer drug within 3 hours after onset of stroke symptoms, but only after excluding intracranial hemorrhage by computed tomography scan or other diagnostic imaging methods.
■ Treatment with drug should be performed only in facilities that can provide appropriate evaluation and management of intracranial hemorrhage.
■ Heparin is usually administered during or after alteplase as part of treatment regimen for acute MI or pulmonary embolism.
■ Use of anticoagulant or antiplatelet therapy for 24 hours is contraindicated when alteplase is used for acute ischemic stroke.
■ Prepare alteplase solution using supplied sterile water, not bacteriostatic water, for injection.
■ Don't mix other drugs with alteplase. Use 18G needle for preparing solution — aim water stream at lyophilized cake. Expect a slight foaming to occur and don't use if vacuum isn't present.

■ Drug may be further diluted with NSS injection or D_5W to yield a concentration of 0.5 mg/ml. Reconstituted or diluted solutions are stable for up to 8 hours at room temperature.

■ Altered results with drug may be expected in coagulation and fibrinolytic tests. The use of aprotinin (150 to 200 U/ml) in the blood sample may attenuate this interference.

■ Excessive I.V. dosage of drug can lead to bleeding problems. Doses of 150 mg have been associated with intracranial bleeding.

■ Discontinue infusion of drug immediately if signs or symptoms of bleeding occur.

Anistreplase

Anistreplase (Eminase; anisoylated plasminogen streptokinase activator complex [APSAC]) is a fibrinolytic agent indicated for acute MI.

Action

Anistreplase is derived from lysplasminogen and streptokinase. It's formulated into a fibrinolytic enzyme plus activator complex with the activator temporarily blocked by an anisoyl group. It's activated in vivo by a nonenzymatic process that removes the anisoyl group. The active drug converts plasminogen to plasmin, resulting in thrombolysis.

Dosage

■ Give 30 IU I.V. over 2 to 5 minutes after reconstitution of 30 U in 5 ml sterile water or D_5W

Special considerations

■ Drugs that alter platelet function, including aspirin, dipyridamole, heparin, or oral anticoagulants, may increase risk of bleeding with anistreplase.

■ Drug prolongs partial thromboplastin time, prothrombin time, and thrombin time.

■ Drug remains active in vivo and can cause degeneration of fibrinogen in blood samples drawn for analysis.

■ Decreases in alpha$_2$-antiplasmin, factor V, factor VII, fibrinogen, and plasminogen, as well as hemoglobin level and hematocrit have been reported with drug.

■ Drug efficacy may be limited if antistreptokinase antibodies are present.

Reteplase

Reteplase (recombinant, Retavase) is a fibrinolytic agent indicated for acute MI.

Action

Reteplase enhances cleavage of plasminogen to generate plasmin, which leads to fibrinolysis.

Dosage

- Give first 10 U I.V. bolus over 2 minutes; 30 minutes later, give a second 10 U I.V. bolus over 2 minutes
- Give NSS flush before and after each bolus

Special considerations

- Heparin, oral anticoagulants, platelet inhibitors (abciximab, aspirin, or dipyridamole) may increase risk of bleeding with drug.
- Drug may alter coagulation studies.
- Potency is expressed in terms of units specific for reteplase and isn't comparable to other thrombolytic drugs.
- Drug is given I.V. as a double-bolus injection.
- Heparin and reteplase are incompatible in solution.

Streptokinase

Streptokinase (Streptase) is a fibrinolytic agent indicated for acute MI, thrombosis, or pulmonary embolism.

Action

Streptokinase activates plasminogen in two steps. First, plasminogen and streptokinase form a complex that exposes the plasminogen-activating site. Plasminogen is then converted to plasmin by cleavage of the peptide bond, which leads to fibrinolysis. In patients with acute MI, streptokinase may decrease infarct size, improve ventricular function, and decrease risk of heart failure.

Dosage

- Give 1.5 million IU I.V. in a 1-hour infusion

Special considerations

- Anticoagulants, as well as aspirin, dipyridamole, drugs affecting platelet activity, indomethacin, and phenylbutazone increase the risk of bleeding with drug.
- Discontinue concomitant heparin and antiplatelet therapy if bleeding occurs.
- Streptokinase activity is inhibited and reversed by antifibrinolytic drugs such as aminocaproic acid; avoid concomitant use.
- Therapeutic effect of drug may be lessened if patient has had either a recent streptococcal infection or previous recent treatment with streptokinase.

Tenecteplase

Tenecteplase (TNKase) is a fibrinolytic agent recently approved by the Food and Drug Administration in the treatment of acute MI.

Key points

Streptokinase
- Indications: acute MI, venous or arterial thrombosis, pulmonary embolism
- Causes plasminogen to be converted to plasmin by cleavage of the peptide bond, which leads to fibrinolysis
- For MI, give 1.5 million IU I.V. in a 1-hour infusion

Key points

Tenecteplase
- Promotes the activity of plasmin to produce fibrinolysis
- Indications: acute MI
- 30 to 50 mg I.V. as a one-time bolus injection

Action

Tenecteplase is as effective as conventional fibrinolytics, but differs in that it's given in a single shot injection. It promotes the activity of plasmin to produce fibrinolysis. Tenecteplase targets established clots and, therefore, doesn't impair the natural clotting process throughout the body.

Dosage

- Give as a bolus injection of 30 to 50 mg I.V.

Special considerations

- Discontinue concomitant heparin and antiplatelet therapy if bleeding occurs.

Glycoproteins

Glycoproteins are conjugated proteins that contain covalently linked carbohydrate residues and inhibit platelet aggregation. They're indicated for acute coronary syndromes without ST-segment elevation, as well as being approved for non-Q wave MI or unstable angina with planned percutaneous coronary intervention (PCI).

Action

As the Fab fragment of the chimeric human-murine monoclonal immunoglobulin antibody 7E3, abciximab binds selectively to platelet glycoprotein (GP) IIb/IIIa receptors and inhibits platelet aggregation. Glycoproteins inhibit the integrin GP IIb/IIIa receptor in the membrane of platelets, which results in the inhibiting of platelet aggregation.

Be aware of bleeding precautions and other general precautions for using glycoproteins. (See *Bleeding precautions for glycoproteins.*)

Abciximab

Abciximab (ReoPro) is an antiplatelet aggregator that binds to the GP IIb/IIIa receptor of human platelets and inhibits platelet aggregation.

Action

See above.

Dosage

- As adjunct to PCI or percutaneous transluminal coronary angioplasty (PTCA): give 0.25 mg/kg as an I.V. bolus 10 to 60 minutes before start of procedure; then a continuous I.V. infusion of 0.125 mcg/kg/minute (maximum dose 10 mcg/min) for 12 hours
- Unstable angina with planned PCI only: give 0.25 mg/kg I.V. bolus; then an 18 to 24 hour 10 mcg/minute I.V. infusion concluding 1 hour after PCI

Key points

Abciximab

- An antiplatelet aggregator that functions as a platelet aggregation inhibitor
- Indications: prevention of acute cardiac ischemic complications related to invasive cardiac procedures, adjunct to PCI or PTCA: give 0.25 mg/kg as an I.V. bolus 10 to 60 minutes before start of procedure; then a continuous I.V. infusion of 0.125 mcg/kg/minute
- Unstable angina with planned PCI only: give 0.25 mg/kg I.V. bolus; then 10 mcg/minute I.V. infusion concluding 1 hour after PCI

Bleeding precautions for glycoproteins

The patient may experience bleeding at the arterial access site for cardiac catheterization, or internal bleeding involving the GI, genitourinary, or retroperitoneal areas. Follow these precautions:

■ maintain patient on bed rest for 6 to 8 hours after sheath removal or drug discontinuation, whichever is later
■ discontinue heparin at least 4 hours before sheath removal
■ minimize or avoid, if possible, arterial and venous punctures, and I.M. injections
■ avoid invasive procedures (if possible), such as nasotracheal intubation, use of urinary catheters, and nasogastric tubes
■ avoid use of constrictive devices, such as automatic blood pressure cuffs and tourniquets
■ remember that antiplatelet drugs, heparin, nonsteroidal anti-inflammatory drugs, thrombolytics, and other anticoagulants may increase risk of bleeding.
    In addition, follow these precautions when administering glycoproteins.
■ Administer drug in a separate I.V. line (don't add other drugs to infusion solution).
■ Monitor patient closely for bleeding.
■ Keep emergency medications available in case of anaphylaxis.
■ Monitor platelet counts before treatment, 2 to 4 hours after treatment, and at 24 hours after treatment or before discharge.
■ Before infusion, measure platelet count, prothrombin time, activated clotting time, and activated partial thromboplastin time to identify preexisting hemostatic abnormalities.

Special considerations
■ Bradycardia and hypotension may occur with drug.
■ Drug is intended for use with heparin and aspirin.
■ If opaque particles are present, discard solution and obtain new vial.
■ Withdraw necessary amount of drug for bolus injection through a sterile, nonpyrogenic, low-protein-binding, 0.2- or 0.22-millipore filter into a syringe. Administer bolus 10 to 60 minutes before procedure.
■ For continuous I.V., inject drug into 250 ml of sterile NSS or D_5W and infuse at 17 ml/hour for 12 hours through a continuous infusion pump equipped with an in-line filter. Discard unused portion at end of 12-hour infusion.
■ Platelet function recovers in about 48 hours but drug remains in circulation for up to 10 days in a platelet-bound state.

Eptifibatide
Eptifibatide (Integrilin) is an antiplatelet aggregator that functions as a platelet aggregation inhibitor.

Action
See "Glycoproteins," page 134.

Key points

Eptifibatide

■ An antiplatelet aggregator that functions as a platelet aggregation inhibitor

■ Indications: acute coronary syndrome, prevention of acute cardiac ischemic complications related to invasive cardiac procedures

■ For acute coronary syndromes: give 180 mcg/kg I.V. bolus, then 2 mcg/kg/minute I.V. infusion for up to 72 hours

■ For PCI: give 135 mcg/kg I.V. bolus, then begin 0.5 mcg/kg/minute I.V. infusion, for 24 hours

Key points

Tirofiban

■ An antiplatelet aggregator that functions as a platelet aggregation inhibitor

■ Indications: acute coronary syndrome, prevention of acute cardiac ischemic complications related to invasive cardiac procedures

■ For acute coronary syndromes or PCI: give 0.4 mcg/kg/minute I.V for 30 minutes, then 0.1 mcg/minute I.V. infusion

Dosage

■ In acute coronary syndromes: give 180 mcg/kg I.V. bolus, then 2 mcg/kg/minute I.V. infusion for up to 72 hours

■ In PCI: give 135 mcg/kg I.V. bolus, then begin 0.5 mcg/kg/minute I.V. infusion for 24 hours

Special considerations

■ Platelet function recovers within 4 to 8 hours after discontinuation of drug.

■ Drug is intended for use with heparin and aspirin.

■ If patient is undergoing coronary artery bypass graft surgery, infusion of drug should be stopped before surgery.

■ Drug may be administered in same I.V. line as alteplase, atropine, dobutamine, heparin, lidocaine, meperidine, metoprolol, midazolam, morphine, nitroglycerin, verapamil, NSS, or D_5NSS. Main infusion may also contain up to 60 mEq/L of potassium chloride. Don't administer drug in I.V. line with furosemide.

Tirofiban

Tirofiban (Aggrastat) is an antiplatelet aggregator that functions as a platelet aggregation inhibitor.

Action

See "Glycoproteins," page 134.

Dosage

■ For acute coronary syndromes or PCI: give 0.4 mcg/kg/minute I.V. for 30 minutes, then 0.1 mcg/minute I.V. infusion

Special considerations

■ Platelet function recovers within 4 to 8 hours after discontinuation of drug.

■ Bradycardia, coronary artery dissection, bleeding, and thrombocytopenia may occur with drug.

■ Hemoglobin, hematocrit, and platelets are monitored before starting tirofiban therapy, 6 hours following loading dose, and at least daily during therapy.

■ Drug is intended for use with aspirin and heparin.

■ Heparin and tirofiban can be administered through the same I.V. catheter.

Inotropics

Inotropic agents, which include the subcategories of chronotropics and dromotropics, are medications that influence the force of muscular contractions. They're typically used in treating heart failure and are described as having either positive or negative effects. For example, positive inotropes increase the force of cardiac contraction. Chronotropic agents influence heart rate. (Negative chronotropic agents slow the heart rate.) Dromotropic agents influence the conductivity of cardiac muscle and action of cardiac nerves. (Negative dromotropic agents slow the electrical impulse conduction through the nodal pathway [AV node].)

Inamrinone lactate

Inamrinone lactate (Inocor) is an inotropic agent indicated for short-term management of heart failure.

Action

Inamrinone produces inotropic action by increasing cellular levels of cAMP. It produces vasodilation through a direct relaxant effect on vascular smooth muscle.

Dosage

■ Give an I.V. bolus of 0.75 mg/kg over 2 to 3 minutes, followed by a maintenance infusion of 5 to 15 mcg/kg/minute; titrate to clinical effect

Special considerations

■ Cardiac glycosides enhance the drug's inotropic effect. Excessive hypotension may occur with concomitant use of disopyramide.
■ Dosage depends on clinical response, including assessment of pulmonary artery wedge pressure and cardiac output.
■ Don't dilute drug with solutions containing dextrose.
■ Don't administer furosemide and inamrinone through the same I.V. line as drug because precipitation occurs.
■ Drug can increase myocardial ischemia, arrhythmias, and thrombocytopenia.

Digoxin

Digoxin (Lanoxin) is an inotropic and antiarrhythmic indicated in heart failure, atrial flutter and fibrillation, and PSVT.

Action

Digoxin depresses the SA node and increases the refractory period of the AV node. It also indirectly increases intracellular calcium by inhibiting sodium-potassium activated adenosine triphosphatase.

Dosage

■ Loading dose — 0.5 to 1 mg I.V. or P.O. in divided doses over 24 hours; maintenance dose — 0.0625 to 0.5 mg daily

Special considerations

■ Avoid electrical cardioversion with drug unless condition is life-threatening; if necessary, use lower current setting (10 to 20 joules).

Key points

Inamrinone lactate
■ Produces inotropic action by increasing cellular levels of cAMP; produces vasodilation through a direct relaxant effect on vascular smooth muscle
■ Indications: short-term management of heart failure
■ I.V. bolus of 0.75 mg/kg over 2 to 3 minutes, followed by a maintenance infusion of 5 to 15 mcg/kg/minute; titrate to clinical effect

Key points

Digoxin
■ Depresses the SA node and increases the refractory period of the AV node; also indirectly increases intracellular calcium
■ Indications: heart failure, atrial flutter and fibrillation, and PSVT
■ Loading dose: 0.5 to 1 mg I.V. or P.O. in divided doses over 24 hours; maintenance dose: 0.0625 to 0.5 mg daily

- Don't use drug with dobutamine.
- Don't mix digoxin with other drugs or give in the same I.V. line.
- Drug may cause increased risk of arrhythmias and hypotension.
- Drug is contraindicated in digoxin toxicity, AV block, profound sinus bradycardia, VT, atrial and junctional tachycardia, or PVCs.
- Amiodarone, captopril, diltiazem, nifedipine, quinidine, spironolactone, and verapamil increase digoxin levels with drug.
- Drug given with calcium salts can cause severe arrhythmias caused by effects on cardiac contractility and excitability. Don't use together.
- Drug's therapeutic serum levels are 0.5 to 2 ng/ml and are based on body weight and response.
- Digoxin-immune FAB can be used to treat digoxin toxicity.

Test your knowledge

Take the following quiz to test your knowledge of cardiovascular pharmacology.

1. You're administering digoxin to a patient as part of his treatment for atrial fibrillation. You're to give a loading dose. Which dosage would be most appropriate?

  A. 1 mg I.V. bolus
  B. 0.25 mg I.V. bolus, followed by 0.5 mg I.V. $\times$ 2
  C. 1 mg I.V. initially, followed by 0.125 mg
  D. 0.5 mg initially, followed by 0.25 mg every 6 hours ($\times$ 2)

Correct answer: D
  Loading dose of digoxin should be given 0.5 to 1 mg I.V. or by mouth in divided doses over 24 hours.

2. You're administering an I.V. loading dose of inamrinone (Inocor) to a patient with acute heart failure. How should you administer this dose?

  A. Over 1 minute
  B. Over 2 to 3 minutes
  C. Over 4 to 5 minutes
  D. Over at least 10 minutes

Correct answer: B

After calculating the dosage at mg/kg, the dose should be administered over at least 2 to 3 minutes.

3. Your patient's cardiac monitor reveals frequent premature ventricular contractions. The patient becomes symptomatic and a bolus of lidocaine is ordered followed by a continuous infusion. How should the bolus dose be calculated?

A. 5 to 75 mg/kg
B. 10 to 20 mg/kg
C. 0.5 to 0.75 mg/kg
D. 1 gm/kg

Correct answer: C

Lidocaine bolus is calculated as 0.5 to 0.75 mg/kg I.V. push.

4. You've just administered propafenone (Rythmol) to treat a life-threatening ventricular arrhythmia. You should monitor the patient for which adverse reaction?

A. Seizures
B. Confusion
C. Hypertensive crisis
D. Bronchospasm

Correct answer: D

Because of its beta-adrenergic blocking properties, propafenone may cause bronchospasm.

5. When administering amiodarone, you should monitor for which of the following electrocardiogram abnormalities?

A. Inverted P waves
B. Prolonged PR interval
C. Narrowed QRS complex
D. Shortened QT interval

Correct answer: B

During amiodarone therapy, the PR and QT intervals may be prolonged and the QRS complex may widen.

6. You are administering metoprolol (Lopressor) to a patient with hypertension. How does metoprolol lower blood pressure?

A. It causes vasoconstriction or increased venous return.
B. It decreases venous return or vasoconstriction.
C. It increases cardiac output or venous return.
D. It causes peripheral vasodilation and decreases cardiac output.

Correct answer: D

Like other sympatholytics, metoprolol lowers blood pressure by causing peripheral vasodilation or decreased cardiac output.

7. Your patient is prescribed the loop diuretic furosemide (Lasix) for treatment of hypertension. Which statement best describes furosemide?

A. It's a sulfonamide derivative.
B. It's less potent than other diuretics.
C. It's a highly potent diuretic.
D. It's typically used to lower intraocular pressure.

Correct answer: C

Furosemide is one of the most potent diuretic agents available.

8. Indications for the administration of atropine include:

A. Symptomatic bradycardia, bradyarrythmia, asystole, bradycardia pulseless electrical activity (PEA)
B. Ventricular fibrillation, atrial fibrillation
C. Asystole, atrial fibrillation
D. third-degree heart block, PEA, ventricular tachycardia

Correct answer: C

Atropine sulfate is an antiarrhythmic indicated for symptomatic bradycardia and bradyarrhythmias (junctional or escape rhythm), asystole (after epinephrine or vasopressin) or bradycardia PEA.

9. Use of which medication may precipitate torsades de pointes?

A. Procainamide
B. Diltiazem
C. Atenolol
D. Atropine

Correct answer: A

Procainamide can precipitate torsades de pointes secondary to its effect on the QT interval (prolongs it).

10. Which therapy is usually considered inappropriate for the treatment of asystole?

A. Isoproterenol
B. Atropine
C. Epinephrine
D. Lidocaine

Correct answer: A

The only indications for isoproterenol are refractory torsades de pointes, asymptomatic bradycardia, and counteraction of beta-adrenergic blockers. Atropine may be given to patients in asystole whose rhythms haven't responded to epinephrine.

CHAPTER SIX

Electrical therapy

Electrical therapy, an integral part of ACLS, is used to quickly terminate or control potentially lethal arrhythmias. Electrical therapy can be administered by defibrillation, cardioversion, or pacemaker.

Defibrillation

Defibrillation delivers large amounts of electric current to a patient over brief periods of time. It's the standard treatment for ventricular fibrillation (VF) and is also used to treat ventricular tachycardia (VT), in which the patient doesn't have a pulse.

A defibrillation shock aims to temporarily depolarize the irregularly beating heart and allow more coordinated contractile activity to resume. It does so by completely depolarizing the myocardium, producing a momentary asystole. This provides opportunity for the natural pacemaker centers of the heart to resume normal activity.

Principle of early defibrillation

The most frequent initial rhythm in sudden cardiac arrest is VF, which leads to death if not corrected. Cardiopulmonary resuscitation (CPR), performed while waiting for defibrillation, appears to prolong VF and preserve heart and brain function. But basic CPR can't convert VF to a normal rhythm. The only way to end VF and restore normal rhythm is electrical defibrillation.

Defibrillation is significantly more effective when VF is recognized and treated quickly. When defibrillation is provided within the first 5 minutes of a cardiac arrest, the survival rate is 50%. This survival rate decreases by 7% to10% for each minute that the patient is in VF.

For this reason, communities have embraced the principle of early defibrillation, which seeks to make the procedure available to patients as quickly as possible, even if cardiac arrest occurs outside the hospital. Law enforcement and fire-fighting personnel are trained to perform early defibrillation, and defibrillators (the devices used to administer controlled electrical shocks to patients) are becoming more common in such places as casinos, malls, and amusement parks. There are two main types of defibrillators: automated external defibrillators (AEDs) and conventional defibrillators.

Automated external defibrillators

AEDs have cardiac rhythm analysis systems. The AED interprets the patient's cardiac rhythm and gives the operator step-by-step directions on how to proceed if defibrillation is indicated. Most AEDs have a "quick-look" feature that allows visualization of the rhythm with the paddles before electrodes are connected.

The AED is equipped with a microcomputer that senses and analyzes a patient's heart rhythm at the push of a button. Then it audibly or visually prompts you to deliver a shock. All models have the same basic functions but offer different operating options. For example, all AEDs communicate directions by displaying messages on a screen, giving voice commands, or both. Some AEDs simultaneously display a patient's heart rhythm.

All devices record your interactions with the patient during defibrillation, either on a cassette tape or in a solid-state memory module. Some AEDs have an integral printer for immediate event documentation.

There are two types of AEDs:

■ fully automated, in which the machine automatically delivers a shock if VF is present

■ semiautomatic, in which the rescuer must press an ANALYZE control to start the rhythm analysis and press a SHOCK control to deliver the shock. (See *Automated external defibrillator.*)

In either device, the electrical shock is delivered through two adhesive electrode pads applied to the patient (upper-right sternal border, lower-left ribs over the cardiac apex). The adhesive pads have two functions: to act as electrodes to transmit the patient's rhythm and to deliver the shock.

How AEDs sense rhythm

The accuracy of AEDs in rhythm analysis is considered very high. A microprocessor analyzes features of the patient's electrocardiogram (ECG) signal for frequency, amplitude, and integration of frequency and amplitude. A safety filter checks for false signals, such as those deriving from radio transmissions, poor electrode contact, 60-cycle interference, or loose electrodes.

In addition, AEDs take multiple looks at the rhythm being analyzed—each lasting a few seconds. Several analyses must confirm the presence of a rhythm for which a shock is indicated, and other checks must be consistent with a nonperfusing cardiac status. A fully automated AED will then charge and deliver a shock, or a semiautomated AED will signal the operator that a shock is advised.

Procedure

The American Heart Association recommends that an AED be attached only to patients who have no pulse and no respirations. In addition, AEDs shouldn't be put in analysis mode until all movement, especially the move-

Automated external defibrillator

Automated external defibrillators (AEDs) vary with the manufacturer, but the basic components for each device are similar. This illustration shows a typical AED and proper electrode placement.

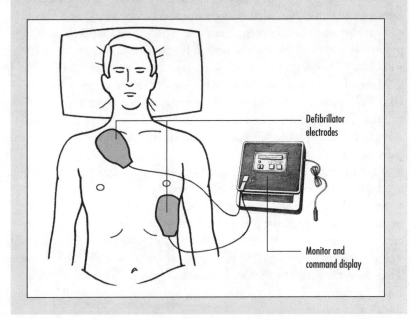

Defibrillator
electrodes

Monitor and
command display

ment of patient transport, has stopped and until full cardiac arrest has been confirmed.

To perform defibrillation with an AED:

■ Open the packets containing the two electrode pads.

■ Attach the white electrode cable connector to one pad and the red electrode cable connector to the other. (The electrode pads themselves aren't site specific.)

■ Expose the patient's chest.

■ Remove the plastic backing film from the electrode pads.

■ Place the electrode attached to the white cable connector on the right upper portion of the patient's chest, just beneath the clavicle; place the pad attached to the red cable connector to the left of the heart's apex. (To remember proper placement, think "white-right," "red-ribs.")

■ Press the ON button and wait while the machine performs a self-test. (Most AEDs signal their readiness by a computerized voice that says, "stand clear" or by emitting a series of loud beeps. When that occurs, the machine is ready to analyze the patient's heart rhythm.)

■ Ask all personnel to stand clear, and press the ANALYZE button when the machine prompts; don't touch or move the patient while the AED is in analysis mode. (The AED will analyze the patient's rhythm in 15 to 30 seconds.)

■ When the patient needs a shock, the AED will display a "stand clear" message and emit a beep that changes to a steady tone as it's charging.

■ When an AED is fully charged and ready to deliver a shock, it will prompt you to press the SHOCK button. If a shock isn't needed, the AED will display "No shock indicated" and prompt you to "Check patient."

■ Make sure no one is touching the patient or bed and call out "Stand clear." Then press the SHOCK button on the AED.

■ After the first shock, the AED will automatically reanalyze the rhythm. If no additional shock is needed, the machine will prompt you to check the patient.

■ If the patient is still in VF, the AED will automatically begin recharging at a higher joule level to prepare for a second shock.

■ Repeat the steps you performed before shocking the patient. According to the AED algorithm, the patient can be shocked up to three times at increasing energy levels (200, 200 to 300, and 360 joules; see *AED algorithm*).

■ If the patient is still in VF after three shocks, resume CPR for 1 minute. Then press the ANALYZE button on the AED to identify the heart rhythm. If the patient is still in VF, continue the algorithm sequence until the code team leader arrives.

■ After the code, remove and transcribe the AED's computer memory module or tape, or prompt the AED to print a rhythm strip with code data.

Special considerations

■ Less training is required to operate and maintain skill levels with the AED than with the conventional defibrillator.

■ The speed of operation and delivery of the first shock is faster than with the conventional defibrillator.

■ The AED permits a hands-free defibrillation technique.

■ The liquid crystal display may not be as easy to read as the display of the conventional defibrillator.

■ The lowest energy setting for the AED is 200 joules, which is relatively high for patients weighing less than 110.2 lb (50 kg).

■ The patient can't be touched while the AED analyzes the rhythm, charges its capacitors, and delivers the shocks.

■ Chest compressions and ventilations must stop while the device is operating.

AED algorithm

Use this algorithm for patients with ventricular fibrillation or pulseless ventricular tachycardia who need to be defibrillated with an automated external defibrillator (AED).

When a patient is unresponsive
- Confirm that he's unresponsive.
- Activate the emergency response system.
- Get the AED.
- Identify and respond to special situations.
- Open his airway.
- See if he's breathing (look, listen, and feel).

When a patient isn't breathing
- Give him two slow breaths (2 seconds per breath).
- Check his pulse.

When a patient is breathing
- Place him in a recovery position if his breathing is adequate.
- Start rescue breathing (one breath every 5 seconds) if his breathing is inadequate.
- Check his pulse every 30 to 60 seconds.

When a patient has no pulse
- Administer cardiopulmonary resuscitation (CPR) until AED arrives and is ready to attach.
- Begin defibrillating as soon as AED is on scene.
- Make sure AED power is on.
- Stop chest compressions as you secure AED electrode pads
- ANALYZE ("Clear!")
- SHOCK ("Clear!") as many as three times, if advised.
  After three shocks or after any "no shock indicated":
- Check the patient's pulse.
- If he has no pulse, perform CPR for 1 minute.
  Check for pulse. If he has no pulse:
  — Press ANALYZE.
  — Try to defibrillate.
  — Repeat as many as three times.

When a patient has a pulse
- Start rescue breathing (one breath every 5 seconds).
- Check his pulse every 30 to 60 seconds.

Special situations

Precautions must be taken when defibrillating a patient with an implantable cardioverter-defibrillator (ICD), a pacemaker, or a transdermal medication patch or when he's in contact with water.

Defibrillating a patient with an ICD or pacemaker
Application of automated external defibrillator (AED) electrodes must be modified so the electrode pad isn't placed directly over the implanted device. Place the AED pad at least 1″ (2.54 cm) away from the device.

Defibrillating a patient with a transdermal medication patch
AED electrodes shouldn't be placed directly on top of a transdermal medication patch, such as nitroglycerin, nicotine, analgesics, or hormone replacements, because the patch can block delivery of energy from the electrode pad to the heart and cause a small burn to the skin. Remove the medication patch and wipe the area clean before attaching the electrode pad.

Defibrillating a patient near water
Water is a conductor of electricity and may provide a pathway for energy from the AED to the rescuers treating the victim. Therefore, be sure to remove the patient from freestanding water and dry his chest before using an AED. You should also dry the patient's chest because wet skin can provide a direct path of energy between one electrode pad and the other, which can decrease the effectiveness of the shock delivered to the heart.

■ The time between activation of the rhythm analysis system and delivery of an electrical shock (which is when CPR must stop) is approximately 10 to 15 seconds.

■ Actions need to be modified for patients with implanted pacemakers, implantable cardioverter-defibrillators, or transdermal medication patches or for those being resuscitated around water. (See *Special situations.*)

Conventional defibrillators

Conventional defibrillators are commonly used in most health care facilities. They require the operator to be able to analyze the rhythm, select the energy level to be administered, apply the paddles to the patient's chest, and discharge the current by pressing both paddle buttons simultaneously.

Procedure

To determine if the patient has a shockable rhythm, follow these steps:
■ If the defibrillator has "quick look" capability, place the paddles on the patient's chest to quickly view his cardiac rhythm.
■ If the defibrillator doesn't have a "quick look" capability, connect the monitoring leads of the defibrillator to the patient and assess the rhythm.
   If defibrillation is appropriate:

■ Expose the patient's chest and apply conductive pads at the paddle placement positions. For anterolateral placement, place one paddle to the right of the upper sternum, just below the right clavicle, and the other over the fifth or sixth intercostal space at the left anterior axillary line. For anteroposterior placement, place the anterior paddle directly over the heart at the precordium to the left of the lower sternal border. Place the flat posterior paddle under the patient's body beneath the heart and immediately below the scapula (but not under the vertebral column).

■ Turn on the defibrillator and set the energy level for 200 joules for an adult patient.

■ Charge the paddles by pressing the CHARGE buttons, which are located either on the machine or on the paddles themselves.

■ Place the paddles over the conductive pads, and press firmly against the patient's chest using 25 lb (11.3 kg) of pressure

■ Reassess the patient's cardiac rhythm.

■ If the patient remains in VF or pulseless VT, instruct all personnel to stand clear of the patient and the bed.

■ Discharge the current by pressing both paddles' CHARGE buttons simultaneously.

■ Leave the paddles in position on the patient's chest to reassess the patient's cardiac rhythm; have someone else assess the pulse.

■ If necessary, prepare to defibrillate a second time. Instruct someone to reset the energy level on the defibrillator to 200 to 300 joules. Announce that you're preparing to defibrillate, and follow the procedure described above.

■ Reassess the patient. If defibrillation is again necessary, instruct someone to reset the energy level to 360 joules. Then follow the same procedure as before.

■ Perform the three countershocks in rapid succession, reassessing the patient's rhythm before each defibrillation.

■ If the patient still has no pulse after the three initial defibrillations, resume CPR, give supplemental oxygen, and begin administering appropriate medications.

■ If defibrillation restores a cardiac rhythm, check the patient's central and peripheral pulses. Obtain a blood pressure reading, heart rate, and respiratory rate. Assess the patient's level of consciousness (LOC), cardiac rhythm, breath sounds, skin color, and urine output. Obtain baseline arterial blood gas levels and a 12-lead ECG. Provide supplemental oxygen, ventilation, and medications as needed.

■ Check the patient's chest for electrical burns and treat them, as ordered.

■ Use a shift checklist to prepare the defibrillator for immediate reuse.

Key points

Understanding conventional defibrillators

■ Cardiac rhythm must be analyzed by operator

■ Emergency procedure for patients with no pulse and no respirations

■ Paddle must be positioned by operator

■ 25 lb (11.3 kg) of pressure must be used when delivering shocks

■ Energy levels = 50 to 360 joules

Cardioversion

Cardioversion (synchronized countershock) is an elective or emergency procedure used to treat tachyarrhythmias (such as atrial tachycardia, atrial flutter, atrial fibrillation, and symptomatic VT). Cardioversion is also the treatment of choice for arrhythmias that don't respond to drug therapy or vagal massage. (See *Location and technique for carotid sinus massage.*)

Cardioversion delivers electric current to the heart to correct an arrhythmia, but unlike defibrillation, it uses much lower energy levels and is synchronized to discharge at the peak of the R wave.

How cardioversion works

Cardioversion delivers an electric charge to the myocardium at the peak of the R wave. This causes immediate depolarization, interrupting reentry circuits and allowing the sinoatrial node to resume control. Synchronizing the electric charge with the R wave ensures that the current won't be delivered on the vulnerable T wave and disrupt repolarization.

Procedure

Explain an elective procedure to the patient and make sure signed consent is obtained. Also withhold all food and fluids for 6 to 12 hours before the procedure or, if cardioversion is urgent, withhold food beginning as soon as possible.

To perform cardioversion:
- Obtain a 12-lead ECG to serve as a baseline.
- Connect the patient to a pulse oximeter and blood pressure cuff, if available.
- If the patient is awake and time permits, administer a sedative as ordered.
- Place the leads on the patient's chest and assess his cardiac rhythm to see if cardioversion is appropriate.
- Apply conductive material (gel to the paddles or defibrillation pads to the chest wall); position the pads so that one pad is to the right of the sternum, just below the clavicle, and the other is at the fifth or sixth intercostal space in the left anterior axillary line.
- Turn on the defibrillator.
- Select the appropriate energy level—usually between 50 and 100 joules.
- Activate the synchronized mode by depressing the synchronizer switch.
- Check that the machine is sensing the R wave correctly.
- Place the paddles on the chest and apply firm pressure.
- Charge the paddles.
- Instruct other personnel to stand clear of the patient and the bed to avoid the risk of an electric shock.

Location and technique for carotid sinus massage

When a patient suffers sinus, atrial, or junctional tachyarrhythmias, vagal maneuvers, such as Valsalva's maneuver and carotid sinus massage, can slow his heart rate. These maneuvers stimulate the autonomic nervous system to increase vagal tone and decrease the heart rate. Vagal maneuvers are contraindicated for patients with severe coronary artery disease, acute myocardial infarction, or hypovolemia. Carotid sinus massage is contraindicated for patients with digoxin toxicity or cerebrovascular disease and for patients who have had carotid artery surgery.

Valsalva's maneuver

A patient who holds his breath, bears down, or coughs while sitting with the upper body bent forward is performing Valsalva's maneuver. This increases intrathoracic pressure. When this pressure increase is transmitted to the heart and great vessels, venous return, stroke volume, and systemic blood pressure decrease. The baroreceptors respond to these changes, increase the heart rate, and cause peripheral vasoconstriction. When the patient exhales at the end of this maneuver, blood pressure rises to the previous level. This increase, combined with the peripheral vasoconstriction caused by bearing down, stimulates the vagus nerve, decreasing the heart rate.

Carotid sinus massage

Carotid sinus massage is also used to slow the heart rate. Before applying manual pressure to the patient's right carotid sinus, locate the bifurcation of the carotid artery on the right side of the neck. Turn the patient's head slightly to the left and hyperextend the neck. Using a circular motion, gently massage the right carotid sinus between your fingers and transverse processes of the spine for 3 to 5 seconds. To avoid the risk of life-threatening complications, don't massage for more than 5 seconds.

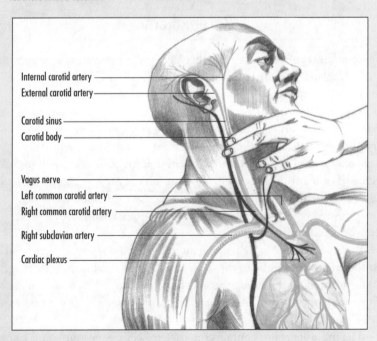

- Internal carotid artery
- External carotid artery
- Carotid sinus
- Carotid body
- Vagus nerve
- Left common carotid artery
- Right common carotid artery
- Right subclavian artery
- Cardiac plexus

■ Discharge the current by pushing both paddles' DISCHARGE buttons simultaneously; don't remove the paddles from the chest until the device discharges. (Unlike in defibrillation, the discharge won't occur immediately; you'll notice a slight delay while the defibrillator synchronizes with the R wave.)

■ If cardioversion is unsuccessful, repeat the procedure two or three times, as ordered, gradually increasing the energy with each additional countershock.

■ If normal rhythm is restored, continue to monitor the patient and provide supplemental ventilation as long as needed.

■ If the patient's cardiac rhythm changes to VF, switch the mode to defibrillate (change it from the synchronized mode) and defibrillate the patient immediately after charging the machine.

Amperage

Use the following amperage sequences for cardioversion:

■ unstable VT with a pulse: 100, 200, 300, 360 joules

■ unstable paroxysmal supraventricular tachycardia (PSVT): 50, 100, 200, 300, 360 joules

■ atrial fibrillation with a rapid ventricular response and an unstable patient: 100, 200, 300, 360 joules

■ atrial flutter with a rapid ventricular response and an unstable patient: 50, 100, 200, 300, 360 joules.

Pacemakers

A pacemaker is an artificial device that electrically stimulates the myocardium to depolarize, producing myocardial contraction. The device can correct abnormal electrical rhythm in patients who have had a myocardial infarction or open-heart surgery. It may also be used to complete the cardiac cycle when the heart is unable to do so itself. A pacemaker may be temporary or permanent, depending on the patient's condition. A temporary pacemaker is used in an emergency situation if the patient shows signs of decreased cardiac output, such as hypotension or syncope; it's often required in patients with unstable bradycardia that's unresponsive to drug therapy. A temporary pacemaker can also serve as a bridge until a permanent pacemaker is inserted.

Pacemakers work by generating an impulse from a power source and transmitting that impulse to the heart muscle. The impulse flows throughout the heart and causes the heart muscle to depolarize. Pacemakers consist of two components: the pulse generator and the pacing leads with electrode tips.

The pulse generator contains the pacemaker's power source and circuitry. The lithium batteries in a permanent or implanted pacemaker serve

Understanding pacing leads

Pacing leads have either one electrode (unipolar) or two (bipolar). These illustrations show the difference between the two leads.

Leads for a pacemaker may be designed to stimulate a single heart chamber and are placed in either the atrium or the ventricle. For dual-chamber, or atrioventricular, pacing, the leads are placed in both chambers, generally on the right side of the heart.

In a unipolar system, electrical current moves from the pulse generator through the leadwire to the negative pole. From there, it stimulates the heart and returns to the pulse generator's metal surface (the positive pole) to complete the circuit.

In a bipolar system, current flows from the pulse generator through the leadwire to the negative pole at the tip. At that point, it stimulates the heart and then flows back to the positive pole to complete the circuit.

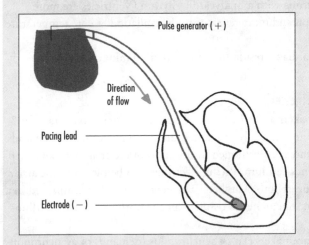

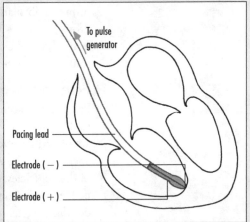

as its power source and last about 10 years. The circuitry of the pacemaker is a microchip that guides heart pacing.

A temporary pacemaker, which isn't implanted, is about the size of a small radio or a telemetry box and is powered by alkaline batteries. These pacemakers also contain a microchip and are programmed by a touch pad or dials.

An electrical stimulus from the pulse generator moves through wires or pacing leads to the electrode tips. The leads for a pacemaker designed to stimulate a single heart chamber are placed in either the atrium or the ventricle. For dual-chamber, or atrioventricular (AV), pacing, the leads are placed in both chambers, usually on the right side of the heart. (See *Understanding pacing leads*.)

The electrodes — one on a unipolar lead or two on a bipolar lead — send information about electrical impulses in the myocardium back to the pulse generator. The pulse generator senses the electrical stimulus and then delivers it to the heart muscle.

Pacemakers are typically used for the following conditions:

■ hemodynamically unstable bradycardia, especially if the patient doesn't respond to drug therapy; symptoms include hypotension, change in mental status, angina, and pulmonary edema

■ bradycardia in which the heart rate is so slow that it leads to pause-dependent ventricular rhythms (wide-complex ventricular beats that can precipitate VT, or VF)

■ malignant PSVTs and VTs

■ cardiac arrest due to drug overdose, acidosis, or electrolyte abnormalities.

Pacemakers are contraindicated in patients with:

■ severe hypothermia with a bradycardic rhythm (Ventricles are more prone to fibrillation and more resistant to defibrillation as core temperature drops.)

■ bradysystolic cardiac arrest lasting more than 20 minutes, due to poor resuscitation rate.

Permanent pacemakers

Permanent pacemakers are self-contained devices designed to operate for 3 to 20 years. They are surgically implanted under local anesthesia. The leads are placed transvenously, positioned in the appropriate chambers, and then anchored to the endocardium. Pacing electrodes can be placed in the atria, in the ventricles, or in both chambers. The generator is then implanted in a pocket made from subcutaneous tissue, which is normally constructed under the clavicle.

Permanent pacemakers can be synchronous (demand) or asynchronous (fixed rate). A synchronous pacemaker monitors the heart's rhythm and paces the heart only when the heart fails to do so itself. An asynchronous pacemaker fires at a preset heart rate regardless of the heart's intrinsic cycle. This type of pacemaker is used more rarely than a synchronous one.

Temporary pacemakers

Several types of temporary pacemakers are available: transcutaneous, transvenous, transthoracic, and epicardial.

Transcutaneous pacemaker

A transcutaneous pacemaker, also known as external pacing, is a temporary pacemaker that's the best choice for life-threatening situations when time is critical. It's a noninvasive pacing method that works by sending electrical impulses from the pulse generator to the patient's heart by way of two electrodes placed on the front and back of the patient's chest.

Transcutaneous pacemakers are used only until a doctor can institute transvenous pacing. They are typically used with unconscious patients because most alert patients can't tolerate the uncomfortable sensations produced by the high energy levels needed to pace externally.

Proper transcutaneous electrode placement

For a noninvasive temporary pacemaker, place the two pacing electrodes at heart level on the patient's chest and back, as shown. This placement ensures that the electrical stimulus must travel only a short distance to the heart.

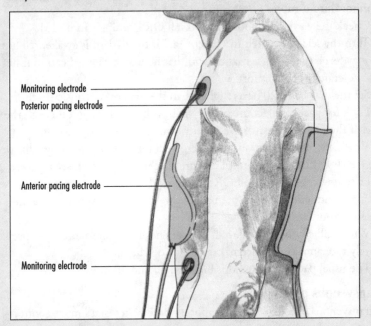

Monitoring electrode

Posterior pacing electrode

Anterior pacing electrode

Monitoring electrode

Procedure

■ If necessary, clip the hair over the areas of electrode placement.

■ Attach monitoring electrodes to the patient in lead I, II, or III position.

■ Plug the patient cable into the ECG input connection on the front of the pacing generator.

■ Set the selector switch to the "Monitor On" position.

■ An ECG waveform should be visible on the monitor.

■ Adjust the R-wave beeper volume to a suitable level.

■ Activate the ALARM ON button; set the alarm for 10 to 20 beats lower and 20 to 30 beats higher than the intrinsic rate.

■ Press the START/STOP button for a printout of the waveform.

■ Make sure the patient's skin is clean and dry to ensure good skin contact.

■ Pull the protective strip from the posterior electrode marked "Back" and apply the electrode on the left side of the back, just below the scapula and to the left of the spine. (See *Proper transcutaneous electrode placement.*)

■ The anterior pacing electrode marked "Front" has two protective strips. Apply the one covering the jellied area to the skin in the anterior position, to the left of the precordium in the V_2 to V_5 position. Move this electrode around to get the best waveform. Expose the electrode's outer rim and firmly press it to the skin.

■ The device can then begin to pace the heart. Make sure the OUTPUT control is on 0 milliamperes (mA), and connect the electrode cable to the monitor output cable.

■ Check the waveform, looking for a tall QRS complex in lead II.

■ Turn the selector switch to "Pacer On." If the patient is awake, tell him he may feel a twitching sensation and that he may have medication if he can't tolerate the discomfort.

■ Set the dial 10 to 20 beats higher than the patient's intrinsic rhythm.

■ Look for pacer artifact or spikes, which will appear as you increase the rate. If the patient doesn't have an intrinsic rate, set the rate to 60.

■ Slowly increase the amount of energy delivered to the heart by adjusting the OUTPUT dial. Do this until capture is achieved — you'll see a pacer spike followed by a widened QRS complex that resembles a premature ventricular contraction. This is the pacing threshold. To ensure capture, increase output by 10%.

■ When full capture is achieved, the patient's heart rate should be approximately the same as the pacemaker rate set on the machine.

■ The usual pacing threshold is between 40 and 80 mA.

Transvenous pacemaker

A transvenous pacemaker is a temporary pacemaker that's more comfortable for the patient than a transcutaneous pacemaker. It's the most commonly used type of temporary pacemaker.

With a transvenous pacemaker, an electrode catheter is threaded through a vein into the patient's right atrium or right ventricle. The electrode is then attached to a pulse generator. You'll notice several types of settings on the pulse generator. (See *A look at a pulse generator.*) The pulse generator can provide an electrical stimulus directly to the endocardium.

Procedure

■ Attach a cardiac monitor to the patient and obtain a baseline assessment, including the patient's vital signs, skin color, LOC, heart rate and rhythm, and emotional state.

■ Insert a peripheral I.V. line if the patient doesn't already have one.

■ Insert a new battery into the external pacemaker generator, and test it to make sure it has a strong charge.

■ Connect the bridging cable to the generator, and align the positive and negative poles.

■ Place the patient in a supine position.

■ Open the supply tray and maintain a sterile field. Using an antibacterial solution, clean the insertion site and cover it with a drape.

A look at a pulse generator

Here's an illustration of a temporary pulse generator with brief descriptions of its parts.

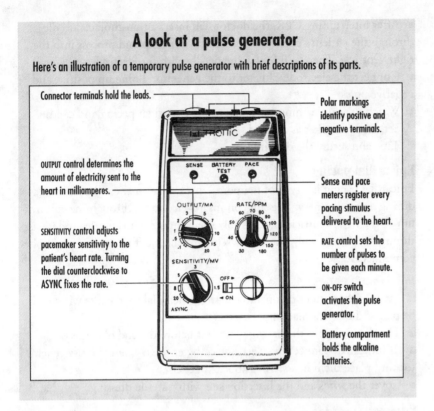

Connector terminals hold the leads.

Polar markings identify positive and negative terminals.

OUTPUT control determines the amount of electricity sent to the heart in milliamperes.

Sense and pace meters register every pacing stimulus delivered to the heart.

SENSITIVITY control adjusts pacemaker sensitivity to the patient's heart rate. Turning the dial counterclockwise to ASYNC fixes the rate.

RATE control sets the number of pulses to be given each minute.

ON-OFF switch activates the pulse generator.

Battery compartment holds the alkaline batteries.

■ Puncture the brachial, femoral, subclavian, or jugular vein; insert the guide wire or introducer; and advance the electrode catheter.

■ Watch the cardiac monitor as the catheter is advanced, and treat any arrhythmias appropriately.

■ When the electrode catheter is in place, attach the catheter leads to the bridging cable, lining up positive and negative poles.

■ Check the battery's charge by pressing the BATTERY TEST button.

■ Set the pacemaker as ordered.

Transthoracic pacemaker

A transthoracic pacemaker is a temporary pacemaker used as an elective surgical procedure or as an emergency measure. To attach it, the doctor performs a procedure similar to pericardiocentesis, using a needle to pass an electrode through the chest wall and into the right ventricle. This procedure carries significant risk of coronary artery laceration and cardiac tamponade; therefore, it's used only if it's the only possible option.

Procedure

■ Clean the skin to the left of the xiphoid process, working quickly because CPR must be interrupted for this procedure.

■ After interrupting CPR, the doctor will insert a transthoracic needle through the patient's chest wall to the left of the xiphoid process into the right ventricle. Then he'll follow the needle with the electrode catheter.
■ Connect the electrode catheter to the generator, lining up positive and negative poles.
■ Watch the cardiac monitor for signs of ventricular pacing and capture.
■ Set the pacemaker as ordered.
■ Tape and secure the dressing.

Epicardial pacing

Epicardial pacing is a type of temporary pacemaker that can be instituted during cardiac surgery. The surgeon inserts electrodes through the epicardium of the right ventricle and possibly the right atrium. The electrodes pass through the chest wall, where they remain available if temporary pacing becomes necessary.

Procedure

■ Instruct the patient preoperatively that epicardial pacemaker wires will be placed during cardiac surgery.
■ The doctor hooks the pacing wires just before the end of surgery.
■ If indicated, connect the electrode catheter to an external pulse generator. and place them in a sterile rubber finger cot.
■ Cover the wires and the insertion site with a sterile dressing.

Pacemaker modes

Pacemaker systems are usually named according to the location of the electrodes and the pathway the electrical stimulus travels to the heart. The capabilities of pacemakers are described by a five-letter coding system, though the first three letters are the most commonly used. (See *Pacemaker coding systems.*)

The four most commonly used pacemaker modes are:
■ AAI—a single-chamber device that paces and senses the atria
■ VVI—a single-chamber device that paces and senses the ventricle; often used for patients with complete heart block and for patients who only need intermittent pacing
■ DVI—a device that paces both the atria and the ventricles but senses only the ventricles; typically used for patients with AV block or sick sinus syndrome
■ DDD—a device that senses and paces the atria and the ventricles at the same time; used with severe AV block.

Evaluating pacemaker function

As part of performing ACLS, you may need to evaluate a patient's pacemaker. Follow these steps:

Pacemaker coding systems

The capabilities of pacemakers are described by a five-letter coding system, though typically only the first three letters are used.

First letter
The first letter identifies which heart chambers are paced. Here are the letters used to signify these options:
- V = Ventricle
- A = Atrium
- D = Dual (ventricle and atrium)
- O = None.

Second letter
The second letter signifies the heart chamber where the pacemaker senses the intrinsic activity:
- V = Ventricle
- A = Atrium
- D = Dual
- O = None.

Third letter
The third letter shows the pacemaker's response to the intrinsic electrical activity it senses in the atrium or ventricle:
- T = Triggers pacing
- I = Inhibits pacing
- D = Dual; can be triggered or inhibited depending on the mode and where intrinsic activity occurs
- O = None; doesn't change mode in response to sensed activity.

Fourth letter
The fourth letter denotes the pacemaker's programmability; it tells whether the pacemaker can be modified by an external programming device:
- P = Basic functions programmable
- M = Multiprogrammable parameters
- C = Communicating functions such as telemetry
- R = Rate responsiveness — rate adjusts to fit the patient's metabolic needs and achieve normal hemodynamic status.

Fifth letter
The fifth letter denotes the pacemaker's response to a tachyarrhythmia:
- P = Pacing ability — the pacemaker's rapid burst paces the heart at a rate above its intrinsic rate to override the tachycardia source
- S = Shock — an implantable cardioverter-defibrillator identifies ventricular tachycardia and delivers a shock to stop the arrhythmia
- D = Dual ability to shock and pace
- O = None.

- Determine the pacemaker's mode and settings.
- Review the patient's 12-lead ECG.
- Select a monitoring lead that clearly show the pacemaker spikes.
- When evaluating the ECG tracing, consider the pacemaker mode and whether symptoms of decreased cardiac output are present.
- Look for information that tells you which chamber is paced. Ask:
– Is there capture?
– Is there a P wave or QRS complex after each atrial or ventricular spike? (See *Pacemaker spikes*, page 158.)
– Do P waves and QRS complexes stem from intrinsic activity?
– If intrinsic activity is present, what's the pacemaker's response?
- Determine the rate by quickly counting the number of complexes in a 6-second ECG strip or, more accurately, by counting the number of small boxes between complexes and dividing by 1,500.

Pacemaker spikes

Pacemaker impulses, the stimuli that travel from the pacemaker to the heart, are visible on the patient's electrocardiogram tracing as spikes. Whether large or small, the spikes appear above or below the isoelectric line. This example shows an atrial and a ventricular pacemaker spike.

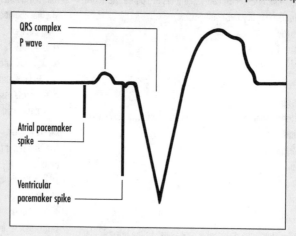

Common pacemaker problems

After you have evaluated the pacemaker, you can then determine if the pacemaker is suffering from one of the four common pacemaker problems: failure to capture, failure to pace, failure to sense, or oversensing.

Failure to capture

Failure to capture is indicated on an ECG by a pacemaker spike without the appropriate atrial or ventricular response (a spike without a complex). Failure to capture indicates the pacemaker's inability to stimulate the chamber. (See *Failure to capture.*)

Causes of failure to capture include:

- acidosis
- electrolyte imbalance
- fibrosis
- incorrect lead position
- low mA setting
- depletion of battery
- broken or cracked leadwire
- perforation of the leadwire through the myocardium.

To treat failure to capture:

- Check all connections.
- Change the battery.
- Gradually increase mA, as per facility protocol, to see if capture occurs.

Failure to capture

This illustration shows failure to capture, in which the pacemaker spike is seen but there's no response from the heart.

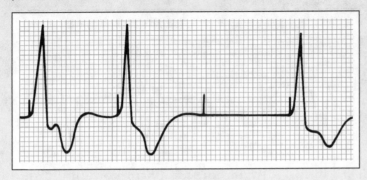

- Turn the patient from side to side.
- Reverse the cables in the pulse generator so the positive wire is in the negative terminal and vice versa.
- Obtain a chest X-ray to determine lead placement.

Failure to pace

Failure to pace is seen as no pacemaker activity on an ECG (see *Failure to pace*, page 160). It can lead to asystole.

Causes of failure to pace include:
- battery or circuit failure
- cracked or broken leads
- interference between atrial and ventricular sensing in a dual-chambered pacemaker.

To treat failure to pace:
- If the pacing or indicator light flashes, check the connections to the cable and the position of the pacing electrode (done by X-ray).
- If the pulse generator is turned on but the indicators aren't flashing, change the battery.
- Use a different pulse generator.

Failure to sense

Failure to sense is indicated by a pacemaker spike that occurs abnormally when intrinsic cardiac activity is already present. (See *Failure to sense intrinsic beats*, page 161.) When spikes fall on the T wave, they can indicate VT or VF.

Causes of failure to sense include:
- electrolyte imbalances
- disconnection of a lead

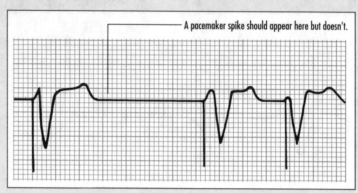

Failure to pace

This illustration shows failure to pace, in which the pacemaker spike isn't seen and no electrocardiogram complex occurs.

A pacemaker spike should appear here but doesn't.

- improper lead placement
- increased sensing threshold from edema or fibrosis at the electrode tip
- drug interactions
- ineffective pacemaker battery.

    To treat failure to sense:
- If the pacemaker is undersensing (it fires but at the wrong times or for the wrong reasons), turn the SENSITIVITY control completely to the right.
- Change the battery or pulse generator.
- Remove items in the room that might be causing electromechanical interference.
- Check that the equipment is grounded.
- If the pacemaker is firing on the T wave and all corrective actions have failed, turn it off. Be prepared to initiate ACLS protocol, depending on the resulting rhythm.

Oversensing

If the pacemaker is too sensitive, it can misinterpret muscle movement or other events in the cardiac cycle as depolarization. It then won't pace the patient when needed, and heart rate and AV synchrony won't be maintained.

    Causes of oversensing include:
- pacemaker not programmed accurately
- improper lead placement
- disconnection of a lead.

    If the pacemaker is oversensing (it incorrectly senses depolarization and refuses to fire when it should), turn the SENSITIVITY control slightly to the left.

Failure to sense intrinsic beats

This illustration shows failure to sense intrinsic beats, in which the pacemaker spike is seen firing at the wrong time or for the wrong reason.

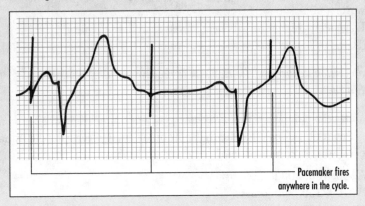

Pacemaker fires anywhere in the cycle.

Test your knowledge

Test your knowledge of electrical therapy with the following questions.

1. The AED should be used in which situation?

    A. By paramedics only in situations outside of the hospital
    B. For a pulseless, motionless, apneic patient
    C. For a patient needing cardioversion
    D. After a precordial thump

Correct answer: B.

The American Heart Association recommends that an AED be attached only to patients who have no pulse or respirations when all movement has stopped.

2. When using an AED, the correct position for the adhesive pads is:

    A. below the left clavicle at the cardiac apex.
    B. anterior to the chest and posterior to the thorax.
    C. below the right nipple and below the left nipple.
    D. upper-right sternal border and lower-left ribs over the cardiac apex.

Correct answer: D

The correct position for the pads is at the upper-right sternal border and at the lower-left ribs over the cardiac apex.

3. Cardioversion is used to:

    A. deliver a shock on the T wave.

    B. treat atrial arrhythmias only.

    C. deliver an electric charge to the myocardium at the peak of the R wave.

    D. generate higher initial energy levels than defibrillation.

Correct answer: C

Cardioversion delivers an electric shock to the myocardium during the peak of the R wave.

4. A 68-year-old male is found by emergency personnel in his home. He's apneic with no pulse. What are the appropriate energy levels for the initial "stacked" shocks to this patient?

    A. 50, 100, 200 joules

    B. 100, 200, 300 joules

    C. 100, 300, 360 joules

    D. 200, 200 to 300, 360 joules

Correct answer: D

The correct treatment algorithm for "stacked shocks" is 200, 200 to 300, 360 joules.

5. With a malfunctioning pacemaker, how does failure to capture appear on the ECG?

    A. Spikes occurring where they shouldn't be

    B. A spike without a complex

    C. No pacemaker activity

    D. Spikes on T waves

Correct answer: B

A spike without a complex indicates that the pacemaker isn't capturing or stimulating the chamber.

6. With a malfunctioning pacemaker, how does failure to sense appear on the ECG?

    A. Lack of a pacemaker spike

    B. A pacemaker spike in the presence of intrinsic activity

    C. A pacemaker spike with no cardiac stimulation

    D. No pacemaker activity

Correct answer: B

Failure to sense is indicated by a pacemaker spike that occurs abnormally in the presence of intrinsic cardiac activity. When spikes fall on a T wave, they can indicate VT or VF.

7. When utilizing an external temporary pacemaker, the energy level should be set at:

A. the lowest mA setting the patient can tolerate.

B. the lowest mA setting that ensures capture of the myocardium.

C. an mA setting midway between the setting that causes capture of the myocardium and the setting at which symptoms first appear.

D. a preset mA setting designated by the manufacturer.

Correct answer: B

Choose the lowest mA setting that causes capture of the myocardium. Higher energy levels may be too irritating for the patient.

8. The purpose of defibrillation is to:

A. "jump start" the heart.

B. increase the heart rate.

C. produce momentary asystole.

D. awaken the patient.

Correct answer: C

The purpose of defibrillation is to produce momentary asystole. This provides an opportunity for the natural pacemaker of the heart to resume normal activity.

9. The strength (energy) of a countershock is expressed in:

A. joules.

B. volts.

C. watts.

D. ohms.

Correct answer: A

The energy of a countershock is expressed in joules.

10. When defibrillating a patient with a permanent pacemaker, where should the electrodes be placed in relation to the pulse generator?

A. At least 2" from the generator

B. At least 1" from the generator

C. Less than 1" from the generator

D. On the pulse generator

Correct answer: B

The electrodes should be placed at least 1" away from the pulse generator because it's possible for defibrillation to cause pacemaker malfunction.

CHAPTER SEVEN

Therapeutic and monitoring techniques

ACLS demands knowledge of a variety of therapeutic and monitoring techniques. Some of these techniques involve I.V. access, which is necessary to effectively administer medications and monitor the patient. Other techniques, such as pericardiocentesis and needle thoracostomy, are more invasive but are sometimes necessary in ACLS-related emergencies.

I.V. access: An overview

I.V. access is necessary to gain peripheral or central access to the venous circulation. An I.V. line is inserted to:
- administer drugs and fluids
- administer blood and blood products
- obtain blood for laboratory tests
- provide a way to insert a catheter into the central circulation for hemodynamic monitoring and electrical pacing.

Choosing an access site
The site you choose for I.V. access is based on the patient's needs and condition. Factors include:
- availability and condition of adequate peripheral veins
- volume of fluid required and time available to administer fluids
- type of fluid to be administered
- purpose and duration of I.V. therapy.

   During resuscitation attempts, you should obtain venous access at the site of the largest vein available that doesn't require interrupting resuscitation (such as the antecubital or femoral vein).

I.V. safety
Regardless of the site you choose, certain precautions must be taken for patient and provider safety. These include:
- the use of standard precautions
- antiseptic cleaning of the site
- appropriate disposal of needles
- changing the I.V. site within 3 days.

It's also important to note that I.V. lines placed in the field (outside the hospital setting) should be changed within 24 hours if possible. They usually aren't inserted under the most ideal circumstances, so they're more likely to cause infection or complications.

Basic venipuncture devices

There are three major types of venipuncture devices: over-the needle catheter, through-the-needle catheter, and winged steel needle set.

Over-the-needle catheter

The over-the-needle catheter can be used for long-term therapy and is often useful for the active or agitated patient. Advantages of the over-the-needle catheter include:

- Inadvertent puncture of the vein is less likely than with a winged steel needle set.
- Patients are more comfortable.
- Radiopaque thread makes location easy.
- The syringe attached to some units permits easy check of blood return and prevents air from entering the vessel on insertion.
- An activity-restricting device, such as an arm board, is rarely required.

One disadvantage of the over-the-needle catheter is that the device is difficult to insert and requires expertise. In addition, extra care is required to ensure that the needle and catheter are inserted into the vein.

Through-the-needle catheter

The through-the-needle catheter can be used for long-term therapy and with an active or agitated patient. Advantages of the through-the-needle catheter include:

- Infiltration is less likely than with a winged steel needle set.
- Patients are more comfortable.
- Many lengths are available.
- Radiopaque thread is present in most types for easy location.
- An activity-restricting device, such as an arm board, is rarely required.

A disadvantage of the through-the-needle catheter is that leaking at the site can occur, especially in an elderly patient, because the needle produces a skin puncture larger than the catheter. In addition, a severed catheter is possible if a needle guard isn't used.

Winged steel needle set

The winged steel needle set is used for short-term I.V. therapy for any cooperative adult patient. It's also used for therapy of any duration for an infant or child or for an elderly patient with fragile or sclerotic veins. Advantages of the winged steel needle set include:

■ It's the easiest intravascular device to insert because the needle is thin-walled and extremely sharp.
■ It's ideal for I.V. push drugs.
■ It's available with a catheter that can be left in place such as an over-the-needle catheter.

The disadvantage of the winged steel needle set is that infiltration can easily occur if a rigid needle winged infusion device is used.

Establishing peripheral I.V. lines

Peripheral venipuncture sites — those located in the hand, forearm, foot, and leg — offer various advantages and disadvantages. Potential peripheral I.V. access veins include the antecubital, external jugular, femoral, hand, and saphenous veins. (See *Veins used in I.V. therapy*, and *Comparing peripheral venipuncture sites*, pages 168 and 169.) Here are some general suggestions for selecting the vein:
■ Keep in mind that the most prominent veins aren't necessarily the best veins; they're frequently sclerotic from previous use.
■ Avoid selecting a vein in an edematous or impaired arm if at all possible.
■ Never select a vein in the arm closest to an area that's surgically compromised, such as veins compromised by a mastectomy or placement of dialysis access.
■ Never select a vein in the affected arm of a patient following cerebrovascular accident.
■ Select a vein in the nondominant arm or hand.
■ For subsequent venipunctures, select sites above the previously used or injured vein.
■ Make sure you rotate access sites. (See *Complications of peripheral I.V. therapy*, pages 170 to 173.)

Antecubital veins

The largest veins of the arm are in the antecubital fossa. Of these veins, the median cephalic and median basilic veins are often selected for I.V. access. This site is useful when rapid I.V. access is desired and for patients in circulatory collapse or cardiac arrest. The veins of this site are large and easily accessed.

Disadvantages of this site include:
■ I.V. insertion here may restrict movement of the patient's arm.
■ The site can't be used to draw blood if I.V. access is obtained and the vein is being used for I.V. fluid administration.
■ If the I.V. infiltrates, sites below this one may be unusable.
■ Accessing a peripheral vein may be difficult if the patient is in circulatory collapse.
■ Drugs given peripherally take longer to reach the central circulation in cardiac arrest. For this reason, raise the arm after drug administration dur-

Veins used in I.V. therapy

This illustration shows the veins commonly used for peripheral I.V. and central venous therapy.

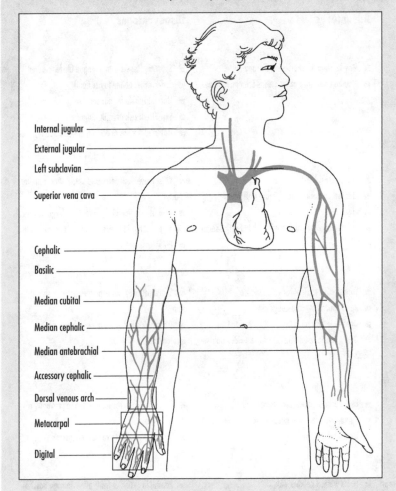

Internal jugular
External jugular
Left subclavian
Superior vena cava
Cephalic
Basilic
Median cubital
Median cephalic
Median antebrachial
Accessory cephalic
Dorsal venous arch
Metacarpal
Digital

ing cardiopulmonary resuscitation (CPR) and follow with a 20-ml bolus of I.V. fluid.

■ Hypertonic or irritating solutions shouldn't be administered through a peripheral vein.

Required equipment

■ alcohol sponges or other approved antimicrobial solution, such as 10% povidone-iodine
■ gloves
■ tourniquet

Comparing peripheral venipuncture sites

This chart includes some of the major benefits and drawbacks of several common venipuncture sites.

Site	Advantages	Disadvantages
Digital veins Run along lateral and dorsal portions of fingers	■ May be used for short-term therapy ■ May be used when other means aren't available	■ Splinting fingers with a tongue blade required, which decreases ability to use hand ■ Uncomfortable for patient ■ Significant risk of infiltration ■ Not used if veins in dorsum of hand already used
Metacarpal veins On dorsum of hand; formed by union of digital veins between the knuckles	■ Easily accessible ■ Lies flat on back of hand; more difficult to dislodge ■ In adult or large child, bones of hand act as splint	■ Wrist movement decreased unless short catheter is used ■ Painful insertion likely because of large number of nerve endings in hands ■ Phlebitis likely at site
Accessory cephalic vein Runs along radial bone as a continuation of metacarpal veins of thumb	■ Large vein excellent for venipuncture ■ Readily accepts large-gauge needles ■ Doesn't impair mobility ■ Doesn't require an arm board in an older child or adult	■ Some difficulty positioning catheter flush with skin ■ Discomfort during movement due to device located at bend of wrist
Cephalic vein Runs along radial side of forearm and upper arm	■ Large vein excellent for venipuncture ■ Readily accepts large-gauge needles ■ Doesn't impair mobility	■ Decreased joint movement due to proximity of device to elbow ■ Tendency of vein to roll during insertion
Median antebrachial vein Arises from palm and runs along ulnar side of forearm	■ Holds winged needles well ■ A last resort when no other means are available	■ Painful insertion or infiltration damage possible due to large number of nerve endings in area ■ High risk of infiltration in area
Basilic vein Runs along ulnar side of forearm and upper arm	■ Readily accepts large-gauge needles ■ Straight, strong vein suitable for large-gauge venipuncture devices	■ Uncomfortable position for patient during insertion ■ Painful insertion due to penetration of dermal layer of skin where nerve endings are located ■ Tendency of vein to roll during insertion

Comparing peripheral venipuncture sites *(continued)*

Site	Advantages	Disadvantages
Antecubital veins Located in antecubital fossa (median cephalic, on radial side; median basilic, on ulnar side; median cubital, which rises in front of elbow joint)	■ Large vein; facilitates drawing blood ■ Often visible or palpable in children when other veins won't dilate ■ May be used in an emergency or as a last resort	■ Difficult to splint elbow area with arm board ■ Veins may be small and scarred if blood has been drawn frequently from site
Dorsal venous network Located in dorsal portion of foot	■ Suitable for infants and toddlers	■ Difficult to see or find vein if edema is present ■ Difficult to walk with device in place ■ Increased risk of deep vein thrombosis

■ I.V. cannula
■ I.V. solution with attached and primed administration set
■ I.V. pole
■ sharps container
■ transparent semipermeable dressing
■ 1″ hypoallergenic tape
■ I.V. start kits (prepared by some facilities)

Procedure
■ Select the site.
■ Apply a tourniquet about 6″ (15.2 cm) above the desired site to dilate the vein.
■ Leave the tourniquet in place for no longer than 3 minutes. If you can't locate a vein and prepare the site in that time, release the tourniquet and reapply after the site is prepared.
■ Put on gloves.
■ Clean the site with alcohol or povidone-iodine. *Note:* Don't apply alcohol after applying povidone-iodine because alcohol negates the beneficial effect of povidone-iodine.
■ If the patient is conscious, ask him to open and close his fist a few times to enhance visualization of the veins.
■ Stabilize the vein by stretching the skin taut above and below the intended insertion site.
■ Puncture the skin with the bevel of the needle up. Check the flash-back chamber behind the hub for blood return, signifying that the vein has been accessed.

(Text continues on page 174.)

Complications of peripheral I.V. therapy

Peripheral I.V. therapy complications may be local or systemic. This chart lists some common complications along with their signs and symptoms, possible causes, and nursing interventions, including preventive measures.

Signs and symptoms	Possible causes	Nursing interventions
Local complications		
Phlebitis		
■ Tenderness at tip of device and above ■ Redness at tip of catheter and along vein ■ Puffy area over vein ■ Vein hard on palpation ■ Elevated temperature	■ Poor blood flow around device ■ Friction from catheter movement in vein ■ Device left in vein too long ■ Clotting at catheter tip (thrombophlebitis) ■ Solution with high or low pH or high osmolarity	■ Remove device. ■ Apply warm pack. ■ Notify doctor if patient has fever. ■ Document patient's condition and your interventions. ***Prevention:*** ■ Restart infusion using larger vein for irritating infusate, or restart with smaller-gauge device to ensure adequate blood flow. ■ Use filter to reduce risk of phlebitis. ■ Tape device securely to prevent dislodgment.
Infiltration		
■ Swelling at and above I.V. site (may extend along entire limb) ■ Discomfort, burning, or pain at site ■ Feeling of tightness at site ■ Decreased skin temperature around site ■ Blanching at site ■ Continuing fluid infusion even when vein is occluded, although rate may decrease ■ Absent backflow of blood ■ Slower flow rate	■ Device dislodged from vein or perforated vein	■ Remove device. ■ Apply ice (early) or warm soaks (later) to aid absorption. ■ Elevate limb. ■ Periodically assess circulation by checking for pulse and capillary refill. ■ Restart infusion above infiltration site or in another limb. ■ Document patient's condition and your interventions. ***Prevention:*** ■ Check I.V. site frequently (especially when using I.V. pump). ■ Don't obscure area above site with tape. ■ Teach patient to observe I.V. site and report discomfort, pain, or swelling.
Catheter dislodgment		
■ Catheter partly backed out of vein ■ Infusate infiltrating	■ Loosened tape or tubing snagged in bedclothes, resulting in partial retraction of catheter	■ If no infiltration occurs, retape without pushing catheter back into vein. ***Prevention:*** ■ Tape device securely on insertion.
Occlusion		
■ No increase in flow rate when I.V. container is raised ■ Blood backup in line ■ Discomfort at insertion site	■ I.V. flow interrupted ■ Intermittent device not flushed ■ Blood backup in line when patient walks ■ Hypercoagulable patient ■ Line clamped too long	■ Use mild flush pressure during injection. Don't force. If unsuccessful, remove and reinsert I.V. device. ***Prevention:*** ■ Maintain I.V. flow rate. ■ Flush promptly after intermittent piggyback administration. ■ Have patient walk with arm folded to chest to reduce risk of blood backup.

Complications of peripheral I.V. therapy (continued)

Signs and symptoms	Possible causes	Nursing interventions
Local complications (continued)		
Vein irritation or pain at I.V. site ■ Pain during infusion ■ Possible blanching if vasospasm occurs ■ Red skin over vein during infusion ■ Rapidly developing signs of phlebitis	■ Solution with high or low pH or high osmolarity, such as 40 mEq/L of potassium chloride, phenytoin, some antibiotics (vancomycin and nafcillin)	■ Slow flow rate. ■ Try using electronic flow device to achieve steady regulated flow. **Prevention:** ■ Dilute solutions before administration. For example, give antibiotics in 250-ml solution rather than 100 ml. If drug has low pH, ask pharmacist if drug can be buffered with sodium bicarbonate. (Refer to facility policy.) ■ If long-term therapy of irritating drug is planned, ask doctor to insert central I.V. line.
Severed catheter ■ Leakage from catheter shaft	■ Catheter inadvertently cut by scissors ■ Reinsertion of needle into catheter	■ If broken part is visible, attempt to retrieve it. If unsuccessful, notify doctor. ■ If portion of catheter enters bloodstream, place tourniquet above I.V. site to prevent progression of broken portion. ■ Notify doctor and radiology department. ■ Document patient's condition and your interventions. **Prevention:** ■ Don't use scissors around I.V. site. ■ Never reinsert needle into catheter. ■ Remove unsuccessfully inserted catheter and needle together.
Hematoma ■ Tenderness at venipuncture site ■ Bruising around site ■ Inability to advance or flush I.V. line	■ Vein punctured through ventral wall at time of venipuncture ■ Leakage of blood from needle displacement	■ Remove device. ■ Apply pressure and warm soaks to affected area. ■ Recheck for bleeding. ■ Document patient's condition and your interventions. **Prevention:** ■ Choose vein that can accommodate size of intended venous access device. ■ Release tourniquet as soon as successful insertion is achieved.
Venous spasm ■ Pain along vein ■ Sluggish flow rate when clamp is completely open ■ Blanched skin over vein	■ Severe vein irritation from irritating drugs or fluids ■ Administration of cold fluids or blood ■ Very rapid flow rate (with fluids at room temperature)	■ Apply warm soaks over vein and surrounding area. ■ Slow flow rate. **Prevention:** ■ Use blood warmer for blood or packed red blood cells when appropriate.

(continued)

Complications of peripheral I.V. therapy (continued)

Signs and symptoms	Possible causes	Nursing interventions
Local complications (continued)		
Thrombosis ■ Painful, reddened, and swollen vein ■ Sluggish or stopped I.V. flow	■ Injury to endothelial cells of vein wall, allowing platelets to adhere and thrombus to form	■ Remove device; restart infusion in opposite limb if possible. ■ Apply warm soaks. ■ Watch for I.V. therapy-related infection (thrombi provide excellent environment for bacterial growth). ***Prevention:*** ■ Use proper venipuncture techniques to reduce injury to vein.
Thrombophlebitis ■ Severe discomfort ■ Reddened, swollen, and hardened vein	■ Thrombosis and inflammation	■ Remove device; restart infusion in opposite limb if possible. ■ Apply warm soaks. ■ Watch for I.V. therapy-related infection (thrombi provide an excellent environment for bacterial growth). ***Prevention:*** ■ Check site frequently. Remove device at first sign of redness and tenderness.
Nerve, tendon, or ligament damage ■ Extreme pain (similar to electric shock when nerve is punctured) ■ Numbness and muscle contraction ■ Delayed effects, including paralysis, numbness, and deformity	■ Improper venipuncture technique, resulting in injury to surrounding nerves, tendons, or ligaments ■ Tight taping or improper splinting with arm board	■ Stop procedure. ***Prevention:*** ■ Don't repeatedly penetrate tissues with venipuncture device. ■ Don't apply excessive pressure when taping or encircle limb with tape. ■ Pad arm board and, if possible, pad tape securing arm board.
Systemic complications		
Circulatory overload ■ Discomfort ■ Neck vein engorgement ■ Respiratory distress ■ Increased blood pressure ■ Crackles ■ Large positive fluid balance (Intake is greater than output.)	■ Roller clamp loosened to allow run-on infusion ■ Flow rate too rapid ■ Miscalculation of fluid requirements	■ Raise head of bed. ■ Administer oxygen as needed. ■ Notify doctor. ■ Administer medications (probably furosemide) as ordered. ***Prevention:*** ■ Use pump, controller, or rate minder for elderly or compromised patients. ■ Recheck calculations of fluid requirements. ■ Monitor infusion frequently.

Complications of peripheral I.V. therapy (continued)

Signs and symptoms	Possible causes	Nursing interventions
Systemic complications (continued)		
Systemic infection (septicemia or bacteremia) ■ Fever, chills, and malaise for no apparent reason ■ Contaminated I.V. site, usually with no visible signs of infection at site	■ Failure to maintain aseptic technique during insertion or site care ■ Severe phlebitis, which can set up ideal conditions for organism growth ■ Poor taping that permits access device to move, which can introduce organisms into bloodstream ■ Prolonged indwelling time of device ■ Immunocompromised patient	■ Notify doctor. ■ Administer medications as prescribed. ■ Culture site and device. ■ Monitor vital signs. **Prevention:** ■ Use scrupulous aseptic technique when handling solutions and tubings, inserting venipuncture device, and discontinuing infusion. ■ Secure all connections. ■ Change I.V. solutions, tubing, and access device at recommended times. ■ Use I.V. filters.
Air embolism ■ Respiratory distress ■ Unequal breath sounds ■ Weak pulse ■ Increased central venous pressure ■ Decreased blood pressure ■ Loss of consciousness	■ Empty solution container ■ Solution container empties; next container pushes air down line	■ Discontinue infusion. ■ Place patient in Trendelenburg's position to allow air to enter right atrium and disperse through pulmonary artery. ■ Administer oxygen. ■ Notify doctor. ■ Document patient's condition and your interventions. **Prevention:** ■ Purge tubing or air completely before infusion. ■ Use air-detection device on pump or air-eliminating filter proximal to I.V. site. ■ Secure connections.
Allergic reaction ■ Itching ■ Tearing eyes and runny nose ■ Bronchospasm ■ Wheezing ■ Urticarial rash ■ Edema at I.V. site ■ Anaphylactic reaction (within minutes or up to 1 hour after exposure), including flushing, chills, anxiety, agitation, generalized itching, palpitations, paresthesia, throbbing in ears, wheezing, coughing, seizures, and cardiac arrest	■ Allergens such as medications	■ If reaction occurs, stop infusion immediately. ■ Maintain patent airway. ■ Notify doctor. ■ Administer antihistaminic steroid, anti-inflammatory, and antipyretic drugs, as ordered. ■ Give 0.2 to 0.5 ml of 1:1,000 aqueous epinephrine subcutaneously. Repeat at 3-minute intervals and as needed and ordered. ■ Administer cortisone if ordered. **Prevention:** ■ Obtain patient's allergy history. Be aware of cross-allergies. ■ Assist with test dosing. ■ Monitor patient carefully during first 15 minutes of administration of new drugs.

■ Advance the catheter either over or through the needle, depending on the type of catheter used. Remove the tourniquet.

■ Remove the needle and attach the primed I.V. administration tubing. Dispose of the needle in a sharps container.

■ Clean the area and apply the transparent semipermeable dressing. Label the site per facility protocol.

External jugular vein

The external jugular vein is large and easily accessible. This site is indicated when rapid I.V. access is desired. It's often used for patients in circulatory collapse or cardiac arrest, when peripheral insertion in other places isn't appropriate.

I.V. insertion into the external jugular vein takes more skill than insertion into other peripheral veins.

Required equipment

■ alcohol sponges or other approved antimicrobial solution, such as 10% povidone-iodine

■ gloves

■ I.V. cannula

■ I.V. solution with attached and primed administration set

■ I.V. pole

■ sharps container

■ transparent semipermeable dressing

■ 1″ hypoallergenic tape

■ I.V. start kits (prepared by some facilities)

Procedure

■ Position the patient in Trendelenburg's position to enhance visualization of the vein. Turn the patient's head to the opposite side.

■ Put on gloves.

■ Clean the site with alcohol or povidone-iodine. *Note:* Don't apply alcohol after applying povidone-iodine because alcohol negates the beneficial effect of povidone-iodine.

■ Anesthetize the skin if the patient is conscious.

■ With the bevel side up, aim the catheter toward the ipsilateral (same side) shoulder.

■ Insert the catheter midway between the angle of the jaw and the midclavicular line. Stabilize the vein by holding the skin taught right above the clavicle.

■ Check the flash-back chamber behind the hub for blood return, signifying that the vein has been accessed.

■ Advance the catheter either over or through the needle, depending on the type of catheter used.

■ Remove the needle and attach the primed I.V. administration tubing. Dispose of the needle in a sharps container.

■ Clean the area and apply the transparent semipermeable dressing. Label the site per facility protocol.

Veins of the hand

A series of easily accessible veins exist on the dorsum of the hand. These veins can be used when rapid I.V. access is desired, and the site is adequate for patients in circulatory collapse or cardiac arrest. In addition, these veins shouldn't interfere with future blood drawing or I.V. access.

Here are some disadvantages of this site:

■ Accessing these veins may be difficult in cases of circulatory collapse or cardiac arrest.

■ I.V. access here may restrict movement in a conscious patient.

■ These veins may be short and difficult to stabilize.

■ Drugs given from this site take longer to reach the central circulation in cardiac arrest. For this reason, raise the arm after drug administration during CPR and follow with a 20-ml bolus of I.V. fluid.

■ Hypertonic or irritating solutions shouldn't be administered through a peripheral vein.

Required equipment

■ alcohol sponges or other approved antimicrobial solution, such as 10% povidone-iodine
■ gloves
■ tourniquet
■ I.V. cannula
■ I.V. solution with attached and primed administration set
■ I.V. pole
■ sharps container
■ transparent semipermeable dressing
■ 1″ hypoallergenic tape
■ I.V. start kits (prepared by some facilities)

Procedure

■ Select the site.

■ Apply a tourniquet about 6″ (15.2 cm) above the desired site to dilate the vein.

■ Leave the tourniquet in place for no longer than 3 minutes. If you can't locate a vein and prepare the site in that time, release the tourniquet and reapply after the site is prepared.

■ Put on gloves.

■ Clean the site with alcohol or povidone-iodine. *Note:* Don't apply alcohol after applying povidone-iodine because alcohol negates the beneficial effect of povidone-iodine.

■ If the patient is conscious, ask him to open and close his fist a few times to enhance visualization of the veins.

■ Stabilize the vein by stretching the skin taut above and below the intended insertion site.

■ Puncture the skin with the bevel of the needle up. Check the flash-back chamber behind the hub for blood return, signifying that the vein has been accessed.

■ Advance the catheter either over or through the needle, depending on the type of catheter used. Remove the tourniquet.

■ Remove the needle and attach the primed I.V. administration tubing. Dispose of the needle in a sharps container.

■ Clean the area and apply the transparent semipermeable dressing. Label the site per facility protocol.

Saphenous veins

Saphenous veins are lower extremity veins that may be used for I.V. access; These veins are large, which allows for easy access.

Here are some disadvantages of this site:

■ As with other peripheral veins, accessing a saphenous vein may be difficult if the patient is in circulatory collapse.

■ Drugs given peripherally take longer to reach the central circulation in cardiac arrest. For this reason, raise the leg after drug administration during CPR and follow with a 20-ml bolus of I.V. fluid.

■ Hypertonic or irritating solutions shouldn't be administered through a peripheral vein.

■ Phlebitis is more common when the veins of the lower extremities are used.

■ I.V. access here may restrict movement in a conscious patient.

Required equipment

■ alcohol sponges or other approved antimicrobial solution, such as 10% povidone-iodine

■ gloves

■ tourniquet

■ I.V. cannula

■ I.V. solution with attached and primed administration set

■ I.V. pole

■ sharps container

■ transparent semipermeable dressing

■ 1″ hypoallergenic tape

■ I.V. start kits (prepared by some facilities)

Procedure

- Select the site.
- Apply a tourniquet about 6″ (15.2 cm) above the desired site to dilate the vein.
- Leave the tourniquet in place for no longer than 3 minutes. If you can't locate a vein and prepare the site in that time, release the tourniquet and reapply after the site is prepared.
- Put on gloves.
- Clean the site with alcohol or povidone-iodine. *Note:* Don't apply alcohol after applying povidone-iodine because alcohol negates the beneficial effect of povidone-iodine.
- Stabilize the vein by stretching the skin taut above and below the intended insertion site.
- Puncture the skin with the bevel of the needle up. Check the flash-back chamber behind the hub for blood return, signifying that the vein has been accessed.
- Advance the catheter either over or through the needle, depending on the type of catheter used. Remove the tourniquet.
- Remove the needle and attach the primed I.V. administration tubing. Dispose of the needle in a sharps container.
- Clean the area and apply the transparent semipermeable dressing. Label the site per facility protocol.

Establishing central I.V. lines

You can use the internal jugular, subclavian, and femoral veins to establish central I.V. access. In central venous (CV) therapy, drugs or fluids are infused directly into a major vein. This access may be used in emergencies or when a patient's peripheral veins are inaccessible. Central I.V. access is used for:

- large volumes of fluid
- multiple infusions
- long-term I.V. therapy
- drawing blood samples
- measuring central venous pressure (CVP), an important indicator of circulatory function
- administering medications that may be caustic to peripheral veins.

Central I.V. access also reduces the need for repeated venipunctures. Fewer venipunctures decrease the patient's anxiety and help to preserve or restore the peripheral veins.

Using a CV catheter also has disadvantages. A CV catheter:
- requires more time and skill to insert than a peripheral I.V. catheter

Key points

Understanding central I.V. lines
- Access important in emergencies or when peripheral access inaccessible or inappropriate
- Usually inserted by doctor or specially trained professional
- Allows hemodynamic monitoring
- Complication rate higher than with peripheral access
- Appropriate for hypertonic or irritating solutions, blood samples, and multiple infusions

- costs more to maintain than a peripheral I.V. catheter
- carries a risk of air embolism.

  Certain situations may preclude the use of central I.V. access. These include:

- presence of scar tissue
- interference with surgical site or other therapy
- configuration of the lung apices
- patient's lifestyle or daily activities. (See *Complications of CV therapy.*)

Internal jugular vein

The internal jugular vein is lateral and anterior to the common carotid artery. The right side is preferred for I.V. access because the lung and pleura are lower on the right, and there's a fairly straight line to the superior vena cava. Accessing the internal jugular vein doesn't depend on visualization of the vein.

The internal jugular vein is indicated when peripheral venous access is unsuccessful and for the measurement of CVP. It's useful for administering hypertonic or irritating solutions and for inserting catheters into the heart and pulmonary circulation. It allows direct access to the central circulation and also allows for rapid administration of large volumes of fluid. Multiple blood samples can be withdrawn through the catheter.

Disadvantages to this site include:

- Accessing this site requires more experience than accessing peripheral veins.
- Nearby structures (carotid artery, apical pleura, lymphatic ducts, and nerves) can be damaged.
- It's more costly than peripheral I.V. access.
- The complication rate is higher than with peripheral access.
- CPR may need to be interrupted to access this vein.

Required equipment

- CV catheter
- central line introducer kit (used at most facilities)
- sterile gloves and gown
- sterile towel or sterile drape
- masks
- alcohol sponges
- 10% povidone-iodine solution
- normal saline solution
- antibiotic ointment
- 3-ml syringe with 25G 1″ needle
- 1% injectable lidocaine
- suture material

Complications of CV therapy

As with any invasive procedure, central venous (CV) therapy can have complications, including pneumothorax, air embolism, thrombosis, and infection. This chart outlines how to recognize, manage, and prevent these complications.

Signs and symptoms	Possible causes	Nursing interventions	Prevention
Pneumothorax, hemothorax, chylothorax, or hydrothorax			
■ Chest pain ■ Dyspnea ■ Cyanosis ■ Decreased breath sounds on affected side ■ With hemothorax, decreased hemoglobin because of blood pooling ■ Abnormal chest X-ray	■ Lung puncture by catheter during insertion or exchange over a guide wire ■ Large blood vessel puncture with bleeding inside or outside of lung ■ Lymph node puncture with leakage of lymph fluid ■ Infusion of solution into chest area through infiltrated catheter	■ Notify doctor. ■ Remove catheter or assist with removal. ■ Administer oxygen as ordered. ■ Set up and assist with chest tube insertion. ■ Document interventions.	■ Position patient's head down, with a towel roll between the scapulae, to dilate and expose the internal jugular or subclavian vein as much as possible during catheter insertion. ■ Assess for early signs of fluid infiltration, such as swelling in shoulder, neck, chest, and arm area. ■ Ensure immobilization of patient with adequate preparation for procedures and restraint during procedure; active patients may need to be sedated or taken to the operating room for CV catheter insertion. ■ Minimize patient activity after insertion, especially if peripheral CV catheter is used.
Air embolism			
■ Respiratory distress ■ Unequal breath sounds ■ Weak pulse ■ Increased central venous pressure (CVP) ■ Decreased blood pressure ■ Churning murmur over precordium ■ Change in level of consciousness	■ Intake of air into CV system during catheter insertion or tubing changes; inadvertent opening, cutting, or breaking of catheter	■ Clamp catheter immediately. ■ Turn patient on his left side, head down, so air can enter right atrium and be dispersed via pulmonary artery. Maintain position for 20 to 30 minutes. ■ Don't have patient perform Valsalva's maneuver. (A large intake of air would worsen the situation.) ■ Administer oxygen. ■ Notify doctor. ■ Document interventions.	■ Purge all air from tubing before hookup. ■ Teach patient to perform Valsalva's maneuver during catheter insertion and tubing changes (bear down or strain and hold breath to increase CVP). ■ Use air-eliminating filters proximal to patient. ■ Use infusion-control device with air detection capability. ■ Use luer-lock tubing, tape connections, or use locking devices for all connections.

(continued)

Complications of CV therapy *(continued)*

Signs and symptoms	Possible causes	Nursing interventions	Prevention
Thrombosis			
■ Edema at puncture site ■ Erythema ■ Ipsilateral swelling of arm, neck, and face ■ Pain along vein ■ Fever, malaise ■ Tachycardia	■ Sluggish flow rate ■ Composition of catheter material (some materials such as polyvinyl chloride are more thrombogenic) ■ Hematopoietic status of patient ■ Preexisting limb edema ■ Infusion of irritating solutions ■ Repeated or long-term use of same vein ■ Preexisting cardiovascular disease	■ Notify doctor. ■ Possibly, remove catheter. ■ Possibly, infuse anticoagulant doses of heparin. ■ Verify thrombosis with diagnostic studies. ■ Apply warm, wet compresses locally. ■ Don't use limb on affected side for subsequent venipuncture. ■ Document interventions.	■ Maintain flow through catheter at steady rate with infusion pump, or flush at regular intervals. ■ Use catheters made of less thrombogenic materials or catheters coated to prevent thrombosis. ■ Dilute irritating solutions. ■ Use 0.22-micron filter for infusions.
Local infection			
■ Redness, warmth, tenderness, and swelling at insertion or exit site ■ Possible exudate of purulent material ■ Local rash or pustules ■ Fever, chills, malaise	■ Failure to maintain aseptic technique during catheter insertion or care ■ Failure to comply with dressing change protocol ■ Wet or soiled dressing remaining on site ■ Immunosuppression ■ Irritated suture line	■ Monitor temperature frequently. ■ Culture site. ■ Re-dress aseptically. ■ Possibly, use antibiotic ointment locally. ■ Treat systemically with antibiotics or antifungals, depending on culture results and doctor's order. ■ Catheter may be removed and tip sent for culture. ■ Document interventions.	■ Maintain strict aseptic technique. Use gloves, masks, and gowns when appropriate. ■ Adhere to dressing change protocols. ■ Teach patient about restrictions on swimming, bathing, and so on. (Patients with adequate white blood cell counts can do these activities if doctor allows.) ■ Change wet or soiled dressing immediately. ■ Change dressing more frequently if catheter is located in femoral area or near tracheostomy. ■ Complete tracheostomy care after catheter care.

Complications of CV therapy *(continued)*

Signs and symptoms	Possible causes	Nursing interventions	Prevention
Systemic infection			
■ Fever, chills without other apparent reason ■ Leukocytosis ■ Nausea, vomiting ■ Malaise ■ Elevated urine glucose level	■ Contaminated catheter or infusate ■ Failure to maintain aseptic technique during solution hookup ■ Frequent opening of catheter or long-term use of single I.V. access ■ Immunosuppression	■ Draw central and peripheral blood cultures; if same organism, catheter is primary source of sepsis and should be removed. ■ If cultures don't match but are positive, catheter may be removed or infection may be treated through catheter. ■ Treat patient with antibiotic regimen, as ordered. ■ Culture tip of catheter if removed. ■ Assess for other sources of infection. ■ Monitor vital signs closely. ■ Document interventions.	■ Examine infusate for cloudiness and turbidity before infusing, and check fluid container for leaks. ■ Monitor urine glucose level in patients receiving total parenteral nutrition; if greater than 2+, suspect early sepsis. ■ Use strict sterile technique for hookup and disconnection of fluids. ■ Use 0.22-micron filter. ■ Catheter may be changed frequently to decrease chance of infection. ■ Keep the system closed as much as possible. ■ Teach patient aseptic technique.

■ I.V. solution with administration set primed
■ infusion pump
■ heparin or normal saline flushes
■ transparent semipermeable dressing

Procedure

■ Explain the procedure to the patient and obtain consent as required.
■ Place the patient in Trendelenburg's position to dilate the vein and reduce the risk of air embolism.
■ Place a rolled towel under the opposite shoulder to extend the neck, making anatomic landmarks more visible.
■ Turn the patient's head in the opposite direction to make the site more accessible.
■ Clean the site with alcohol or povidone-iodine. *Note:* Don't apply alcohol after applying povidone-iodine because alcohol negates the beneficial effect of povidone-iodine.
■ Anesthetize the area with 1% lidocaine.
■ Open the catheter or central line insertion tray.
■ Locate the suprasternal notch and move laterally until the clavicular head of the sternomastoid muscle is located. Trace the course of the carotid artery by locating the carotid pulse. The vein will run just lateral.

■ Insert the needle bevel up at the apex of the triangle formed by the two heads of the sternomastoid muscle and the clavicle. (See *The central approach.*)

■ Maintain negative pressure on the syringe as the needle is advanced. The vein is normally at a depth of 2 to 4 cm.

■ After you access the vein and as you prepare to attach the primed I.V. tubing, ask the conscious patient to perform Valsalva's maneuver. This increases intrathoracic pressure, reducing the possibility of an air embolus.

■ Flush any unused ports with heparin or saline solution.

■ Suture the catheter in place. Obtain a chest X-ray film to confirm placement.

■ Most facilities require that all central lines be infused via an infusion pump.

■ Clean the area and apply a dressing per facility protocol.

Subclavian vein

The subclavian vein lies beneath the clavicle and is frequently used for I.V. access. The subclavian vein can be used when peripheral venous access is unsuccessful. It offers the opportunity to measure CV access and is also indicated for administering hypertonic or irritating solutions and for inserting catheters into the heart and pulmonary circulation. More neck movement is possible with this site than with the internal jugular approach.

Disadvantages of accessing the subclavian site include:

■ Accessing this site requires more experience than is needed to access peripheral veins.

■ Nearby structures (carotid artery, apical pleura, lymphatic ducts, and nerves) can be damaged.

■ It's more costly than peripheral I.V. access.

■ The complication rate is higher than with peripheral access.

■ It carries a higher risk of pleural puncture than the internal jugular approach.

■ Hematomas may not be readily visible and aren't easily compressible.

■ CPR may need to be interrupted for insertion.

Required equipment

■ CV catheter
■ central line kit (used at most facilities)
■ sterile gloves and gown
■ sterile towel or sterile drape
■ masks
■ alcohol sponges
■ 10% povidone-iodine solution
■ normal saline solution

The central approach

The central approach to accessing the internal jugular vein is shown here. The patient lies in a supine position with his head turned toward the left side. The practitioner stands at the patient's head and locates the vessel from this position. The needle is inserted bevel side up into the internal jugular vein.

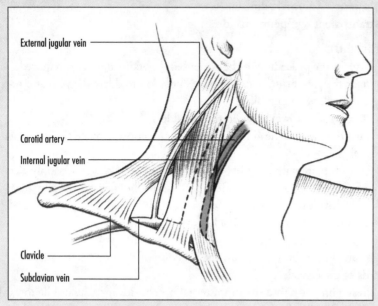

- External jugular vein
- Carotid artery
- Internal jugular vein
- Clavicle
- Subclavian vein

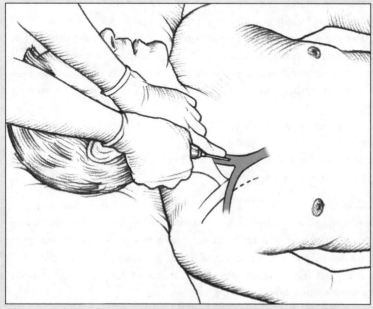

- antibiotic ointment
- 3-ml syringe with 25G 1″ needle
- 1% injectable lidocaine
- suture material
- I.V. solution with administration set primed
- infusion pump
- heparin or normal saline flushes
- transparent semipermeable dressing

Procedure

- Explain the procedure to the patient and obtain consent as required.
- Place the patient in Trendelenburg's position to dilate the vein and re-duce the risk of air embolism.
- Place a rolled towel between the shoulders.
- Turn the patient's head in the opposite direction to make the site more accessible.
- Clean the site with alcohol or povidone-iodine. *Note:* Don't apply alco-hol after applying povidone-iodine because alcohol negates the beneficial effect of povidone-iodine.
- Anesthetize the area with 1% lidocaine.
- Open the catheter or central line insertion tray.
- Insert the needle 1 cm below the junction of the middle and medial thirds of the clavicle.
- Press a fingertip into the suprasternal notch. Advance the needle toward a point immediately above and behind the fingertip.
- The vein is usually accessed at a depth of 3 to 4 cm.
- After the vein is accessed and as you prepare to attach the primed I.V. tubing, ask the conscious patient to perform Valsalva's maneuver. This in-creases intrathoracic pressure, reducing the possibility of an air embolus.
- Suture the catheter in place. Obtain a chest X-ray film to confirm place-ment.
- Most facilities require that all central lines be infused via an infusion pump.
- Clean the area and apply a dressing per facility protocol. (See *Wire-guided catheter technique.*)

Femoral vein

The femoral vein lies medial to the femoral artery below the inguinal liga-ment. If you're able to palpate the femoral artery pulse, the femoral vein will lie just medial to the pulsation. Its use is indicated when rapid I.V. ac-cess is desired. The femoral vein is used primarily for patients in circulatory collapse or cardiac arrest.

Wire-guided catheter technique

Central venous lines can be inserted with wire-guided catheters; this is known as the Seldinger technique. A wire-guided catheter allows use of a smaller needle than those used with other techniques. In addition, a venodilator may be employed to utilize large-bore catheters. This technique also allows you to exchange catheters without repeated "sticks."

An advantage of the femoral site is that CPR doesn't need to be interrupted during insertion. The femoral vein may be easily accessed when peripheral veins have collapsed. In addition, a long catheter can be passed through this site above the diaphragm to access the central circulation.

Disadvantages of selecting this site include:
- The site shouldn't be used unless a long catheter has been threaded above the diaphragm.
- The site may be difficult to locate if the femoral artery pulse isn't palpable.
- More skill is required to access this site.
- Keeping dressings clean in this area may be difficult.

Also, accidental access to the femoral artery may not be readily apparent in a patient in cardiac arrest due to low arterial pressure. Infusion of certain drugs into the femoral artery may cause ischemic injury to the leg.

Required equipment
- alcohol sponges or other approved antimicrobial solution, such as 10% povidone-iodine
- sterile gloves
- CV catheter
- central line introducer kit (used at most facilities)
- sterile towel or sterile drape
- I.V. solution with attached and primed administration set
- I.V. pole
- sharps container
- transparent semipermeable dressing
- 1" hypoallergenic tape
- 10-ml syringe
- suture material
- masks
- heparin or normal saline flushes

Procedure
- Explain the procedure and obtain consent if the patient is conscious.

■ The patient should be in a supine position with the hip on the desired side in a neutral or slightly externally rotated position.

■ Locate the femoral artery and vein as described above.

■ Put on gloves.

■ Clean the site with alcohol or povidone-iodine. *Note:* Don't apply alcohol after applying povidone-iodine because alcohol negates the beneficial effect of povidone-iodine.

■ Anesthetize the skin if the patient is conscious (1% injectable lidocaine is in the introducer kit).

■ Open the central catheter.

■ Attach the 10-ml syringe to the needle. Align the needle with the vein and point it toward the head. Insert the needle bevel up, at a 45-degree angle with the skin.

■ Maintain suction with the syringe until blood appears.

■ Lower the needle to be more parallel with the leg and advance or insert the catheter, depending on the type of device used.

■ Connect I.V. solution or flush with heparinized or saline solution.

■ Secure the catheter with a suture.

■ Dispose of the needle in a sharps container.

■ Clean the area and apply the transparent semipermeable dressing. Label the site per facility protocol.

Blood samples and infusion pumps

Once you've established either peripheral or central I.V. access, the next step is often to collect a blood sample or set up an infusion pump to maintain a steady flow of liquid.

Collecting a blood sample

After inserting an I.V. line, blood may be collected immediately and sent for studies, avoiding the need for another needle stick to obtain the specimen. To collect a blood sample smoothly and safely, follow these step-by-step techniques after assembling your equipment:

■ Place a pad underneath the site to protect the bed linens.

■ When the venipuncture device is correctly placed, remove the inner needle if you're using an over-the-needle device.

■ Keep the tourniquet tied.

■ Attach the syringe to the venipuncture device's hub, and withdraw the appropriate amount of blood.

■ Release the tourniquet and disconnect the syringe.

■ Quickly attach the saline or heparin lock or I.V. tubing, regulate the flow rate, and stabilize the device.

■ Attach a 19G needle to the syringe, and insert the blood into the evacuated tubes (or use equipment for drawing samples with evacuated devices).

■ Properly dispose of the needle and syringe.

Setting up and monitoring an infusion pump

Infusion pumps help maintain a steady flow of liquid at a set rate over a specified time. After gathering your equipment, follow these step-by-step directions to smoothly set up an infusion pump for peripheral I.V. therapy.

■ Attach the controller to the I.V. pole. Insert the administration spike into the I.V. container.

■ Fill the drip chamber completely to prevent air bubbles from entering the tubing. To avoid fluid overload, clamp the tubing whenever the pump door is open.

■ Follow the manufacturer's instructions for priming the tubing and for placing the I.V. tubing.

■ Be sure to flush all air out of the tubing before connecting it to the patient; this lowers the risk of air embolism.

■ Place the infusion pump on the same side as the I.V. setup and the intended venipuncture site.

■ Set the appropriate controls to the desired infusion rate or volume.

■ Check the patency of the I.V. device, watch for infiltration, and monitor the accuracy of the infusion rate.

■ Be sure to explain the alarm system to the patient so he isn't frightened when a change in the infusion rate triggers the alarm.

■ Be prepared to disengage the device if infiltration occurs; otherwise, the pump will continue to infuse medication in the infiltrated area.

■ Frequently check the infusion pump to make sure it's working properly; especially note the flow rate. Monitor the patient for signs of infiltration and other complications, such as infection and air embolism.

Invasive techniques

Emergent invasive techniques, such as pericardiocentesis and needle thoracostomy, are sometimes needed to restore cardiac function or prevent cardiac arrest.

Pericardiocentesis

Pericardiocentesis is the aspiration of fluid or blood with a needle from the pericardial sac surrounding the heart. Pericardiocentesis is indicated to relieve cardiac tamponade (fluid or blood in the pericardial sac) and to obtain fluid for diagnostic studies. (See *Cardiac tamponade,* page 188.)

Pericardiocentesis is contraindicated in cardiac tamponade without evidence of hemodynamic instability; surgical treatment is safer.

Cardiac tamponade

Pericardiocentesis is typically used to treat cardiac tamponade, a condition in which fluid or blood fills the pericardial sac, causing a decrease in ventricular filling.

Causes

Cardiac tamponade is most commonly caused by the following factors:

- trauma
- infection
- neoplastic disease
- myocardial rupture
- uremia
- collagen-vascular disease
- cardiopulmonary resuscitation
- complications following cardiac surgery
- radiation or drug reactions
- perforation of the heart or its vessels by a vascular catheter.

Signs and symptoms

Signs and symptoms of cardiac tamponade include:

- hypotension (due to decreased ventricular filling and decreased contractility of heart)
- jugular venous distention (hypovolemia may mask this symptom)
- muffled heart sounds (blood in the pericardial sac muffles the sounds)
- pulsus paradoxus (a decline greater than 10 mm Hg in systolic pressure with normal inspiration)
- dyspnea
- cyanosis
- signs of shock
- decreasing voltage of electrocardiogram complexes.

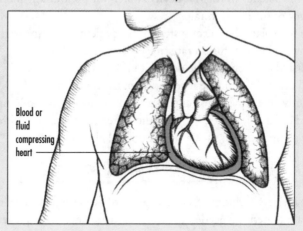

Blood or fluid compressing heart

Complications of pericardiocentesis include:

- cardiac arrhythmias
- puncture of the heart or its vessels
- inadvertent introduction of air into the heart chambers
- hemothorax
- pneumothorax
- hemorrhage from myocardial or coronary artery puncture or laceration.

Pericardiocentesis technique

Pericardiocentesis is an emergency procedure performed for cardiac tamponade. The needle is inserted at the left fifth intercostal space when pericardiocentesis is performed. Because the needle can easily touch the epicardium of the heart, stimulating arrhythmias, it's important to monitor the patient closely for electrocardiogram changes.

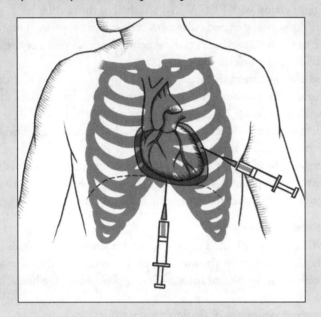

Required equipment
- electrocardiogram (ECG) monitor
- resuscitative equipment
- sterile alligator clip connected to ECG V lead
- short-bevel, large-bore needle (at least 16G and 9 cm long)
- 30- or 50-ml syringe
- povidone-iodine solution
- syringe with 1% lidocaine for anesthesia
- sterile gloves, drapes, gowns, and masks

Procedure
- Give I.V. bolus to transiently increase filling pressures while preparing to perform pericardiocentesis, if appropriate.
- Explain the procedure to the patient and ensure that a consent form is signed as appropriate.
- Place the patient in a supine position or with the head elevated 20 to 30 degrees.

- Clean the area with povidone-iodine.
- The left fifth intercostal approach will probably be used because most studies recommend it as the safest approach. (See *Pericardiocentesis technique,* page 189.)
- Anesthetize the area with 1% lidocaine.
- Attach the large-bore needle to the 30- or 50-ml syringe, and connect the alligator clamp with ECG V lead attached to the needle.
- Insert the needle perpendicular to the chest while applying negative pressure to the syringe. If the needle touches the epicardium of the heart, PR and ST-segment elevations may occur.
- Blood obtained from the pericardial space won't clot. (Blood is defibrinated from agitation during myocardial contraction. In addition, this blood will have a lower hematocrit than venous blood.)
- Be alert to the possibility that emergency thoracotomy may be needed.
- Prepare the patient for surgery.
- Removal of fluid from the pericardial sac should produce immediate improvement in the patient's symptoms. Removing as little as 5 to 10 ml of fluid can improve cardiac performance.

Needle thoracostomy

Needle thoracostomy is used to treat tension pneumothorax. Tension pneumothorax is caused when air enters the pleural space. Needle thoracostomy removes air from the pleural space, relieving pressure on the lungs, heart, trachea, and great vessels.

Signs and symptoms of tension pneumothorax include:
- dyspnea
- chest pain
- tachypnea
- tachycardia
- distended neck veins (may not be evident if hypovolemia is present)
- deviated trachea (away from the affected side)
- initial hypertension, followed by hypotension
- decreased or absent breath sounds on affected side
- hyperresonance on injured side
- increasing difficulty when bagging intubated patient.

When tension pneumothorax occurs, needle thoracostomy must be performed as soon as possible to ensure the patient's survival.

Complications of needle thoracostomy include:
- misdiagnosis of tension pneumothorax. If the patient has suffered only a simple pneumothorax, needle thoracostomy will convert it to an open pneumothorax. If the patient had no pneumothorax at all, needle thoracostomy will produce a pneumothorax. The following conditions will need to be treated with a chest tube:

Landmarks for needle thoracostomy

Needle thoracostomy is an emergency procedure performed when the patient has a hemothorax or pneumothorax. Typically, the second intercostal space is accessed if a pneumothorax is suspected, and the fifth intercostal space is accessed if hemothorax is suspected.

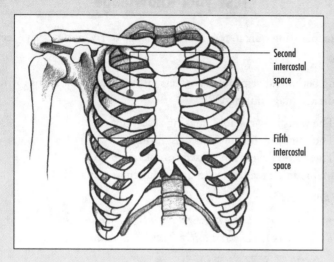

Second intercostal space

Fifth intercostal space

– laceration of the lung causing injury or hemothorax
– puncture of the internal mammary artery
– puncture of the intercostal vessels.

Required equipment
■ povidone-iodine solution
■ 14G catheter-over-needle device

Procedure
■ Explain the procedure to the patient. Tell him he may feel some discomfort and a sensation of pressure during the needle insertion.
■ A sedative may be ordered and given.
■ Obtain baseline vital signs and assess respiratory function.
■ Remind the patient not to cough, breathe deeply, or move suddenly during the procedure to avoid puncture of the visceral pleura or lung.
■ Expose the patient's entire chest or back as appropriate.
■ Using sterile technique, open the equipment and clean the site.
■ Insert the needle into the second intercostal space in the midclavicular line. This is just above the top of the third rib on the injured side.
■ Alternatively, insert the needle into the fifth intercostal space in the midaxillary line on the injured side. (See *Landmarks for needle thoracostomy*.)

■ When the pleural space is entered, you'll hear the air escape.
■ Remove the needle and dispose of it properly.
■ The catheter may be left in place, disposed of, or replaced with chest tubes if the patient's condition warrants.

Test your knowledge

Take the following quiz to test your knowledge of I.V. and invasive techniques.

1. Using peripheral veins for I.V. access rather than central veins carries which disadvantage during CPR?

    A. The veins may collapse, making access difficult.
    B. The veins are difficult to access during CPR.
    C. These sites have an increased complication rate.
    D. Maintaining aseptic technique is difficult during CPR.

Correct answer: A

Peripheral veins may collapse during a low blood-flow state, such as occurs during CPR. This may make access difficult and time-consuming.

2. One local complication of I.V. therapy is:

    A. phlebitis.
    B. sepsis.
    C. air embolism.
    D. catheter-fragment embolism.

Correct answer: A

Phlebitis is a local complication of I.V. therapy. The other options are considered systemic complications.

3. Which technique for inserting an external jugular I.V. is correct?

    A. Place the patient in Trendelenburg's position with the head turned toward the side you'll cannulate.
    B. Point the cannula in the direction of the vein and aim it toward the shoulder on the same side.
    C. Use the Seldinger technique when cannulating the vein.
    D. Introduce the needle under the sternomastoid muscle near the junction of the middle and lower thirds of the lateral border.

Correct answer: B

After positioning the patient in Trendelenburg's position with the head turned to the opposite side of insertion, insert the cannula in the direction of the vein with the point aimed toward the shoulder on the same side.

4. You're performing CPR on a patient with a peripheral I.V. line. Which intervention would best help get medications to the central circulation?

    A. Give a 20-ml bolus of I.V. fluid and raise the arm.
    B. Increase the rate of chest compressions for 1 to 2 minutes after drug administration.
    C. Give all I.V. medications over 1 to 2 seconds.
    D. Pause respirations for the patient during I.V. medication administration.

Correct answer: A

Medications administered peripherally take a longer time to reach the central circulation than those given through a central vein. To assist drugs in reaching the central circulation sooner, give a 20-ml bolus of I.V. fluid and raise the arm after medication administration.

5. After inserting a subclavian line, it's necessary to obtain a chest X-ray film to:

    A. confirm correct placement.
    B. identify hematomas.
    C. rule out air embolism.
    D. check for fluid overload.

Correct answer: A

A chest X-ray can confirm that the subclavian line catheter tip is in the superior vena cava. If the catheter tip is in the right atrium or ventricle instead, it may cause cardiac arrhythmias or perforation. A chest X-ray is also done to check for a pneumothorax — a complication of CV therapy.

6. The preferred peripheral access site for a patient in cardiac arrest is the:

    A. antecubital fossa.
    B. most distal site (usually the hand).
    C. external jugular vein.
    D. saphenous vein.

Correct answer: A

During cardiac arrest, peripheral veins in the upper extremities are preferred. The largest and easiest to access are typically those in the antecubital fossa.

7. Which venous access site carries the greatest risk of pleural puncture?

    A. External jugular
    B. Internal jugular
    C. Subclavian
    D. Femoral

Correct answer: C

Because of its anatomic location, I.V. access through the subclavian vein carries the highest risk of pleural puncture (pneumothorax).

8. Cardiac tamponade causes:

    A. increase in ventricular filling.
    B. decrease in ventricular filling.
    C. increase in cardiac output.
    D. increased contractility of the heart.

Correct answer: B

Cardiac tamponade, which results from a rapid accumulation of blood or fluid in the pericardial sac, causes a decrease in ventricular filling, a decrease in cardiac output, and decreased contractility of the heart.

9. Immediate treatment for cardiac tamponade involves:

    A. pericardiocentesis.
    B. emergency thoracotomy.
    C. needle thoracostomy.
    D. emergency pericardial window.

Correct answer: A

Immediate, lifesaving treatment for cardiac tamponade is pericardiocentesis. It may be necessary for the patient to go to surgery following the procedure to fully correct the condition.

10. Correct positioning of the patient undergoing pericardiocentesis is:

    A. head elevated 20 to 30 degrees.
    B. Trendelenburg's position.
    C. left lateral decubitus position.
    D. flat, with the head turned to the left.

Correct answer: A

A patient undergoing pericardiocentesis should be positioned with the head elevated 20 to 30 degrees.

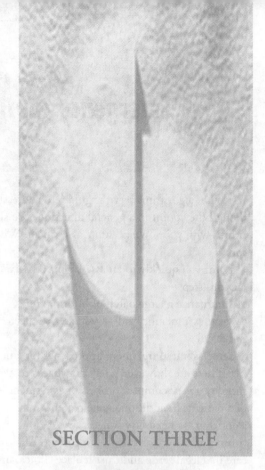

SECTION THREE

ACLS
in action

CHAPTER EIGHT

Emergency cardiac care

In ACLS, algorithms serve as guides to addressing the patient's needs. Although they point in a general direction, you should always couple algorithms with your own accurate assessment. When used properly, algorithms can:

- point you quickly to an assessment (observation) step or an intervention (action) step
- summarize a large batch of information
- serve as a memory aid — you aren't expected to memorize algorithms in full detail
- serve as initial treatment approaches for a broad range of patients.

There are, however, a few drawbacks to algorithms. They tend to oversimplify a very complex process of assessment, intervention, and evaluation of a patient. In addition, some patients may require care not covered by an algorithm, so flexibility is necessary. It's also important not to let an algorithm limit your treatment of a patient. Algorithms also aren't standards of care in a legal sense and can't replace clinical understanding.

Although algorithms appear sequential, they aren't. Most resuscitations require multiple and simultaneous assessments and interventions. It also isn't unusual to "jump" between several algorithms during a cardiac arrest, depending on a patient's rhythm, vital signs, level of consciousness, and response to treatment. In any patient care situation, the rule is always to treat the patient, not the algorithm. (See *Classes of interventions*.)

Adult cardiac arrest algorithm

The adult cardiac arrest algorithm begins with basic step-by-step assessment of the patient and the interventions that follow. The basic ABCD assessment provided by this algorithm applies to all adult patients, and you should note that it's recommended as the initial step in all ACLS situations.

This approach helps organize the health care providers' thoughts, because the team leader must often pay attention to various activities simultaneously. The approach provided by this algorithm is not only useful during resuscitation but also before and after resuscitation as the team provides care for the patient.

Key points

Using the adult cardiac arrest algorithm

- Contains basic ABCD assessment that applies to all ACLS situations
- Treatment for a collapsed patient
- Goal: Secure airway, provide breathing, establish circulation

Classes of interventions

Algorithms may contain "class" notations that relate to a particular therapy. These classes rank interventions based on current research data:

■ Class I — considered a universal standard of care.

■ Class II — considered a generally accepted standard of care but may be controversial in some circumstances.

■ Class IIa — indicated when the data support its usefulness and efficacy.

■ Class IIb — less accepted than higher classes of actions but hasn't been proven harmful.

■ Class III — considered inappropriate and doesn't have research to support its use.

Basic concepts underlying the algorithm

Here are some basic concepts you should remember when using the adult cardiac arrest algorithm:

■ When a patient is in cardiac arrest, cerebral resuscitation is of utmost importance.

■ When caring for a patient, you should maintain standard precautions. At minimum, this requires gloved hands and usually a barrier device for cardiopulmonary resuscitation (CPR).

■ Reassessment is always key after an intervention. After you perform an intervention, assess the patient to see what effect your action has caused, and adjust later actions accordingly.

■ The ABCD survey, which is broken down into primary and secondary surveys, forms the basis of the adult cardiac arrest algorithm.

Following the cardiac arrest algorithm

You're now ready for a step-by-step guide to the adult cardiac arrest algorithm (see *Adult cardiac arrest algorithm,* page 199).

Initial finding

The initial finding occurs when you suspect that a person has collapsed due to cardiac arrest. Remember that individuals can lose consciousness for a multitude of reasons, though cardiac arrest is a likely cause. When you confront a patient you suspect is unconscious, follow these steps:

■ Assess responsiveness by shaking and shouting or touching and shouting, "Are you OK?" Responsiveness is always the first step. A patient may only be sleeping or may have fainted.

■ If you identify that the patient is responsive (a "yes" finding), then you should observe the patient and support hemodynamic stability. Access into the Emergency Medical System (EMS) is still warranted for follow-up because the patient may be responsive but may still require oxygen, an I.V., or medications to maintain stability.

■ If the finding is "no" (the patient isn't responsive), it's crucial to enter the patient into the EMS. Call "911" or an in-hospital "cardiac arrest" pager. This gives the patient the best chance for early access to defibrillation, advanced airway management, and I.V. medications.

Primary Survey

Airway

Begin the primary ABCD survey by assessing the airway. Open and assess the airway using the head-tilt, chin-lift maneuver unless you suspect a neck or spinal injury. In that case, use the jaw-thrust technique.

Breathing

Next, assess for breathing by looking for chest movement, listening, and feeling for air movement for 10 seconds. If breathing is present, place the person in the recovery position because this position helps facilitate breathing.

If breathing isn't present, give two rescue breaths with a pocket face mask, preferably a mask with a one-way valve. Deliver two rescue ventilations over 2 to 4 seconds and allow adequate time to exhale. Exhalation is important in airway management because it reduces the likelihood of gastric distention.

Circulation

The next step is assessing the circulation. Palpate 5 to 10 seconds for a carotid pulse. The pulse may be weak, irregular, or rapid, so taking the full period to assess for a pulse is very important.

If a pulse is present, continue rescue breathing by delivering one ventilation every 5 to 6 seconds. Continue to monitor the patient by periodically checking the pulse, and wait for the emergency medical team to arrive.

If a pulse isn't present, begin CPR and assess the rhythm (if a monitor is available). Compression to ventilation ratio is 15 compressions followed by 2 ventilations. Continue this cycle. When a monitor or defibrillator is available, attach the patient to it.

Defibrillation

If ventricular fibrillation (VF) or ventricular tachycardia (VT) is present on the monitor, immediately defibrillate with 200 joules and follow the VF algorithm. If the rhythm isn't VF or VT, follow the specific algorithm for pulseless electrical activity (PEA) or asystole.

Secondary survey

If you have performed defibrillations or are waiting for the arrival of a defibrillator, begin the secondary ABCD survey. Follow these steps:

Adult cardiac arrest algorithm

Follow the adult cardiac arrest algorithm whenever you find a patient collapsed.

- Person collapses
- Possible cardiac arrest
- Assess responsiveness

Unresponsive

Begin primary ABCD survey.
- Activate emergency response system.
- Call for defibrillator.
- **A** Assess breathing (open airway; look, listen, and feel).

Not Breathing

- **B** Give two slow breaths.
- **C** Assess pulse; if no pulse, start chest compressions.
- **D** Attach monitor/defibrillator when available.

No Pulse

- Perform cardiopulmonary resuscitation (CPR).
- Assess rhythm.

VF and VT

- Attempt defibrillation (up to three shocks if VF persists).
- Continue CPR for 1 minute.

Non-VF and Non-VT (asystole or PEA)

- Perform CPR for up to 3 minutes.

Secondary ABCD Survey

- **Airway:** Attempt to place airway device.
- **Breathing:** Confirm and secure airway device, ventilation, oxygenation.
- **Circulation:** Gain I.V. access; give adrenergic agent; consider antiarrhythmics, buffer agents, pacing.
- **Differential diagnosis:** Search for and treat reversible causes.

NON-VF AND NON-VT PATIENTS
- epinephrine 1 mg I.V.; repeat every 3 to 5 minutes

VF AND VT PATIENTS
- vasopressin 40 U I.V. single dose, one time only (or)
- epinephrine 1 mg I.V.; repeat every 3 to 5 minutes (if no response after single dose of vasopressin, may resume epinephrine 1 mg I.V. push; repeat every 3 to 5 minutes)

■ airway — secure an airway. Choose an airway based on the alertness of the patient and your abilities and knowledge. (Advanced rescuers typically secure an airway using an endotracheal tube.)

■ breathing — administer oxygen if spontaneous breathing returns or, if the patient has an alternative airway, ensure that the device is placed appropriately and is functional; administer positive pressure ventilation through the device, as appropriate.

■ circulation — establish I.V. access as quickly and efficiently as possible. (I.V. lines are a lifeline for a patient in serious condition and provide a way to treat the patient that might otherwise not be possible.) Place the patient on a cardiac monitor or electrocardiograph (ECG) if available and determine the patient's cardiac rhythm. Administer medications as indicated and as the patient's condition permits.

■ differential diagnosis — monitoring the patient is essential in this step. Perform a 12-lead ECG, if the device is available, and obtain a patient history. After assessing the patient, determine a suspected cause and follow the specific algorithm for that cause.

In practice, if the patient is successfully resuscitated but his rhythm deteriorates, repeat the primary and secondary ABCD surveys until airway, breathing, and basic circulation are again secured.

Medication during CPR

If defibrillation is unsuccessful, CPR should be performed and medications administered. These medications may include:

■ epinephrine (1 mg I.V. every 3 to 5 minutes) to induce peripheral vasoconstriction, which will improve cardiac and cerebral perfusion pressure

■ vasopressin (40 mg I.V. in a one-time dose); this adrenergic agent has an effect equivalent to epinephrine.

Acute coronary syndrome algorithm

Acute myocardial infarction (MI) (Q-wave and non–Q-wave) and unstable angina are now recognized as part of a group of clinical diseases called acute coronary syndromes (ACSs). Rupture or erosion of plaque — an unstable and lipid-rich substance — initiates all coronary syndromes. The rupture results in platelet adhesions, fibrin clot formation, and activation of thrombin.

Early thrombus doesn't necessarily block coronary blood flow. When the thrombus does progress and occludes blood flow, an ACS results.

The degree of blockage and the time that the affected vessel remains occluded are major determinants for the type of infarct that occurs. (See *Viewing the coronary vessels.*)

Viewing the coronary vessels

If an occlusion in a coronary artery causes a myocardial infarction (MI), the amount of damage to the myocardium depends on several factors. The area of the heart supplied by the affected vessel is a concern as well as the demand for oxygen in the affected area of the heart. In addition, the collateral circulation in the affected area of the heart influences the outcome. Collateral circulation is an alternate circulation that develops when blood flow to a tissue is blocked. The illustration below shows the major coronary vessels that may be affected in an MI.

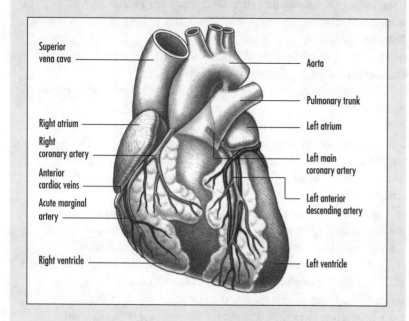

For patients with unstable angina, a thrombus partially occludes a coronary vessel. This thrombus is full of platelets. The partially occluded vessel may have distal microthrombi that cause necrosis in some myocytes. The smaller vessels infarct, and patients are at higher risk for MI. These patients may progress to a non–Q-wave MI. Treatment consists of glycoprotein IIb and glycoprotein IIIa inhibitors and aspirin, which affect platelet formation and decrease platelet adhesion. It has been found that fibrinolytics aren't effective in these patients.

If a thrombus fully occludes the vessel for a prolonged time, this is known as a Q-wave MI. In this type of MI, there's a greater concentration of thrombin and fibrin. Administration of fibrinolytics or percutaneous coronary intervention (PCI), which may decrease or limit the amount of necrosis, is the preferred treatment. In many instances, PCI is superior to fibrinolytic administration; restoration of vessel patency occurs in more than 90% of patients. There are also lower rates of reocclusion when PCI is an initial form of therapy.

While other diagnoses may have chest pain as a symptom, retrosternal chest discomfort, pain, or pressure is a prime symptom of infarction.

Patients typically describe the following symptoms of acute ischemia and MI:

■ uncomfortable pressure, squeezing, pain, or fullness in the center of the chest lasting several minutes (usually longer than 15 minutes)

■ pain radiating to the shoulders, neck, arms, or jaws or pain in the back between the blades

■ accompanying symptoms of light-headedness, fainting, sweating, nausea, or shortness of breath; feeling of impending doom.

Three stages occur when there's occlusion of a vessel: ischemia, injury, and infarct:

■ Ischemia occurs first. It indicates that blood flow and oxygen demand are out of balance. Ischemia can be resolved by improving flow or reducing oxygen needs. ECG changes indicate ST-segment depression or T-wave changes (inversion or hyperacute) indicative of non–Q-wave MI or high-risk unstable angina.

■ Injury is the next stage. This occurs when the ischemia is prolonged enough to damage the area of the heart. ECG changes usually reveal ST-segment elevation (usually in two or more contiguous leads).

■ In infarct, the third stage, actual death of myocardial cells has occurred. ECG changes reveal abnormal Q waves. The Q waves are considered abnormal when they appear greater than or equal to 0.04 second wide and their height is greater than 25% of the R wave height in that lead.

The majority of patients with ST-segment elevation will develop Q-wave MI. Fifty-two percent of patients with MI die before reaching the hospital, and another 19% die within the first 24 hours of hospitalization.

The goals for patients experiencing an ACS are to:

■ reduce the amount of myocardial necrosis in those with ongoing infarction

■ prevent major adverse cardiac events

■ provide for rapid defibrillation when VF is present.

Use the ACS algorithm to quickly classify patients so you can direct treatment appropriately (see *ACS algorithm*). The initial step in assessing a patient complaining of chest pain is to obtain an ECG. This should be done within 10 minutes of being seen by a health care professional. It's a crucial component in determining if myocardial ischemia is present. Interpretation of the ECG is the next step in identifying an ACS. The findings will direct the treatment plan. Patients should be classified as having ST-

ACS algorithm

The acute coronary syndrome (ACS) algorithm reviews assessment and actions for the patient complaining of chest pain. It outlines the three different syndromes of which you should be aware along with their respective treatments.

Assess the initial ECG.

↓

The 12-lead ECG is central to triage of an ACS in the emergency department. Classify patients as being in 1 of 3 syndromes within 10 minutes of arrival.

ST-segment elevation or new left-bundle-branch block (LBBB)	ST-segment depression/dynamic T-wave inversion: Strongly suspicious for ischemia	Nondiagnostic or normal ECG
■ ST elevation ≥ 1 mm in two or more contiguous leads ■ New or presumably new LBBB (BBB obscuring ST-segment analysis)	■ ST depression > 1 mm ■ Marked symmetrical T-wave inversion in multiple precordial leads ■ Dynamic ST-T changes with pain	■ ST depression 0.5 to 1 mm ■ T-wave inversion or flattening in leads with dominant R waves ■ Normal ECG
■ More than 90% of patients with ischemic-type chest pain and ST-segment elevation will develop new Q waves or positive serum markers for acute myocardial infarction (MI). ■ Patients with hyperacute T waves benefit when acute MI diagnosis is certain. Repeat ECG may be helpful. ■ Patients with ST depression in early precordial leads who have posterior MI benefit when acute MI diagnosis is certain.	**High-risk subgroup with increased mortality:** ■ Persistent symptoms, recurrent ischemia ■ Diffuse or widespread ECG abnormalities ■ Depressed left ventricular function ■ Heart failure ■ Serum marker release: positive troponin or CK-MB+	**Heterogeneous group: Rapid assessment needed:** ■ Serial ECGs ■ ST-segment monitoring ■ Serum cardiac markers Further risk assessment helpful: ■ Perfusion radionuclide imaging ■ Stress echocardiography
■ Reperfusion therapy ■ Aspirin ■ Heparin (if using fibrin-specific lytics) ■ Beta-adrenergic blockers ■ Nitrates as indicated	■ Antithrombin therapy with heparin ■ Antiplatelet therapy with aspirin ■ Glycoprotein IIb/IIIa inhibitors ■ Beta-adrenergic blockers ■ Nitrates	■ Aspirin ■ Other therapy as appropriate ■ Patients with positive serum markers, ECG changes, or functional study: manage as high risk

segment elevation or new left bundle-branch block (LBBB), ST-segment depression or dynamic T-wave inversion, or nondiagnostic or normal ECG.

ST-segment elevation or new LBBB

■ Patients with an ST-segment elevation greater than or equal to 1 mm in two or more leads or with LBBB need to be treated for acute MI.

■ More than 90% of patients with this presentation will develop new Q waves and have positive serum cardiac markers.

■ Repeating the ECG may be helpful for patients who present with hyper-acute T waves.

■ Patients with ST depression indicating a posterior MI benefit most when an acute MI diagnosis is confirmed.

■ Treatment options include reperfusion therapy, aspirin, heparin (if using fibrin-specific lytics), beta-adrenergic blockers, and nitrates (as indicated).

ST-segment depression or dynamic T-wave inversion

■ Ischemia should be suspected with findings of ST depression greater than 1 mm, marked symmetrical T-wave inversion in multiple precordial leads, and dynamic ST-T changes with pain.

■ Patients who display persistent symptoms and recurrent ischemia, diffuse or widespread ECG abnormalities, heart failure, and positive serum markers are considered high risk.

■ Treatment options include antithrombin therapy with heparin, antiplatelet therapy with aspirin, glycoprotein IIb/IIIa inhibitors, beta-adrenergic blockers, or nitrates.

Nondiagnostic or normal ECG

■ A normal ECG won't show any ST changes or arrhythmias.

■ If the ECG is nondiagnostic, it may show an ST depression of 0.5 to 1 mm or a T-wave inversion or flattening in leads with dominant R waves.

■ Continue assessment of myocardial changes through use of serial ECGs, ST-segment monitoring, and serum cardiac markers.

■ If further assessment is warranted, perform perfusion radionuclide imaging and stress echocardiography.

■ Treatment for the patient is individualized; however, aspirin should be included in all treatment plans. Patients who have ECG changes, positive serum markers, or positive findings on any functional studies need to be managed as high risk.

Ischemic chest pain algorithm

Begin the algorithm for ischemic chest pain when your patient experiences chest discomfort, a symptom that suggests ischemia. (See *Ischemic chest pain algorithm,* pages 206 and 207.) As with any patient, you'll initially follow the adult cardiac arrest algorithm.

MONA

Emergency personnel should begin assessment immediately and follow with treatment using the memory aid "MONA" (morphine, oxygen, nitroglycerin [NTG], and aspirin).

Morphine

Morphine is indicated for central anxiety and is the drug of choice to relieve pain associated with acute MI. The dosage is 2 to 4 mg I.V. push with repeat doses every 5 to 10 minutes until pain relief is obtained. Pain adversely increases myocardial oxygen demand because heart rate, contractility, and systolic blood pressure are affected. Evaluate both the patient's pain response and his vital signs. Frequent blood pressure monitoring is especially important because morphine can cause hypotension.

Oxygen

Oxygen has been proven to reduce ST elevation and limit ischemic myocardial injury and should be administered to anyone experiencing chest discomfort. Oxygen may be administered by nasal cannula or mask. The type and amount of oxygen to be administered is determined by oxygen saturation. Lower concentrations (less than 40%) of oxygen can be delivered by nasal cannula, while higher concentrations (over 40%) can be delivered by mask. If capable of measuring pulse oximetry, oxygen saturation should be maintained at more than 90%.

Nitroglycerin

Sublingual NTG is the initial treatment for a patient with chest pain that suggests ischemia. Nitrates are the preferred drug initially for the treatment of ischemic pain; their administration will result in coronary dilation and allow greater perfusion. Venodilation improves preload because it increases venous capacitance. Systemic arteriolar dilation improves afterload as it reduces the workload of the left ventricle. Both of these actions reduce the heart's oxygen requirements.

A dose of 0.3 to 0.4 mg NTG sublingually may be given three times at 5-minute intervals as long as blood pressure is stable (usually greater than 90 mm Hg systolic). When NTG use will be prolonged, the I.V. route allows active titration. Nitrates are contraindicated with right ventricular infarct or when the heart rate is less than 50 beats per minute.

(Text continues on page 208.)

Ischemic chest pain algorithm

The ischemic chest pain algorithm reviews initial assessment and actions for a patient with possible ischemic chest pain. It also shows electrocardiogram (ECG) changes you may encounter with the patient. Base your treatments on ECG findings and patient status.

Chest pain suggests ischemia.

Immediate assessment (< 10 minutes)
- Measure vital signs.
- Measure oxygen saturation.
- Obtain I.V. access.
- Obtain 12-lead ECG.
- Perform brief assessment; focus on eligibility for fibrinolytics.
- Obtain initial serum cardiac marker levels.
- Evaluate initial electrolyte and coagulation studies.
- Obtain portable chest X-ray (< 30 minutes).

Immediate general treatment
"Mona" greets all patients
(**M**orphine, **O**xygen, **N**itroglycerin [NTG], **A**spirin):
- Oxygen at 4 L/min
- aspirin 160 to 325 mg
- NTG, sublingual or spray
- morphine I.V. (if pain not relieved with NTG).

Assess initial 12-lead ECG.

- ST elevation or new or presumably new left bundle branch block (LBBB): strongly suspicious for injury
- ST elevation: acute myocardial infarction (MI)

Start adjunctive treatments (as indicated; no reperfusion delay).
- Beta-adrenergic blockers
- NTG I.V.
- heparin I.V.
- Angiotensin-converting enzyme inhibitors (after 6 hours or when stable)

What's the time from onset of symptoms?

> 12 hours → Assess clinical status.

< 12 hours

High-risk patient

Select reperfusion strategy
- Angiography
- Percutaneous coronary intervention (PCI)
- Cardiothoracic surgery if necessary

Perform cardiac catheterization.

Yes

Primary PCI selected
- Perform within 60 to 120 minutes of arrival
- Institution is high-volume center with experienced operators and cardiac surgery capability
- Treatment of choice if patient has signs of cardiogenic shock or if fibrinolytics are contraindicated

Fibrinolytic therapy selected (if PCI not available)
- alteplase (Activase), streptokinase (Streptase), reteplase (Retavase), or tenecteplase (TNKase)
- Goal: Administer within 30 minutes of reaching hospital.

PCI or coronary artery bypass graft

- ST depression or dynamic T-wave inversion: strongly suspicious for ischemia
- High-risk unstable angina or non–ST-segment elevation acute MI

- Nondiagnostic ECG: absence of changes in ST segment of T waves
- Intermediate- or low-risk unstable angina

Start adjunctive treatments (as indicated; no contraindications)
- heparin I.V.
- aspirin 160 to 325 mg daily
- Glycoprotein IIB/IIIA receptor inhibitors
- NTG I.V.
- Beta-adrenergic blockers I.V.

Yes ←

Meets criteria for unstable or new-onset angina or troponin positive?

No

Admit to emergency unit or monitored bed.
- Collect serial serum markers.
- Perform serial ECG/continuous ST monitoring.
- Consider imaging study.

Clinically stable

No   **Yes**

Evidence of ischemia or infarction

No

Admit to coronary care unit or monitored bed.
- Adjunctive therapy as appropriate
- Serial ECG
- Serial serum cardiac markers
- Consider imaging study.

Discharge acceptable, arrange follow-up.

Aspirin

Aspirin is considered a Class I action in the treatment of the patient with MI. Aspirin 160 to 325 mg is given by mouth as soon as possible. Chewed aspirin is absorbed the fastest and is preferred.

Prehospital treatment

The patient should be transported at this time to an emergency care facility for more definitive treatment. In addition, a 12-lead ECG can be performed if the rescuer is capable. Because other conditions can mimic the signs and symptoms of acute MI, a 12-lead ECG serves as an important diagnostic tool.

Prehospital screening should be done by EMS personnel, if possible, to determine if a patient is a candidate for thrombolytic therapy. Thrombolytic therapy should begin immediately if the patient meets the criteria and the EMS personnel are able to administer thrombolytics (this depends on the state's or county's specific licensing criteria).

Emergency department

When the patient reaches the emergency department (ED), one doctor assumes the "team leader" role and directs the team. The secondary ABCD survey is reapplied, including vital signs, oxygen saturation, brief and targeted history, 12-lead ECG, I.V. access, and a decision regarding thrombolytic therapy. The focus is on rapid but accurate diagnosis.

In the secondary survey, you may elicit some findings that place the individual at risk for ischemia. High-risk individuals are those who have one or more of the following:

- prior MI
- prior life-threatening arrhythmia episode
- known coronary artery disease
- clinical signs of angina
- significant ECG changes (ST-segment changes with chest symptoms or marked T-wave changes in the anterior precordial leads).

Intermediate-risk individuals lack high-risk features but do have one of the following:

- clinical signs of angina in a young patient
- probable signs of angina in an older patient
- possible signs of angina
- three other risk factors in the patient history
- diabetes
- ECG changes (ST-segment depression or T-wave inversion greater than or equal to 1 mm).

Low-risk individuals lack high- or intermediate-risk features but do have one of the following:

- possible signs of angina
- one risk factor, but not diabetes
- ECG changes (T-wave inversion less than 1 mm)
- normal ECG.

Simultaneous treatment is also performed while the secondary survey is underway. This includes oxygen administration, NTG sublingually (may be followed by I.V.), morphine I.V., aspirin by mouth, thrombolytic agents, heparin I.V., beta-adrenergic blockers, lidocaine if ectopy, magnesium sulfate I.V., and coronary angiography.

Adjunctive therapy can be started while reperfusion strategies are being considered. Adjunctive therapies include:
- beta-adrenergic blockers (decrease the workload of the heart)
- I.V. NTG (dilates coronary arteries, improves preload and afterload)
- heparin (indicated for patients receiving tissue plasminogen activator or reteplase [Retavase] and for patients who are candidates for percutaneous transluminal coronary angioplasty or surgical revascularization)
- angiotensin-converting enzyme inhibitors (block conversion of angiotensin; should be given within 12 to 24 hours of symptoms).

Reperfusion strategies include:
- angiography
- PCI, which includes angioplasty with or without stents
- cardiothoracic surgery
- fibrinolytic therapy.

Asystole algorithm

Asystole usually represents confirmation of death rather than a treatable rhythm. Spontaneous circulation rarely returns after a positive diagnosis of asystole. (See *Asystole algorithm,* page 210.)

However, a mistaken diagnosis of asystole isn't unusual. The most common reason is an operator making a monitor error during cardiac arrest. Aystole can also be mistaken for a fine VF. For these reasons, to positively identify asystole, you must determine its presence in two leads.

First steps
As with any possible cardiac arrest situation, begin with the primary ABCD. If asystole isn't present, follow the appropriate algorithm. If asystole is suspected, evaluate whether resuscitation should be attempted. Factors to consider include:
- an objective indicator of "do not resuscitate" status, such as a bracelet, written documentation, or family statements
- clinical indicators that resuscitation attempts aren't indicated (a pulse is present, the patient is awake).

Key points

Using the asystole algorithm
- Indicates poor survival rate
- Need to consider "Do not resuscitate" status
- Goal: Reestablish adequate heart rhythm

Asystole algorithm

A diagnosis of asystole indicates a poor chance of survival for the patient. Still, after completing the primary and secondary surveys, your goal is to reestablish a heart rhythm. Treatments include pacing and appropriate medications to stimulate impulse conduction.

Primary ABCD survey

Focus: Basic cardiopulmonary resuscitation (CPR) and defibrillation

- Check responsiveness.
- Activate emergency response system.
- Call for defibrillator.
- **A** Airway: Open the airway.
- **B** Breathing: Provide positive-pressure ventilations.
- **C** Circulation: Give chest compressions.
- **C** Confirm true asystole.
- **D** Defibrillation: Assess for ventricular fibrillation (VF) or pulseless ventricular tachycardia (VT); shock if indicated.
- Rapid scene survey: Any evidence personnel should not attempt resuscitation?

Secondary ABCD survey

Focus: More advanced assessments and treatments

- **A** Airway: Place airway device as soon as possible.
- **B** Breathing: Confirm airway device placement by examination plus confirmation device.
- **B** Breathing: Secure airway device; purpose-made tube holders preferred.
- **B** Breathing: Confirm effective oxygenation and ventilation.
- **C** Circulation: Confirm true asystole.
- **C** Circulation: Establish I.V. access.
- **C** Circulation: Identify rhythm via monitor.
- **C** Circulation: Give medications appropriate for rhythm and condition.
- **D** Differential diagnosis: Search for and treat identified reversible causes.

Transcutaneous pacing

If considered, perform immediately.

epinephrine 1 mg I.V. push; repeat every 3 to 5 minutes

atropine 1 mg I.V.; repeat every 3 to 5 minutes up to a total of 0.04 mg/kg

Asystole persists

Withhold or cease resuscitation efforts?

- Consider quality of resuscitation?
- Atypical clinical features present?
- Support for cease-efforts protocols in place?

If either of these factors is present, resuscitation attempts shouldn't be started. If you determine that the asystolic rhythm should be treated, the algorithm continues.

Transcutaneous pacemaker
Apply a transcutaneous pacemaker as soon as it's available. Remember, however, that just because a pacemaker is applied, it doesn't mean the patient is no longer in cardiac arrest. Observe the monitor for pacemaker capture and check for the presence of a pulse.

Medications
Administer epinephrine 1 mg I.V. push every 3 to 5 minutes. Epinephrine is an alpha-adrenergic receptor, which stimulates the sympathetic nervous system and can ultimately restore an electrical rhythm. It's the drug of choice for treating asystole.

Until a transcutaneous pacemaker can be applied, administer atropine 1 mg I.V. push every 3 to 5 minutes up to a total dose of 0.03 to 0.04 mg/kg. Atropine, an anticholinergic agent, inhibits acetylcholine, which causes a blockage of the vagal effects on the sinoatrial and atrioventricular (AV) nodes. This enhances conduction and increases heart rate.

If asystole persists after these measures have been taken, you should consider terminating resuscitative efforts.

Family presence
In a number of patient care areas, families are allowed to remain in the resuscitation area during patient care. If the resuscitation efforts aren't successful, these will be the last moments the family will see the patient alive. Here are some points to consider if you need to convey to the family that their loved one has died:
- If family members aren't present, call them and explain that their relative has been admitted to the ED.
- Never tell the family that the patient is dead over the telephone, but do tell them that the patient's condition is serious.
- Review with the resuscitation team what was done on behalf of the patient and carefully review the events.
- Take the family to a private area.
- Sit down with the family members and introduce yourself, addressing the patient's closest relative. Remember to use eye contact and make sure the family members understand what you're saying.
- Briefly review the events that occurred in the ED.
- Avoid phrases such as "passed on" and "no longer with us." Use concrete terms such as death, dying, or dead: Say, for example, "Your family member died without suffering."

■ Allow time for questions, reflection, and discussion.

■ Check with the individuals caring for the patient's body to make sure it's appropriate to bring in the family. Allow the family to see their loved one.

■ Describe to the family members what they'll see, hear, or smell to prepare them for seeing their loved one, especially if equipment is still connected to the patient's body.

■ Let the family know that they'll have to contact the funeral home and arrange for transportation of their loved one.

■ Also tell the family that the staff may need to call them with questions, or may need help to fill out certificates.

■ It may be helpful to enlist the aid of clergy or social workers to help with the family.

■ Offer to contact the attending or family physician, or give them the phone number of the individual so that they may contact him with any questions or concerns.

Bradycardia algorithm

Bradycardia can be absolute or relative. Absolute bradycardia means that the heart rate is less than 60 beats per minute. Relative bradycardia means that the heart rate produces signs and symptoms of bradycardia, regardless of the actual rate. (See *Bradycardia algorithm*.) As with any ACLS patient, begin by applying the adult cardiac arrest algorithm.

Identify signs and symptoms of bradycardia

In your assessment, look for signs and symptoms of bradycardia, remembering that sometimes patients don't experience any ill effects from bradycardia. Trained athletes, for example, have much slower heart rates and tolerate them without difficulty.

Signs of bradycardia may include hypotension, shock, pulmonary congestion, heart failure, acute MI, and increased ventricular activity. Symptoms may include chest pain, shortness of breath, and decreased level of consciousness.

Identify and treat heart block

Assess for presence of second-degree AV block type II or third-degree AV block in the cardiac rhythm monitor. If no AV block is present and no serious signs are present, observe the patient closely.

If AV block or serious signs are present, administer atropine 0.5 to 1 mg I.V. push every 3 to 5 minutes, if needed, for a total of 0.03 to 0.04 mg/kg. Atropine will decrease vagal tone and increase the heart rate.

Apply a transcutaneous pacemaker immediately upon its arrival. A transcutaneous pacemaker is a Class I intervention for all symptomatic

Bradycardia algorithm

A patient with a bradycardic rhythm may either show few symptoms or show symptoms of decreased cardiac output (CO). If the patient does have decreased CO, determine the cause and initiate appropriate treatment.

Bradycardia
- Slow (absolute bradycardia = rate < 60 beats/minute)

  or
- Relatively slow (rate less than expected relative to underlying condition or cause)

Primary ABCD survey
- Assess ABCs.
- Secure airway noninvasively.
- Ensure monitor or defibrillator is available.

Secondary ABCD survey
- Assess secondary ABCs (invasive airway management needed?).
- Administer oxygen; establish I.V. access; monitor; administer fluids.
- Monitor vital signs, pulse oximetry, blood pressure.
- Obtain and review 12-lead electrocardiogram.
- Obtain and review portable chest X-ray.
- Obtain problem-focused history.
- Obtain problem-focused physical examination.
- Consider causes (differential diagnoses).

Serious signs or symptoms?
Due to the bradycardia?

No

Type II second-degree atrioventricular (AV) block or third-degree AV block?

No

Observe.

Yes

- Prepare for transvenous pacer.
- If symptoms develop, use transcutaneous pacemaker until transvenous pacer placed.

Yes

Intervention sequence
- atropine 0.5 to 1 mg
- Transcutaneous pacing if available
- dopamine 5 to 20 mcg/kg/minute
- epinephrine 2 to 10 mcg/minute

bradycardias. Using a pacemaker allows less medication to be given. Use the monitor to assess pacemaker capture.

Assess blood pressure

If blood pressure is normal, observe the patient. If blood pressure is low, consider using medications.

For low blood pressure, administer a dopamine infusion at 5 to 20 mcg/kg per minute I.V. Dopamine will stimulate beta-receptors, which causes a positive inotropic response (contractility) and a positive chronotropic response (heart rate). If contractility and heart rate are increased, then blood pressure will increase. Dopamine will also stimulate alpha-receptors, which causes vasoconstriction. Again, vasoconstriction will help elevate blood pressure.

If there's no response to dopamine, administer epinephrine infusion at 2 to 10 mcg/minute I.V. Epinephrine is a catecholamine with alpha-adrenergic activity. This will cause vasoconstriction. Vasoconstriction will then elevate blood pressure.

If there's no response with epinephrine, administer an isoproterenol (Isuprel) drip but do so cautiously. Isoproterenol is considered a Class III intervention.

Patients with transplanted hearts don't respond to atropine because their hearts have been denervated. They need a transcutaneous pacemaker or a catecholamine infusion. In addition, patients with bradycardic third-degree block with underlying ventricular escape rhythms should not be treated with lidocaine. Lidocaine's action is to suppress automaticity. This could lead to a worsening of the block and result in asystole.

Acute pulmonary edema, hypotension, and shock algorithm

An MI involving 40% or more of the left ventricular tissue usually causes cardiogenic shock. Mortality for cardiogenic shock is 50% to 70%. Suspect cardiogenic shock if the patient is experiencing hypotension and pulmonary edema. (See *Acute pulmonary edema, hypotension, and shock algorithm*, pages 216 and 217.)

The acute pulmonary edema, hypotension, and shock algorithm begins with the basics. Initiate the adult cardiac arrest algorithm. Perform the primary ABCD survey and assess the patient. The findings may help to distinguish heart failure from acute pulmonary edema.

Depending on your assessment, you'll need to decide what type of problem the patient has. The underlying cause of the problem can be a pump problem, a rate problem, a volume problem, or acute pulmonary edema.

Key points

Using the acute pulmonary edema, hypotension, and shock algorithm

■ Hypotension and pulmonary edema: indicators of cardiogenic shock

■ Determine source of problem: volume, pump, rate, or pulmonary edema

■ Goal: Improve cardiac function

Pulmonary edema

Here are interventions for a patient experiencing pulmonary edema.

First actions

First actions include:

■ Administer oxygen by the least invasive route, but perform intubation, if needed.

■ Administer furosemide, a loop-diuretic, 0.5 to 1 mg/kg I.V. push.

■ Administer morphine for anti-anxiety and pain relief at 2 to 4 mg I.V. push. (Morphine also helps to relieve pulmonary congestion by increasing venous capacity and reducing systemic vascular resistance.)

■ Give sublingual NTG 0.3 to 0.4 mg. (This is a vasodilator that reduces afterload.)

Reassess the patient after each treatment; typically, the patient responds dramatically with reversal of the symptoms.

Second actions

If initial treatment is unsuccessful, systolic blood pressure readings guide second-line actions. Second-line actions include:

■ NTG 10 to 20 mcg/minute I.V. or nitroprusside 0.1 to 5 mcg/kg/ minute I.V. if systolic blood pressure is higher than 100 mm Hg

■ dopamine 5 to 15 mcg/kg/minute I.V. if systolic blood pressure is 70 to 100 mm Hg and signs and symptoms of shock are present

■ dobutamine 2 to 20 mcg/kg/minute I.V. if systolic blood pressure is higher than 100 mm Hg and signs and symptoms of shock are absent.

Sometimes a patient needs the benefit of a vasodilator, but his blood pressure is lower than 100 mm Hg, which contraindicates its use. In that case, a vasopressor and a vasodilator are administered to support blood pressure and to vasodilate; the medications are closely titrated to desired effect, which is to reduce pulmonary and cardiovascular workload.

Use continuous positive airway pressure or positive end-expiratory pressure if the patient is intubated and this option is available on the ventilator. These options keep airways open forcibly, trying to supply oxygen to collapsed alveoli. These measures also indirectly decrease cardiac output.

Third actions

Reassess the patient; if the patient doesn't respond to second-line actions, then third-line actions are used. Third-line actions include:

■ insertion of a pulmonary artery catheter for hemodynamic monitoring

■ use of an intra-aortic balloon pump for more effective myocardial contractions

■ angiography for acute MI or ischemia

■ additional diagnostic studies.

(Text continues on page 218.)

Acute pulmonary edema, hypotension, and shock algorithm

Assess the patient during the primary and secondary ABCD surveys to help determine the cause of acute pulmonary edema, hypotension, and shock. Initiate treatments based on the severity of the hypotension and the underlying cause.

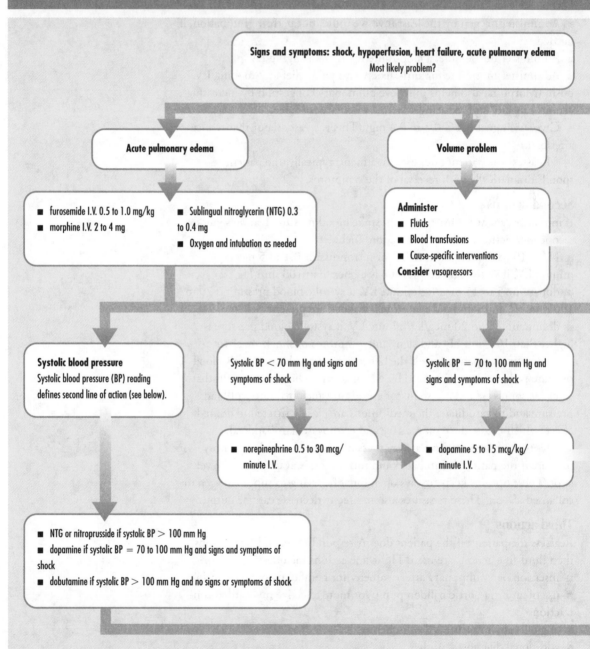

Signs and symptoms: shock, hypoperfusion, heart failure, acute pulmonary edema
Most likely problem?

Acute pulmonary edema

Volume problem

- furosemide I.V. 0.5 to 1.0 mg/kg
- morphine I.V. 2 to 4 mg
- Sublingual nitroglycerin (NTG) 0.3 to 0.4 mg
- Oxygen and intubation as needed

Administer
- Fluids
- Blood transfusions
- Cause-specific interventions
Consider vasopressors

Systolic blood pressure
Systolic blood pressure (BP) reading defines second line of action (see below).

Systolic BP < 70 mm Hg and signs and symptoms of shock

Systolic BP = 70 to 100 mm Hg and signs and symptoms of shock

- norepinephrine 0.5 to 30 mcg/ minute I.V.

- dopamine 5 to 15 mcg/kg/ minute I.V.

- NTG or nitroprusside if systolic BP > 100 mm Hg
- dopamine if systolic BP = 70 to 100 mm Hg and signs and symptoms of shock
- dobutamine if systolic BP > 100 mm Hg and no signs or symptoms of shock

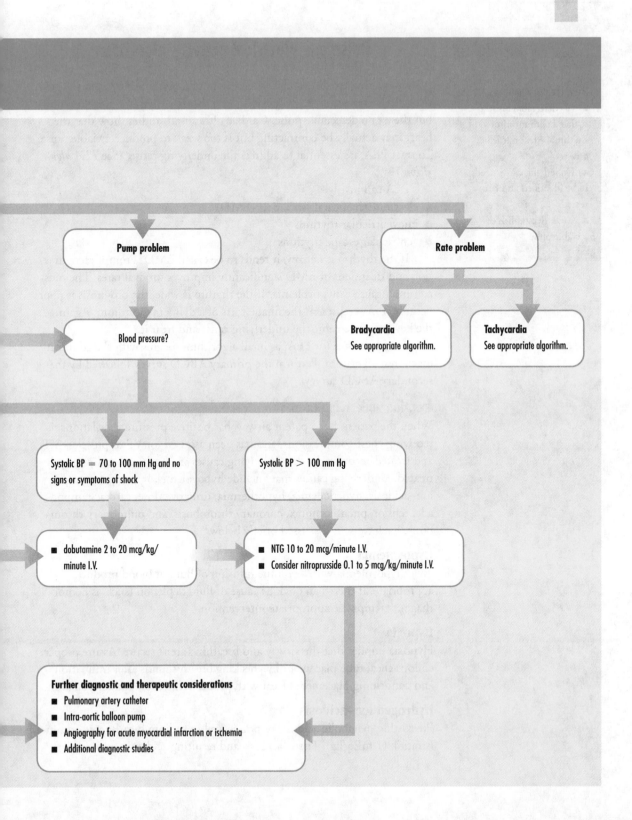

Key points

Using the PEA algorithm
■ No detectable pulse associated with monitored rhythm—treat as cardiac arrest
■ Underlying cause needs to be identified and corrected
■ Goal: Reestablish detectable pulse

Pulseless electrical activity algorithm

PEA isn't a rhythm; it's actually a symptom of a rhythm. However, the patient can be resuscitated. PEA exists when there's a rhythm on the monitor but there's no detectable pulse. Cardiac ultrasound studies show that the heart may actually be contracting but is too weak to produce a viable pulse. To treat PEA, it's essential to address the underlying cause. (See *PEA algorithm*.)

PEA can involve:
■ electromechanical dissociation (EMD)
■ idioventricular rhythms
■ ventricular escape rhythms.

If the rhythm is narrow, it tends to be called EMD. Prompt recognition and treatment of EMD significantly improves survival rates. The most common cause is hypovolemia. If the rhythm is wide, the prognosis is poor because it may represent the final efforts of a dying myocardium. Again, the key is to determine the underlying cause and treat it.

The algorithm for PEA, as in all algorithms, begins with the adult cardiac arrest algorithm. Perform the primary ABCD survey followed by the secondary ABCD survey.

Treating underlying causes

When the patient has a patent airway, has positive pressure ventilations, is receiving chest compressions, and has been assessed for VF or pulseless VT and treated accordingly, the underlying causes are examined and promptly treated. Underlying causes may include hypovolemia, hypoxia, hydrogen ion–acidosis, hyperkalemia, hypothermia, drug overdose, cardiac tamponade, tension pneumothorax, coronary thrombosis, and pulmonary thrombosis. Each cause is discussed briefly below.

Hypovolemia

Treat hypovolemia with a volume infusion of fluid or blood products as appropriate. If there's an obvious cause of fluid depletion (such as hemorrhage), attempt the appropriate intervention.

Hypoxia

Hypoxia implies that the airway and breathing aren't secure. Assure proper endotracheal tube placement by checking breath sounds after intubation and confirming placement. Treat with proper ventilation and oxygenation.

Hydrogen ion–acidosis

Preexisting metabolic acidosis responds well to sodium bicarbonate administration (1 mEq/kg). Tissue acidosis and resulting acidemia from cardiac

PEA algorithm

After you confirm pulseless electrical activity (PEA), you need to determine its cause and treat it rapidly. Supportive measures include epinephrine and atropine.

Pulseless electrical activity
(PEA = rhythm on monitor, without detectable pulse)

Primary ABCD survey
Focus: basic cardiopulmonary resuscitation (CPR) and defibrillation

- Check responsiveness.
- Activate emergency response system.
- Call for defibrillator.
- **A** Airway: Open the airway.

- **B** Breathing: Provide positive-pressure ventilations.
- **C** Circulation: Give chest compressions.
- **D** Defibrillation: Assess for and shock ventricular fibrillation (VF) or pulseless ventricular tachycardia (VT).

Secondary ABCD survey
Focus: more advanced assessments and treatments

- **A** Airway: Place airway device as soon as possible.
- **B** Breathing: Confirm airway device placement by examination plus confirmation device.
- **B** Breathing: Secure airway device; purpose-made tube holders are preferred.
- **B** Breathing: Confirm effective oxygenation and ventilation.

- **C** Circulation: Establish I.V. access.
- **C** Circulation: Identify rhythm and monitor.
- **C** Circulation: Administer drugs appropriate for rhythm and condition.
- **C** Circulation: Assess for occult blood flow.
- **D** Differential diagnosis: Search for and treat identified reversible causes.

Review for most frequent causes

- Hypovolemia
- Hypoxia
- Hydrogen ion (acidosis)
- Hyperkalemia or hypokalemia
- Hypothermia

- "Tablets" (drug overdose, accidents)
- Tamponade, cardiac
- Tension pneumothorax
- Thrombosis, coronary (acute coronary syndrome)
- Thrombosis, pulmonary (embolism)

---

epinephrine 1 mg I.V. push; repeat every 3 to 5 minutes

---

atropine 1 mg I.V. (if PEA rate is slow); repeat every 3 to 5 minutes as needed, to a total dose of 0.04 mg/kg arrest and resuscitation may also be treated with sodium bicarbonate, but the chance of successful defibrillation will be diminished.

Adequate ventilation and restored tissue perfusion and circulation are more effective treatments of acidosis resulting from cardiac arrest.

Hyperkalemia

Sodium bicarbonate administered at 1 mEq/kg may be attempted to correct hyperkalemia.

Hypothermia

Hypothermia is discussed in a later chapter (please see chapter nine, "ACLS in special situations," for specific care guidelines). Primarily, resuscitative efforts must continue while warming procedures are attempted. Body temperature must reach above 30° C (86° F). After this temperature is reached, full advanced life support measures can be performed.

Tablets–drug overdose

Common drugs that produce PEA are tricyclics, beta-adrenergic blockers, calcium channel blockers, and digoxin. The treatment is to clear the drug from the patient's system or to administer medications that combat the effects of the overdosed drug.

Support hemodynamic functioning while other therapies are initiated. Some drugs may be dialyzed out of the patient's renal system in an emergency situation. Other drugs can't be cleared by dialysis.

Cardiac tamponade

Cardiac tamponade is treated with pericardiocentesis. In tamponade, the pericardial space is filled with fluid, and the "space" no longer exists. The heart can't expand correctly or possibly not at all. Pericardiocentesis is an emergency measure used to remove the fluid, allowing the heart to expand.

Tension pneumothorax

In tension pneumothorax, needle thoracostomy is attempted to correct the situation. Adequate ventilation and oxygenation is crucial. If not corrected, tension pneumothorax can be fatal.

Thrombosis, coronary

Coronary thrombosis is considered an ACS. Follow the algorithms for ACS and ischemic chest pain discussed earlier in this chapter.

Thrombosis, pulmonary

With pulmonary embolism, administer thrombolytics, if indicated, or perform surgery.

Other treatments

While treating underlying causes, simultaneously apply other treatments. These treatments include use of a transcutaneous pacemaker and administration of epinephrine or atropine.

Transcutaneous pacemaker

A transcutaneous pacemaker is usually of more value when the heart is contracting and has significant blood flow. In the case of PEA, a healthy heart exists and suffers a temporary disturbance in the cardiac conduction system.

Epinephrine

Give epinephrine 1 mg I.V. push every 3 to 5 minutes and assess its effect.

Atropine

For a bradycardic PEA rhythm, administer atropine 1 mg I.V. push every 3 to 5 minutes for a total of 0.03 to 0.04 mg/kg. Again, this treatment is only indicated for bradycardic PEA rhythms.

Tachycardia algorithm

Tachycardia can stem from many factors. The key is to diagnose which type of tachycardia the patient is experiencing and to identify if the patient has impaired cardiac function. (See *Tachycardia algorithm,* and *Narrow-complex tachycardia algorithm,* pages 222 to 224.)

A potential problem with drug therapy is that many antiarrhythmics are also proarrhythmic, which means that they can cause the same types of rhythm problems that they're intended to relieve. For this reason, the American Heart Association recommends using a total of two drugs to treat tachycardia.

Beginning the algorithm

Initiate the algorithm using the adult cardiac arrest algorithm to perform the primary ABCD survey followed by the secondary ABCD survey. Assess the patient for stability.

If the patient is unstable, synchronized cardioversion at 100 joules is indicated. Synchronization is important so that the energy isn't delivered during the vulnerable period of ventricular repolarization.

If the patient is stable, make a differential rhythm diagnosis and identify if impaired heart function is present. A differential diagnosis that indicates tachycardia includes one of the following four rhythms:
- atrial fibrillation or atrial flutter
- narrow-complex tachycardia

Key points

Using the tachycardia algorithm
- Key to treatment: accurate identification of type of tachycardia
- Impaired heart function affects treatment
- Goal: Reduce heart rate for adequate perfusion

(Text continues on page 225.)

Tachycardia algorithm

The algorithm for tachycardia is quite complex. Remember to base your actions on the type of tachycardia that the patient is experiencing and how the patient is tolerating the rhythm.

Evaluate patient.
- Is patient stable or unstable?
- Are there serious signs or symptoms?
- Are signs and symptoms due to tachycardia?

Stable

Stable patient: no serious signs or symptoms
- Initial assessment identifies one of four types of tachycardia.

Atrial fibrillation or atrial flutter

Narrow-complex tachycardias

Focus evaluation on four clinical features.
- Patient clinically unstable?
- Cardiac function impaired?
- Wolff-Parkinson-White syndrome present?
- Duration < 48 hours or > 48 hours?

Attempt to establish a specific diagnosis.
- 12-lead ECG
- Clinical information
- Vagal maneuvers
- adenosine

Focus treatment on four elements.
- Treat unstable patients urgently.
- Control the rate.
- Convert the rhythm.
- Provide anticoagulation.

Possible diagnoses
- Ectopic atrial tachycardia
- Multifocal atrial tachycardia
- Paroxysmal supraventricular tachycardia (PSVT)

Follow treatment for atrial fibrillation/atrial flutter (in chapter 4).

See narrow-complex tachycardia algorithm for treatment of PSVT.

Unstable

Unstable patient: serious signs or symptoms
- Signs and symptoms are result of rapid heart rate (> 150 beats/minute); prepare for immediate cardioversion.

Stable wide-complex tachycardia: unknown type

Stable monomorphic or polymorphic ventricular tachycardia (VT; see appropriate algorithm)

Attempt to establish a specific diagnosis.
- 12-lead ECG
- Esophageal lead
- Clinical information

Confirmed PSVT

Wide-complex tachycardia of unknown type

Confirmed stable VT (see appropriate algorithm)

Preserved cardiac function

Impaired heart (ejection fraction < 40%), clinical heart failure

Cardioversion, procainamide, or amiodarone

Cardioversion or amiodarone

Narrow-complex tachycardia algorithm

Types of narrow-complex tachycardia include junctional tachycardia, paroxysmal supraventricular tachycardia (PSVT), or multifocal atrial tachycardia. Treatment for each type of rhythm depends on how well the patient tolerates the rhythm.

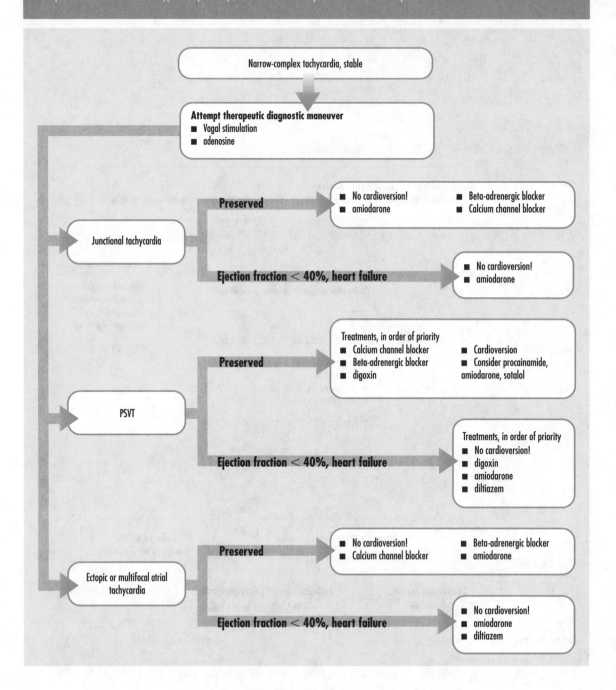

Narrow-complex tachycardia, stable

Attempt therapeutic diagnostic maneuver
- Vagal stimulation
- adenosine

Junctional tachycardia

Preserved
- No cardioversion!
- amiodarone
- Beta-adrenergic blocker
- Calcium channel blocker

Ejection fraction < 40%, heart failure
- No cardioversion!
- amiodarone

PSVT

Preserved

Treatments, in order of priority
- Calcium channel blocker
- Beta-adrenergic blocker
- digoxin
- Cardioversion
- Consider procainamide, amiodarone, sotalol

Ejection fraction < 40%, heart failure

Treatments, in order of priority
- No cardioversion!
- digoxin
- amiodarone
- diltiazem

Ectopic or multifocal atrial tachycardia

Preserved
- No cardioversion!
- Calcium channel blocker
- Beta-adrenergic blocker
- amiodarone

Ejection fraction < 40%, heart failure
- No cardioversion!
- amiodarone
- diltiazem

- stable wide-complex tachycardia
- stable monomorphic or polymorphic VT.

Ventricular fibrillation or ventricular tachycardia algorithm

VF is the most common rhythm for a person in cardiac arrest. For a patient in either VF or pulseless VT, the goal is early access into the EMS followed by prompt use of an automated external defibrillator (AED). Because the value of medications in this situation hasn't been fully determined, the word "consider" is part of the medication portion of the algorithm. (See *VF or VT algorithm,* page 226.)

Treatment begins by applying the adult cardiac arrest algorithm. Begin the primary ABCD survey, performing CPR if appropriate until a defibrillator is available. (See *Stable monomorphic or polymorphic VT algorithm,* page 227.)

When a defibrillator or monitor becomes available and VF or VT is confirmed, the VF or VT algorithm begins.

Defibrillation

Perform immediate defibrillation at 200 joules either by way of an AED or a traditional defibrillator.

If a defibrillator isn't immediately available, a precordial thump may be attempted. However, defibrillation should never be delayed for a precordial thump.

If VF or VT persists, defibrillate again at 200 to 300 joules. If VF or VT still persists, defibrillate at 360 joules.

These three defibrillations are given as a "stacked" response, meaning that the defibrillations occur without a pulse check in between if the monitor shows no change in rhythm. If VF or VT persists, defibrillate at 360 joules within 30 to 60 seconds after administration of medication. Recheck the rhythm on the monitor and recheck the patient for a pulse. If VF or VT persists, repeat the "drug–defibrillation" process until a change in rhythm occurs. If the patient is successfully defibrillated, give a bolus dose of an antiarrhythmic and start a maintenance infusion.

Epinephrine or vasopressin

If VF or VT persists, administer epinephrine at 1 mg I.V. push with repeat doses every 3 to 5 minutes. Epinephrine has beta-adrenergic properties with the action of improving contractility and heart rate; therefore, it restores a rhythm when used with defibrillation.

(Text continues on page 228.)

Key points

Using the VF or VT algorithm
- Most common rhythm in cardiac arrest
- Early defibrillation improves outcomes
- Goal: Reestablish cardiac rhythm

VF or VT algorithm

If a defibrillator is available and you confirm ventricular fibrillation (VF) or pulseless ventricular tachycardia (VT), perform three defibrillations. If this measure is unsuccessful and you complete the secondary survey, follow appropriate guidelines based on continuation of the rhythm.

Primary ABCD survey
Focus: Basic cardiopulmonary resuscitation (CPR) and defibrillation

- Check responsiveness.
- Activate emergency response system.
- Call for defibrillator.
- **A** Airway: Open the airway.
- **B** Breathing: Provide positive-pressure ventilations.
- **C** Circulation: Give chest compressions.
- **D** Defibrillation: Assess for and shock VF or pulseless VT up to three times (200 joules, 200 to 300 joules, or equivalent biphasic) if necessary.

↓

Rhythm after first three shocks?

↓

Persistent or recurrent VF or VT

↓

Secondary ABCD survey
Focus: More advanced assessments and treatments

- **A** Airway: Place airway device as soon as possible.
- **B** Breathing: Confirm airway device placement by examination plus confirmation device.
- **B** Breathing: Secure airway device; purpose-made tube holders preferred.
- **B** Breathing: Confirm effective oxygenation and ventilation.
- **C** Circulation: Establish I.V. access.
- **C** Circulation: Identify rhythm and monitor.
- **C** Circulation: Administer drugs appropriate for rhythm and condition.
- **D** Differential diagnosis: Search for and treat identified reversible causes.

↓

- epinephrine 1 mg I.V. push; repeat every 3 to 5 minutes
  or
- vasopressin 40 U I.V.; single dose, one time only

↓

Resume attempts to defibrillate.
- 1 x 360 joules (or equivalent biphasic) within 30 to 60 seconds

↓

Consider antiarrhythmics.
- amiodarone (Class IIb intervention)
- lidocaine (indeterminate)
- magnesium (IIb if hypomagnesemic state)
- procainamide (IIb for intermittent or recurrent VF or VT)
- Consider buffers.

↓

Resume attempts to defibrillate.

Stable monomorphic or polymorphic VT algorithm

Cardioversion is an appropriate immediate treatment for any stable ventricular tachycardia (VT). Alternatives to this treatment depend on the type of VT, the patient's cardiac function, and the configuration of the QT interval.

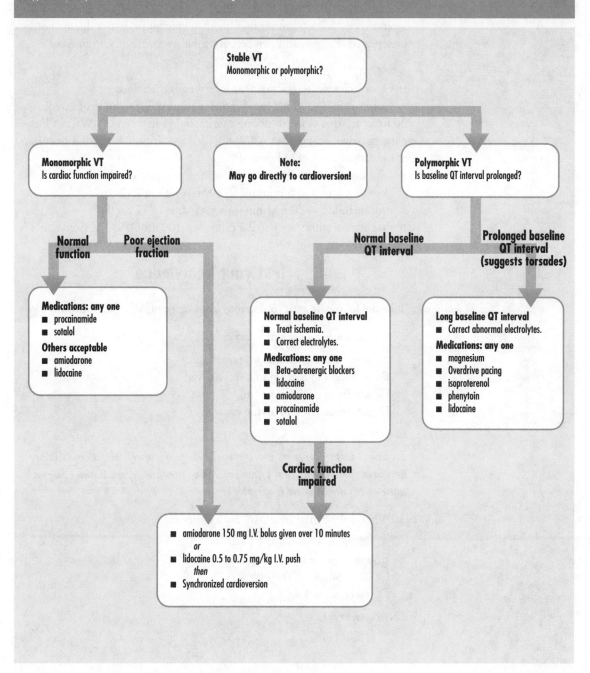

Stable VT
Monomorphic or polymorphic?

Monomorphic VT
Is cardiac function impaired?

Note:
May go directly to cardioversion!

Polymorphic VT
Is baseline QT interval prolonged?

Normal function

Poor ejection fraction

Normal baseline QT interval

Prolonged baseline QT interval (suggests torsades)

Medications: any one
■ procainamide
■ sotalol

Others acceptable
■ amiodarone
■ lidocaine

Normal baseline QT interval
■ Treat ischemia.
■ Correct electrolytes.

Medications: any one
■ Beta-adrenergic blockers
■ lidocaine
■ amiodarone
■ procainamide
■ sotalol

Long baseline QT interval
■ Correct abnormal electrolytes.

Medications: any one
■ magnesium
■ Overdrive pacing
■ isoproterenol
■ phenytoin
■ lidocaine

Cardiac function impaired

■ amiodarone 150 mg I.V. bolus given over 10 minutes
  or
■ lidocaine 0.5 to 0.75 mg/kg I.V. push
  then
■ Synchronized cardioversion

As an alternative to epinephrine, vasopressin 40 U I.V., one time only, may be administered. Vasopressin is a natural antidiuretic hormone that acts as a potent vasoconstrictor when used at much higher doses than normally present in the body. It accentuates epinephrine's positive effects but doesn't accentuate epinephrine's negative effects. It's considered a Class IIb intervention. It has a greater half-life than epinephrine, so it doesn't need to be repeated. Epinephrine can be resumed after a dose of vasopressin.

Antiarrhythmics

If VF or VT persists, consider the following medications:

- amiodarone — 300 mg rapid infusion diluted in a volume of 20 to 30 ml of normal saline solution or dextrose 5% in water (D_5W); if VF recurs, can give second dose at 150 mg I.V. rapid infusion; maximum cumulative daily dose, 2 g/24 hours
- lidocaine — 1 to 1.5 mg/kg I.V. push with repeat doses of 0.5 to 0.75 mg/kg over 3 to 5 minutes for a total of 3 mg/kg
- procainamide — 20 mg/min for a total dose of 17 mg/kg
- magnesium sulfate — 1 to 2 g diluted in 100 ml D_5W I.V. over 1 to 2 minutes.

Test your knowledge

Take the following quiz to test your knowledge of ACLS algorithms.

1. When treating a patient in asystole, it's most important to:

    A. request a transcutaneous pacemaker.
    B. confirm the rhythm in a second lead.
    C. administer atropine 1 mg I.V. push.
    D. determine an underlying cause.

Correct answer: B

Because it isn't uncommon to have a false diagnosis of asystole, it's most important to confirm the rhythm before proceeding to other steps. The most common cause of a "false" asystole is operator error.

2. What is the initial treatment for a patient in VF?

    A. lidocaine 1 mg/kg I.V. push
    B. epinephrine 1 mg I.V. push
    C. Defibrillate at 200 joules
    D. magnesium 1 to 2 g I.V.

Correct answer: C

Defibrillation is the first and most effective treatment for patients with VF and pulseless VT. The faster the defibrillation occurs, the greater the patient's chance of survival.

3. You have a patient with symptomatic bradycardia. You've administered atropine 0.5 mg I.V. push. The patient's pulse has increased to 80 beats/minute, but the blood pressure is 70/40 mm Hg. Your next action is:

    A. infuse a dopamine drip at 5 to 20 mcg/kg/minute.
    B. administer a second bolus of atropine.
    C. infuse an epinephrine drip at 2 to 10 mcg/minute.
    D. apply a transcutaneous pacemaker.

Correct answer: A

Dopamine has alpha-, beta-, and dopaminergic-receptor activity. The alpha activity will cause vasoconstriction, which can raise blood pressure.

4. A patient has stable wide-complex tachycardia at a rate of 210 beats/minute. You should:

    A. administer lidocaine 1 mg I.V. push.
    B. make a differential diagnosis.
    C. administer amiodarone 300 mg I.V. push.
    D. administer adenosine 6 mg I.V. rapid push.

Correct answer: B

For a patient who is stable, making a correct diagnosis for wide-complex tachycardia is essential because it will direct which algorithm to follow for appropriate treatment.

5. A patient is experiencing a wide-complex rhythm of 250 beats/minute with diaphoresis, syncope, and decreased level of consciousness. You should:

    A. defibrillate at 200 joules.
    B. administer lidocaine 1 mg I.V. push.
    C. administer amiodarone 300 mg I.V. push.
    D. perform synchronized cardioversion at 100 joules.

Correct answer: D

These symptoms describe an "unstable" patient. Perform immediate synchronized cardioversion at 100 joules. If synchronization is delayed for any reason and the clinical condition continues to deteriorate, perform unsynchronized cardioversion.

6. You suspect that a patient is experiencing an acute MI. You look at the ECG and expect to see:

    A. ST-segment depression in two or more contiguous leads.
    B. ST-segment elevation in two or more contiguous leads.
    C. T-wave inversion in two or more contiguous leads.
    D. T-wave elevation in two or more contiguous leads.

Correct answer: B

Acute MI is defined as ST-segment elevation in two or more contiguous leads on a 12-lead ECG.

7. A patient is brought to the ED following a motor vehicle accident. He's unresponsive, and EMS personnel are performing CPR. He has been intubated and has I.V. access. You place him on the monitor and his rhythm displays junctional tachycardia at a rate of 120 beats/minute. He has no carotid pulse. Which intervention is appropriate?

    A. epinephrine 1 mg I.V. push
    B. sodium bicarbonate 1 mEq/kg I.V. push
    C. Warming procedures
    D. Fluid bolus infusion

Correct answer: D

Your patient has a heart rhythm but no pulse. This is known as PEA. There are many possible causes for this situation, but one of them is hypovolemia and this is the easiest to treat. A fluid challenge can be rapidly infused while other causes are considered.

8. You're treating a patient whose cardiac rhythm suddenly converts to VF. The patient has no detectable pulse. You:

    A. defibrillate at 200 joules.
    B. administer lidocaine 1 mg/kg I.V. push.
    C. administer epinephrine 1 mg I.V. push.
    D. perform synchronized cardioversion at 200 joules.

Correct answer: A

Early defibrillation significantly increases the chances of survival for a patient in cardiac arrest.

9. The most important treatment for acute MI is:

    A. vasodilators.
    B. I.V. heparin.
    C. reperfusion strategies.
    D. I.V. beta-adrenergic blockers.

Correct answer: C

Reperfusion strategies (because they restore perfusion to the heart) are pivotal in the treatment of acute MI.

10. Your patient has ST-segment depression, recurrent chest pain, and a history of MI. You should treat the patient using:

    A. vasodilators.
    B. cardiac catheterization and revascularization.
    C. beta-adrenergic blockers.
    D. serial ECG and serum markers.

Correct answer: B

This patient is exhibiting signs of unstable angina. A history of MI indicates cardiac catheterization. If revascularization is necessary, it can be performed based on the results of the catheterization.

CHAPTER NINE

ACLS in special situations

Algorithms provide a general approach to treating patients in the most commonly encountered ACLS situations. However, you may encounter situations in which the general guidelines are difficult to apply, such as with patients experiencing acute stroke, cardiac arrest and pregnancy or trauma, submersion or drowning, electric shock or lightning strike, hypothermia, toxicologic emergencies (poisoning), near-fatal asthma, and anaphylaxis. These patients pose challenges and require that you modify the general guidelines. Individualizing the approach to the situation will increase the chances of successful resuscitation.

Acute stroke

Acute stroke, also referred to as a cerebrovascular accident, is a sudden impairment of cerebral circulation in one or more of the blood vessels supplying the brain. Stroke interrupts or diminishes oxygen supply and often causes serious damage or necrosis in brain tissues. About 85% of strokes are ischemic, resulting from thrombus formation in a blood vessel supplying the brain or from embolism (often from the heart). Other strokes are hemorrhagic, resulting from rupture of a cerebral artery or aneurysm. The sooner circulation returns to normal after a stroke, the better the chances are for complete recovery. Therefore, prompt recognition and treatment of a stroke can limit the extent of damage and significantly improve the patient's outcome.

Precipitating events

Some strokes are precipitated by arrhythmia (particularly atrial fibrillation) or by hypertensive crisis. In many cases, no precipitating event is identified. The risk of stroke is increased in patients with a history of:

- transient ischemic attacks
- atherosclerosis
- hypertension
- arrhythmias
- rheumatic heart disease
- diabetes mellitus
- cardiac enlargement

- myocardial infarction (MI)
- cigarette smoking
- oral contraceptive use
- family history of stroke.

Signs and symptoms

Signs and symptoms of stroke vary with the artery affected (and, consequently, the portion of the brain it supplies), the severity of damage, and the extent of collateral circulation that develops to help the brain compensate for decreased blood supply.

Common signs and symptoms of stroke include sudden onset of:
- hemiparesis on the affected side (may be more severe in the face and arm than in the leg)
- unilateral sensory defect (such as numbness, tingling, or abnormal sensation) typically on the same side as the hemiparesis
- slurred or indistinct speech or the inability to understand speech
- blurred or indistinct vision to the same side in both eyes, double vision, or vision loss in one eye (often described as a curtain coming down or gray-out of vision)
- mental status changes or loss of consciousness (particularly if associated with at least one of the above symptoms)
- sudden onset of very severe headache (seen with hemorrhagic stroke).

Management

The essential steps in stroke management can be summarized as the seven D's: detection, dispatch, delivery, door, data, decision, and drug. (See *Treating suspected stroke,* page 234.)

Detection

Early detection of the signs and symptoms of stroke helps ensure the best outcome. Because 85% of strokes occur at home, it's essential for patients at risk for stroke as well as their family members to know the signs and symptoms.

Dispatch

Effective dispatch procedures depend on emergency medical service (EMS) notification at the earliest signs of stroke. When the person calling is confused or unsure, the EMS dispatcher must be able to recognize a possible stroke in order to send the appropriate EMS providers. A patient with suspected stroke should receive the same priority as a patient experiencing an acute MI. EMS providers must respond quickly.

Key points

Acute stroke
- Suddenly impaired cerebral circulation in one or more of the blood vessels supplying the brain
- Prompt recognition and treatment needed to limit the extent of damage and significantly improve the patient's outcome
- May be precipitated by arrhythmia (particularly atrial fibrillation) or by hypertensive crisis
- Essential steps in management: detection, dispatch, delivery, door, data, decision, and drug
- Treatment based on the individual situation, assessment parameters, and type of injury
- Actions and treatments appropriate for all patients with signs and symptoms: maintain patent airway and adequate oxygenation, monitor for and treat hypoglycemia or marked hyperglycemia, monitor blood pressure
- Appropriate antihypertensives, including labetalol (Trandate) and nitroprusside sodium (Nipride)

Treating suspected stroke

This algorithm is used for suspected stroke. The patient's survival depends on prompt recognition of symptoms and treatment.

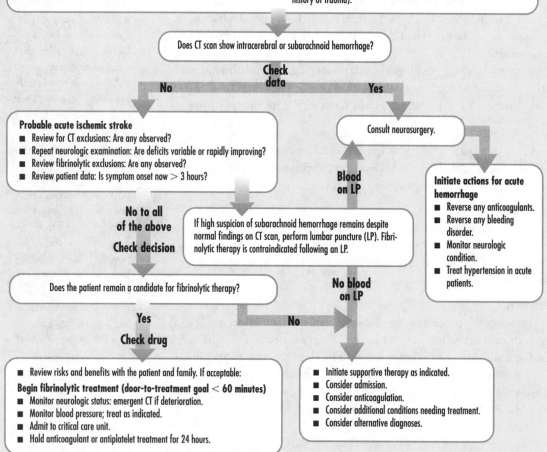

Detection, Dispatch, Delivery to Door

Immediate general assessment: first 10 minutes after arrival
- Assess ABCs and vital signs.
- Provide oxygen by nasal cannula.
- Obtain I.V. access; obtain blood samples (complete blood count, electrolyte levels, coagulation studies).
- Check blood glucose levels; treat if indicated.
- Obtain 12-lead electrocardiogram; check for arrhythmias.
- Perform general neurologic screening assessment.
- Alert stroke team, neurologist, radiologist, computed tomography (CT) technician.

Immediate neurologic assessment: first 25 minutes after arrival
- Review patient history.
- Establish onset (< 3 hours required for fibrinolytics).
- Perform physical examination.
- Perform neurologic examination: Determine level of consciousness (Glasgow Coma Scale) and level of stroke severity (NIH Stroke Scale or Hunt and Hess Scale).
- Order urgent noncontrast CT scan (door-to-CT scan performed: goal < 25 minutes from arrival).
- Read CT scan (door-to-CT scan read: goal < 45 minutes from arrival).
- Perform lateral cervical spine X-ray (if patient is comatose or has a history of trauma).

Does CT scan show intracerebral or subarachnoid hemorrhage?

Check data

No   **Yes**

Probable acute ischemic stroke
- Review for CT exclusions: Are any observed?
- Repeat neurologic examination: Are deficits variable or rapidly improving?
- Review fibrinolytic exclusions: Are any observed?
- Review patient data: Is symptom onset now > 3 hours?

Consult neurosurgery.

Blood on LP

Initiate actions for acute hemorrhage
- Reverse any anticoagulants.
- Reverse any bleeding disorder.
- Monitor neurologic condition.
- Treat hypertension in acute patients.

No to all of the above

Check decision

If high suspicion of subarachnoid hemorrhage remains despite normal findings on CT scan, perform lumbar puncture (LP). Fibrinolytic therapy is contraindicated following an LP.

No blood on LP

Does the patient remain a candidate for fibrinolytic therapy?

Yes   **No**

Check drug

- Review risks and benefits with the patient and family. If acceptable:

Begin fibrinolytic treatment (door-to-treatment goal < 60 minutes)
- Monitor neurologic status: emergent CT if deterioration.
- Monitor blood pressure; treat as indicated.
- Admit to critical care unit.
- Hold anticoagulant or antiplatelet treatment for 24 hours.

- Initiate supportive therapy as indicated.
- Consider admission.
- Consider anticoagulation.
- Consider additional conditions needing treatment.
- Consider alternative diagnoses.

Cincinnati Pre-Hospital Stroke Scale

The Cincinnati Pre-Hospital Stroke Scale is a simplified scale for evaluating stroke patients. Derived from the National Institutes of Health Stroke Scale, it evaluates facial palsy, arm weakness, and speech abnormalities. An abnormality in any one of the categories below is highly suggestive of stroke.

Facial droop (The patient shows teeth or smiles.)
- Normal: Both sides of the face move equally.
- Abnormal: One side of the face doesn't move as well as the other.

Arm drift (The patient closes eyes and extends both arms straight out for 10 seconds.)
- Normal: Both arms move the same or both arms don't move at all.
- Abnormal: One arm either doesn't move or one arm drifts down compared with the other.

Speech (The patient repeats, "The sky is blue in Cincinnati.")
- Normal: The patient says the correct words with no slurring of words.
- Abnormal: The patient slurs words, says the wrong words, or can't speak.

Adapted with permission from: Kothari R.U., et al. "Cincinnati Pre-Hospital Stroke Scale: Reproducibility and Validity," *Annals of Emergency Medicine* 33:373-8, April 1999.

Delivery

As an EMS provider, you should rapidly confirm the signs and symptoms of stroke by performing a quick assessment. You may use the National Institutes of Health (NIH) stroke scale or the Cincinnati Pre-Hospital Stroke Scale, a simplified version of the NIH stroke scale. (See *Cincinnati Pre-Hospital Stroke Scale.*)

Before the patient is transported to the hospital, perform the primary survey by assessing and managing the patient's airway, breathing, and circulation. After completing the primary ABCD survey, immediately transport the patient — don't delay transport for further assessment. The interval between the onset of symptoms and the initiation of treatment is critical.

Communication with the hospital while the patient is en route facilitates prompt action from the emergency department (ED) team when the patient arrives.

Door

As soon as the patient comes through the door of the ED, rapid triage must take place to determine if he's a candidate for fibrinolytic therapy. At this time, the secondary ABCD survey should be completed. Reassess the patient's airway and breathing. If the patient is breathing without assistance, administer oxygen at a minimum rate of 4 L/minute to ensure adequate oxygenation. Next, reassess circulation and make sure that I.V. access has been established. Begin differential diagnosis by obtaining appropriate lab-

Glasgow Coma Scale

The Glasgow Coma Scale provides an easy way to describe the patient's baseline neurologic status. It can also help detect neurologic changes.

A decreased score in one or more categories may signal an impending neurologic crisis. The best response is scored.

Test	Score	Patient's response
Eye opening		
Spontaneously	4	Opens eyes spontaneously
To speech	3	Opens eyes to verbal command
To pain	2	Opens eyes to painful stimulus
None	1	Doesn't open eyes in response to stimulus
Motor response		
Obeys	6	Reacts to verbal command
Localizes	5	Identifies localized pain
Withdraws	4	Flexes and withdraws from painful stimulus
Abnormal flexion	3	Assumes a decorticate posture
Abnormal extension	2	Assumes a decerebrate posture
None	1	No response; just lies flaccid
Verbal response		
Oriented	5	Is oriented and converses
Confused	4	Is disoriented but confused
Inappropriate words	3	Replies randomly with incorrect word
Incomprehensible	2	Moans or screams
None	1	No response

Total score

oratory studies and a 12-lead electrocardiogram (ECG). Assess the patient's neurologic status to determine the extent of his deficits using a standardized tool such as the Glasgow Coma Scale. (See *Glasgow Coma Scale.*)

For the patient with a subarachnoid hemorrhage, you may use the Hunt and Hess Scale to evaluate stroke severity. This scale may also help to predict the patient's risk of complications and chance of survival. (See *Hunt and Hess Scale.*)

Obtain a computed tomography (CT) scan without contrast medium within 25 minutes of the patient's arrival in the ED; results should be available within 45 minutes of arrival to determine whether a subarachnoid hemorrhage is present. If a subarachnoid hemorrhage is present, fibrinolytic therapy is contraindicated. During the first few hours after an ischemic

Hunt and Hess Scale

The Hunt and Hess Scale is used to determine the severity of the patient's symptoms after sub-arachnoid hemorrhage. The higher the grade, the more severe the neurologic deficit.

Category	Criteria
Grade I	Asymptomatic, or minimal headache and slight nuchal rigidity
Grade II	Moderate to severe headache, nuchal rigidity; no neurologic deficit other than third cranial nerve palsy
Grade III	Drowsiness, confusion, or mild focal deficit
Grade IV	Stupor, moderate to severe hemiparesis, possibly early decerebrate posturing and vegetative disturbances
Grade V	Deep coma, decerebrate posturing, and moribund appearance

Adapted with permission from: Hunt W.E.,and Hess, R.M. "Surgical Risk as Related to Time of Intervention in the Repair of Intracranial Aneurysms," *Journal of Neurosurgery* 28:14-20, January 1968.

stroke, the CT scan is typically normal. Those with a subarachnoid hemorrhage will have a normal CT scan only about 5% of the time. If a subarachnoid hemorrhage is suspected despite a normal CT, lumbar puncture should be performed. However, fibrinolytic therapy is contraindicated after lumbar puncture.

Data

Data, such as your assessment, patient history, and CT results, help determine the appropriate treatment plan. The neurosurgical team commonly evaluates the collected data and determines the best treatment plan for the individual patient.

Decision

The type of treatment the patient requires is based on the individual situation, assessment parameters, and the type of injury:

■ Fibrinolytic therapy is indicated for acute ischemic stroke if it can be initiated within the first 3 hours of symptom onset.

■ Emergency angiography may be necessary if the patient has a subarachnoid hemorrhage.

■ If diabetes insipidus is present, treatment may include aneurysm clipping or coiling, nimodipine administration, and correction of hyponatremia and water loss.

■ The patient with intracerebral hemorrhage requires prevention of continued bleeding, management of intracranial pressure (ICP) and, possibly, neurosurgical decompression.

Drug

The goal is to initiate appropriate medical treatment within 60 minutes of arrival in the ED. Fibrinolytics are the drug therapy of choice, but the patient must meet certain criteria to be considered for this type of treatment. (See *Determining who is a candidate for fibrinolytics*.)

ACLS concerns

Because a fall may have accompanied the stroke, the patient may have a head or neck injury. Assess the patient for these injuries. If indicated, apply a cervical collar and logroll the patient to prevent further injury.

Airway

Paralysis of the tongue, mouth, and throat commonly cause partial or complete airway obstruction and hamper the patient's ability to clear secretions. Position the patient in the recovery position to prevent aspiration, or use the head-tilt, chin-lift or jaw-thrust maneuver to open the patient's airway. The patient may also require suctioning to keep the airway patent.

Breathing

Breathing patterns are typically normal except when the patient is comatose. If the patient's breathing pattern is abnormal, an invasive airway such as an endotracheal tube may be necessary. When that's the case, the patient may also need ventilatory assistance provided through a bag-valve device.

Circulation

Assess the patient's circulation. Check the patient's pulse and attach him to a portable cardiac monitor. Be aware that cardiac arrest is uncommon except in cases of intracranial hemorrhage. However, underlying cardiac arrhythmias may be detected with monitoring.

Defibrillation and differential diagnosis

Defibrillate as appropriate.

Hypertension is commonly seen in stroke patients, either as an underlying medical problem or as a result of the stress of the stroke. This often resolves without treatment. Treatments for hypertension that would typically be used should be avoided during ACLS because hypotension may result, impairing cerebral perfusion.

Supportive therapy

Additional actions and treatments appropriate for all patients with signs and symptoms of stroke include:

■ Maintain patent airway and adequate oxygenation (oxygen saturation greater than 90%).

Determining who is a candidate for fibrinolytics

Not every stroke patient is a candidate for fibrinolytic therapy. Each patient must be evaluated to see whether he meets the established criteria.

Criteria that must be present
The following criteria must be present for the patient to be considered for fibrinolytic therapy:
- acute ischemic stroke associated with significant neurologic deficit
- onset of symptoms less than 3 hours before initiation of treatment.

Criteria that can't be present
In addition to meeting the above criteria the patient must *not* have:
- evidence of intracranial hemorrhage during pretreatment evaluation
- suspicion of subarachnoid hemorrhage during pretreatment evaluation
- history of recent (within 3 months) intracranial or intraspinal surgery, serious head trauma, or previous stroke
- history of intracranial hemorrhage
- uncontrolled hypertension at time of treatment
- seizure at stroke onset
- active internal bleeding
- intracranial neoplasm, arteriovenous malformation, or aneurysm
- known bleeding diathesis, including but not limited to:
  – current use of oral anticoagulants such as warfarin sodium, International Normalized Ratio greater than 1.7, or prothrombin time greater than 15 seconds
  – received heparin within 48 hours before the onset of stroke and has elevated activated partial thromboplastin time
  – platelet count less than 100,000/µl.

- Monitor for and treat hypoglycemia or marked hyperglycemia.
- Monitor blood pressure; manage it based on these considerations:
  – If the patient is a candidate for fibrinolytic therapy, keep blood pressure below 185/110 mm Hg to minimize the risk of bleeding complications
  – If the patient isn't a candidate for fibrinolytic therapy, treat only a markedly elevated blood pressure (diastolic blood pressure greater than 140, blood pressure greater than 220/120 mm Hg, or mean blood pressure above 130 mm Hg). Inducing lower perfusion pressures may increase ischemia and worsen the stroke.

The patient's general medical condition also influences treatment. Occurrence of acute MI, severe left ventricular dysfunction, aortic dissection, or hypertensive encephalopathy indicates a need to maintain more normal blood pressure.

Appropriate antihypertensives for the stroke patient include labetalol (Trandate) and nitroprusside sodium (Nipride):
- Administer labetalol 20 mg I.V. push over 1 to 2 minutes; then 40 to 80 mg may be given every 10 minutes to a maximum dose of 300 mg.

■ Administer nitroprusside sodium at 0.25 to 0.3 mcg/kg/minute; may be titrated to keep the patient's blood pressure within an acceptable range, without inducing hypotension.

Additional considerations

Any condition that occurs along with stroke requires additional treatment. Some common examples include:

■ If the patient has a fever, use acetaminophen (Tylenol) and hypothermia blankets to control it.

■ If seizures occur, administer 1 to 4 mg of lorazepam (Ativan) I.V. over 2 to 10 minutes. For a longer-lasting agent, administer 5 mg of diazepam (Valium) I.V. over 2 minutes to a maximum dose of 10 mg.

■ If cerebral edema is suspected (clinically significant in only 10% to 20% of stroke patients), you must maintain ICP sufficient for adequate cerebral perfusion but low enough to avoid brain herniation. Treatments may include:

– elevation of the head of the bed 20 to 30 degrees

– modest fluid restriction

– oxygenation and ventilation support to avoid hypoxemia and hypoventilation (intubation and hyperventilation can rapidly lower ICP in cases of impending herniation)

– hyperosmolar therapy with 1.5 to 2 g/kg of mannitol (Osmitrol) over 30 minutes to lower ICP; effects usually occur about 20 minutes after administration

– high doses of barbiturates — for example, 2 to 4 ml of 2.5% solution of thiopental (Pentothal) — to rapidly lower ICP.

Mechanical ventilation and ICP monitoring are required when a barbiturate coma is induced because of the patient's subsequent respiratory suppression and inability to respond.

Cardiac arrest and pregnancy

Cardiovascular and respiratory systems are altered significantly in pregnancy. As a result, a pregnant woman is more susceptible to the effects of both cardiovascular and respiratory difficulties. When treating a pregnant patient, remember that during pregnancy:

■ circulating blood volume, cardiac output, heart rate, oxygen consumption, and minute ventilation increase

■ systemic and pulmonary vascular resistance, pulmonary functional residual capacity, and colloid oncotic pressure decrease.

Precipitating events

Cardiac arrest in a pregnant woman may be caused by the following precipitating events, some of which may be indirectly attributed to the physiologic changes that occur during pregnancy:

■ pulmonary embolism
■ aortic dissection
■ trauma
■ congenital or acquired cardiac disease
■ peripartum hemorrhage with hypovolemia
■ amniotic fluid embolism
■ eclampsia
■ complications of tocolytic therapy, such as arrhythmias, MI, or heart failure.

Signs and symptoms

When the pregnant woman is in a supine position, the pressure of the uterus on abdominal blood vessels (particularly the inferior vena cava) can inhibit venous return and filling of the abdominal aorta. This can produce hypotension and decreased cardiac output, resulting in signs of shock.

In addition, you must remember that you aren't just treating one patient. Management of cardiac arrest in a pregnant woman includes the need to consider optimal care for the woman and the fetus. If the mother isn't doing well, the fetus will also be affected. The key to resuscitation of the fetus is resuscitation of the mother; the two are inseparable in this situation.

Management

General management of a pregnant patient during ACLS involves applying the primary and secondary ABCD surveys, with some adjustments.

ACLS concerns

A pregnant patient requires displacement of the uterus to the left when placed in a supine position. This action is necessary to relieve pressure on the abdominal blood vessels, preventing positional hypotension. To accomplish this:

■ Place a foam wedge, the backs of overturned chairs, pillows, blankets, or other supporting material under the woman's right torso to displace the uterus to the left (optimally, the torso should be angled 30 to 45 degrees from the floor).
■ Position your knees and thighs under the woman's right hip and back, thus tilting the torso to the left.
■ Manually displace the uterus to the left while resuscitation efforts proceed.

Airway and breathing

Standard procedures for cardiopulmonary resuscitation are appropriate for a pregnant woman in cardiac arrest, as are standard ACLS algorithms. The primary ABCD survey for airway and breathing is mostly unchanged.

The secondary ABCD survey includes no modifications to intubation of the pregnant patient. Concerns may exist about providing adequate ventilation as the gravid uterus pushes up on the diaphragm. This action decreases ventilatory volumes and will make positive-pressure ventilations difficult to provide.

Circulation

Chest compressions may need to be performed slightly higher on the sternum in advanced pregnancy to accommodate the shifting of abdominal contents toward the head. Specific hand position isn't defined. A palpable pulse with compressions indicates adequate circulation, and hand position should be adjusted to achieve a pulse.

Defibrillation and differential diagnosis

Defibrillation requirements are unchanged. Shocks haven't been found to transfer any significant current to the developing fetus.

Differential diagnosis and decision making need to take into account the mother's welfare as well as the fetus's. An emergency cesarean delivery, optimally within 5 minutes of the cardiac arrest, may increase the chance of survival for the mother and the fetus. In a cardiac arrest situation, blood supply to the fetus becomes rapidly hypoxic and acidotic, causing adverse effects in the fetus. Points to consider in this decision include:

- response to appropriate basic life support (BLS) and ACLS care
- the presence of an inevitably fatal injury or condition in the mother
- a cesarean delivery's possible benefit to the mother (removing the fetus and the placenta benefits the mother even if the fetus is too small to compress the inferior vena cava)
- gestational age and viability of the fetus
- time that has elapsed between collapse of the mother and removal of the fetus
- availability of personnel competent to perform the cesarean delivery and to support the mother and neonate after the procedure.

Supportive therapy

In addition to making positional changes to improve circulation, you may administer I.V. fluids. When replacing fluid volume, take into consideration the normal increase in blood volume of up to 50%.

Blood supply to the neonate must be monitored to maintain stability. If a cesarean delivery has been performed, supportive measures should be provided to the mother and neonate as indicated to promote survival.

If either the mother or neonate (or both) hasn't survived, supportive measures should be provided to family members to cope with the loss.

Additional considerations

If persistent arrest is due to an immediately reversible problem (such as excessive anesthesia or analgesia or bronchospasm), cesarean delivery isn't indicated.

If standard BLS and ACLS measures fail and there's a chance that the fetus is viable, consider immediate perimortem cesarean delivery.

Cardiac arrest and trauma

Treatment of the trauma patient with cardiac or respiratory arrest is a complex situation; the best chance for survival occurs with rapid transport to a trauma center rather than with resuscitation attempts in the field. If cardiac arrest is associated with uncontrolled internal hemorrhage or pericardial tamponade, immediate surgical intervention in a capable facility is required. The number of critical patients may exceed the capability of the EMS team. On these occasions, trauma patients without a pulse should be considered lower in priority for care.

Precipitating events

Some of the potential causes of cardiac or respiratory arrest in the trauma patient include:

■ tension pneumothorax or pericardial tamponade causing significant compromise to cardiac output
■ exsanguination with subsequent hypovolemia and inadequate oxygen delivery
■ central neurologic injury causing cardiovascular collapse
■ severe hypothermia complicating injuries occurring in a cold environment
■ hypoxia from airway obstruction, severely lacerated or crushed trachea or bronchi, large open pneumothorax, or neurologic injury
■ severe direct injury to vital organs such as the heart and to such structures as the aorta or pulmonary artery
■ underlying medical problems that led to the injury, such as cardiac arrest precipitating a motor vehicle accident.

Signs and symptoms

The signs and symptoms of cardiac arrest may occur suddenly or insidiously, depending on the mechanism of injury and the age and past medical history of the patient.

Management

The prime consideration is the need for rapid transport to and communication with a hospital capable of managing the trauma patient. Extrication should be performed immediately. It's also important to remember to use standard precautions. If cervical injury is a possibility, the neck must be supported by another rescuer during airway procedures. Immobilize the neck prior to extrication and transport.

Immobilization is usually accomplished by using lateral neck supports, strapping the patient securely, and using a backboard to assist in transporting the patient. A firm cervical collar that has been appropriately sized for the patient should also be applied. These actions minimize neck and spinal cord injury while caring for, moving, and transporting the patient.

ACLS concerns

When performing primary and secondary ABCD surveys on the trauma patient, there are a number of special considerations.

Airway

In suspected head or neck trauma or in multisystem trauma, the spine must be immobilized throughout BLS procedures. This can pose a challenge to providing the care the patient requires.

■ To open the airway, the jaw-thrust maneuver is preferred over the head-tilt, chin-lift.

■ It's recommended that a second rescuer maintain head and neck immobilization until spinal immobilization equipment is applied.

■ The airway should be cleared of secretions, including blood and vomitus, to ensure patency. Use the finger sweep maneuver or suction. Intubation may be indicated to obtain or maintain an adequate airway. To reduce the risk of improper tube location, orotracheal intubation is preferred over nasotracheal intubation if the patient has severe maxillofacial injuries. Confirm proper tube placement initially and with any movement or transfer of the patient.

Cricothyrotomy is indicated when massive facial injury and edema have occurred and if endotracheal intubation is unsuccessful.

Breathing

If ventilation is required, immobilize and maintain the cervical spine. If ventilation attempts don't cause the chest to expand despite repeated attempts to open the airway with a jaw thrust, suspect tension pneumothorax or hemothorax.

When ventilating the patient with a bag-valve device, deliver breaths slowly to reduce the chance of gastric distention and regurgitation, which could easily lead to aspiration.

Ventilation should be provided with high concentrations of oxygen, even if the patient's oxygenation appears adequate. If the patient has suffered chest injury, check for asymmetry of breath sounds or resistance to ventilation. If present, suspect tension pneumothorax or hemothorax; the immediate treatment is needle decompression, followed by insertion of a chest tube. These maneuvers help expand the lung. *If significant flail chest is present, the patient can't maintain adequate oxygenation. Intubation and positive-pressure ventilations are required.*

Circulation

Provide chest compressions as needed to maintain cardiac output. Apply external compression to stop external hemorrhage. A patient with uncontrollable hemorrhage should be transported immediately to a hospital for surgery.

Trauma to the thoracic cage increases the risk that chest compressions may cause a tension pneumothorax. If compressions are necessary, synchronize them with ventilations to minimize the risk to the already traumatized lungs.

Defibrillation and differential diagnosis

Use an automatic ventricular defibrillator (AED) if indicated for ventricular fibrillation (VF) and pulseless ventricular tachycardia (VT).

Identification and treatment of underlying and contributing causes for arrhythmias are essential. Cardiac monitoring may reveal pulseless electrical activity (PEA), bradycardic rhythm, and VT or VF. *Although epinephrine is typically administered to treat these arrhythmias, it may be ineffective if severe hypovolemia is present and left uncorrected.*

Treating PEA requires treating the causes. Treatment may include reversing such situations as hypovolemia, hypothermia, cardiac tamponade, or tension pneumothorax. Bradycardic rhythms are often due to severe hypovolemia, severe hypoxemia, or cardiopulmonary failure. VT or VF in the trauma patient requires immediate defibrillation, regardless of the cause.

Supportive therapy

Assess for open pneumothorax, and seal if present. Assess for subsequent tension pneumothorax and decompress as needed.

Successful resuscitation often depends on restoring adequate circulating blood volume. I.V. access, fluid resuscitation, and medications shouldn't delay transport to the trauma facility and should be initiated at the scene only if extrication of the patient is prolonged. In all other cases, they can be initiated en route to the trauma facility. Aggressive volume replacement may be necessary to obtain adequate perfusion pressures.

Hemothorax may require blood replacement. Surgical exploration may be needed if hemorrhaging is severe.

Control bleeding as quickly as possible. If external pressure doesn't stop bleeding, if bleeding is internal, or if penetrating cardiac injury is suspected, surgical exploration is required.

Emergency open thoracotomy allows direct cardiac massage as well as management of thoracic hemorrhage and cardiac tamponade. Aortic cross-clamping can be done during this procedure. Emergency thoracotomy is a lifesaving action for severe penetrating chest traumas, especially those involving the heart.

Penetrating cardiac injury should be suspected if trauma occurs due to penetrating injury to the left chest and is associated with signs of decreased cardiac output or tamponade (distended neck veins, hypotension, and decreased heart tones).

Myocardial contusion, which is due to blunt chest trauma, can result in significant arrhythmias or impairment in function. Suspect myocardial contusion in patients with extreme tachycardia, arrhythmias, and ST-T wave changes. Diagnosis is confirmed by echocardiography or radionuclide angiography.

Surgical exploration is indicated in trauma patients in the following situations:
- hemodynamic instability despite volume resuscitation
- excessive thoracic drainage (greater than 300 ml/hour for 3 hours or total drainage of 1.5 to 2 L)
- significant hemothorax on X-ray
- cardiac trauma
- gunshot wound to the abdomen
- penetrating injury to the torso
- positive diagnostic peritoneal lavage
- significant solid organ or bowel injury.

Additional considerations

Trauma from a head injury or shock can produce loss of consciousness. Spinal cord injuries can also result in a conscious patient with neurologic deficits. Throughout the primary and secondary surveys, monitor responsiveness closely because deterioration can result from neurologic compromise or cardiorespiratory failure. Use the Glasgow Coma Scale for rapid neurologic examination.

A gastric tube may be indicated to decompress the stomach; however, if the patient has severe maxillofacial injury, the tube should be placed with caution because it can migrate intracranially.

The patient may experience heat loss if clothing is removed to determine the extent of injuries or if blood or other fluids evaporate. Keep the patient warm, if possible.

Submersion or drowning

The outcome of submersion is determined by the duration of the submersion along with the duration and severity of the hypoxia. Hypoxia can cause multisystem complications, such as hypoxic encephalopathy and adult respiratory distress syndrome.

The patient may also develop hypothermia if submersion occurs in icy water. Submersion patients who require resuscitation should be transported to the hospital and evaluated. The hypoxic insult can produce increased pulmonary capillary permeability resulting in pulmonary edema.

If the duration of submersion isn't known (which is generally the case), promptly initiate resuscitation efforts to restore oxygenation, ventilation, and perfusion. Unless there's obvious evidence of death, such as rigor mortis, dependent lividity, or putrefaction, initiate resuscitation at the scene.

Precipitating events

The patient involved in a water incident may be classified according to the type of incident. The patient may be classified as a water rescue, submersion, or drowning patient.

Water rescue applies to a situation in which the patient is alert, experiences distress while swimming, and receives help. Generally, this individual isn't transported to the hospital for further evaluation.

Submersion refers to a patient who requires support in the field and is transported to a facility for observation and treatment.

Drowning is an event in which the patient is pronounced dead, despite resuscitative efforts. Death may occur at the scene or within 24 hours of the event. Up to the time of the drowning-related death, the patient is a submersion patient.

Depending on the condition of the patient, various grades are used to describe the incident. (See *Submersion episodes,* page 248.)

Signs and symptoms

The degree of injury caused by a water incident may vary depending on the amount of time the patient was submerged and the age and past medical history of the patient. Additional considerations include any injury occurring before submersion and the temperature of the water.

Key points

Submersion or drowning
- Outcome determined by duration of the submersion and duration and severity of the hypoxia
- Resuscitation efforts to be promptly initiated to restore oxygenation, ventilation, and perfusion
- Quick retrieval of the patient from the water
- Once rescue breathing established, pulse assessed and compressions initiated
- Chest compressions, as needed, to maintain cardiac output
- If the patient still in the water, no compressions unless special equipment available to support his back
- If the patient is older than age 8 and a shockable rhythm is identified, AED
- No I.V. medications until core temperature increases

Submersion episodes

Numerous terms may be used to describe submersion. The algorithm here was designed to provide for uniform reporting of submersion.

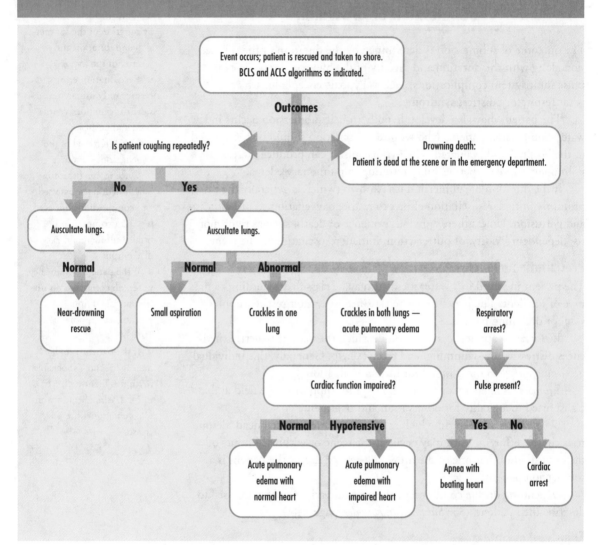

Management

Retrieve the victim from the water as quickly as possible while maintaining the safety of the rescuers. Transport him to a hospital for further evaluation and treatment, even if he has responded very early to resuscitation efforts.

ACLS concerns

Although no change in the primary ABCD survey is necessary, several considerations apply to the submersion or drowning patient. After the primary ABCD survey, institute the secondary ABCD survey.

Airway

Consider all of these patients to have a potential spinal cord injury. Maintain the head and neck in a neutral position while in the water, and immobilize the cervical and thoracic spine before removing the patient from the water. Initiate standard ACLS procedures, including early intubation.

Protection against hypoxia after submersion is generally required only with small patients in icy water where hypothermia develops rapidly.

Don't administer abdominal thrusts (Heimlich maneuver) unless the airway is obstructed by a foreign object. If there's a foreign body airway obstruction, consider using chest compressions instead, which may be superior to abdominal thrusts in clearing an obstruction.

If measures to clear a foreign body airway obstruction are indicated, position the patient's head to the side to avoid aspiration of expelled gastric contents.

Breathing

Initiate rescue breathing as soon as possible. Don't attempt deep-water breathing techniques unless you're specifically trained in their use.

There's no need to clear the patient's airway of water before initiating rescue breathing. In most cases, the volume aspirated is small and is quickly absorbed by the lung tissue.

Once the patient is intubated, deliver positive pressure ventilation with a bag-valve device.

Circulation

After rescue breathing has been established, assess for a pulse, and initiate compressions (if indicated). The pulse of a near-drowning patient may be difficult to palpate because of peripheral vasoconstriction.

Don't attempt compressions while the patient is still in the water unless special equipment (such as a transport board) is available to support his back and rescuers have been specifically trained to use such equipment.

Defibrillation and differential diagnosis

The AED is used in patients older than age 8 if a shockable rhythm is identified. If hypothermia is present — that is, if the patient has a core temperature of 86° F (30° C) or less — a maximum of three defibrillations can be attempted. If these are unsuccessful, return to BLS and ACLS care until the core temperature is greater than 86° F.

After the rescue, the incident should be investigated for any extenuating circumstances, such as drug ingestion or trauma.

Supportive therapy

I.V. medications are withheld until the temperature increases. In moderate hypothermia, I.V. medications are given at longer standard intervals. If hypothermia is a consideration, see "Hypothermia," page 252, for appropriate care. Nearly all drowning patients will experience some degree of hypothermia as a result of the submersion and from evaporation during resuscitation.

Continue oxygen administration to submersion or drowning patients during transport. It may take several hours for pulmonary injury to manifest.

Additional considerations

Despite aggressive care, patients presenting with significant neurologic hypoxia aren't typically affected by attempts to improve outcome. Likewise, VT and VF in children are poor prognostic indicators.

Electric shock or lightning strike

A variety of injuries with different degrees of severity can occur from electric shock or lightning strike. Along with injuries, either cardiac or respiratory arrest may be induced. Institute ACLS measures immediately. While it isn't possible to readily predict the patient's prognosis, those without preexisting cardiopulmonary disease, especially the young, have a good potential for survival when immediate support is provided.

Precipitating events

Although most electric shocks to children occur in the home, most of the incidents involving adults occur in the workplace. Many factors determine the type and severity of injury, including the magnitude of energy received, voltage, duration of contact, resistance to current flow, and path of current flow.

Signs and symptoms

Primary respiratory arrest following electric shock or lightning strike can occur due to:
- inhibition of respiratory center function as the result of electric current passing through the brain
- tetanic contraction of respiratory muscles during the passing of the electric current
- continued paralysis of respiratory muscles even several minutes after the electric current has ended.

Cardiac arrest may take the form of VF, asystole, or VT, which may deteriorate to VF. Myocardial injury can occur as a direct effect of the current and from coronary artery spasm.

Strikes by lightning cause an instantaneous, massive direct current countershock. Depolarization occurs to the entire myocardium resulting in cardiac arrest. In many cases of lightning strike, cardiac cell automaticity restores organized cardiac activity.

Lightning strikes may also affect the cardiovascular system and the neurologic system. Excessive catecholamine release or autonomic nervous system stimulation can result in hypertension, tachycardia, nonspecific ECG changes (including prolongation of the QT interval and T-wave inversion), and myocardial necrosis.

Neurologic injuries may result directly from effects on the brain or secondarily from complications of cardiac arrest and hypoxia. The current may produce such problems as hemorrhages in the brain, edema, small-vessel injury, neuronal injury, hypoxic encephalopathy (from cardiac arrest), and myelin damage to the peripheral nervous system.

Management

Maintain the safety of rescuers at all times. Be certain that electrical current has been turned off before touching the electric shock patient. If there's a chance of head or neck trauma, maintain a neutral head position, and immobilize the spine. Spinal injuries can occur with electric shock due to tetanic contraction of skeletal muscles.

If the patient is caught in a unsafe environment (such as high on a telephone pole), he must be brought to safety prior to treatment.

If rescuers must remain with the patient near live current, only those specially trained to perform in this circumstance should do so.

ACLS concerns

In the primary and secondary ABCD survey, initiate vigorous resuscitative measures, with some modifications.

Airway

Secure an airway if the patient is unable to maintain one naturally. If a head or neck injury is suspected, the jaw-thrust maneuver is favored over the head-tilt, chin-lift technique. Electric burns of the face, mouth, or anterior neck can result in compromised airway. It's important to intubate the patient early, because significant tissue swelling and edema may develop. An endotracheal tube should be inserted before signs of airway obstruction become severe.

Key points

Hypothermia
■ Patients with severe hypothermia (body temperatures lower than 86° F [30° C]) can appear clinically dead, with pulses and respiratory efforts difficult to detect and marked depression of brain function
■ Removal of wet clothing
■ Careful transport of patient to the hospital
■ Monitoring core temperature, cardiac rhythm
■ Gently provided additional supportive measures as needed
■ After securing an airway, assess for breathing for 30 to 45 seconds
■ Assess for a pulse for 30 to 45 seconds
■ Rewarming for any patient with a core temperature lower than 93° F (33.9° C).
■ In passive rewarming, patient placed in a warm room and wrapped in blankets
■ In active external rewarming, careful use of heating devices, such as forced hot air, warm bath water, or warm packs
■ If the core temperature 86° to 93° F, active external rewarming limited to neck, armpits, or groin areas
■ For severe hypothermia, active internal rewarming

Breathing

Initiate rescue breaths if the patient doesn't spontaneously breathe. Provide ventilatory support and supplemental oxygenation.

Circulation

If there are no signs of circulation, initiate chest compressions as soon as possible.

Defibrillation and differential diagnosis

If VT or VF is present, use an AED, when available, to convert the rhythm.

After treatment of injuries, the precipitating event, such as faulty wiring or child neglect, should be evaluated and addressed appropriately.

Supportive therapy

Hypovolemic shock can occur from significant tissue destruction and fluid loss due to increased capillary permeability. Administer adequate I.V. fluids to support circulating blood volume and to produce diuresis. This will promote excretion of myoglobin and potassium, which are by-products of extensive tissue damage.

Electrothermal burns and underlying tissue injury may need surgical treatment, requiring a physician skilled in treatment of electrical injury. Transport the patient as soon as reasonable to allow for a thorough evaluation of injuries.

Additional considerations

In addition to potential spinal injuries, muscular strains or fractures may occur due to tetanic response of skeletal muscles. The patient may also experience thermal damage from smoldering clothing, shoes, and belts. These should be removed to prevent further injury to the patient.

Edema can occur locally at the site of injuries. Jewelry and other constrictive objects that encircle body parts should be removed to promote circulation.

Hypothermia

Patients with severe hypothermia — that is, with a core temperature less than 86° F (30° C) — can appear to be clinically dead, with pulses and respiratory efforts difficult to detect and marked depression of brain function. Don't withhold lifesaving procedures unless the patient has obvious lethal injuries, the body is frozen to the point that chest compressions are impossible, or the nose and mouth are blocked with ice.

Hypothermia has a physiologic effect on vital organs. Severe hypothermia results in depression of cerebral blood flow, diminished oxygen requirements, reduced cardiac output, and decreased arterial pressure. Hypothermia may have a protective effect on the brain and vital organs to some extent in cardiac arrest. Organ ischemia may be reduced if the patient cools rapidly because of decreased oxygen consumption.

Precipitating events

Unintentional hypothermia may be associated with poverty, mental illness, or the use of drugs and alcohol. Hypothermia may also be a secondary occurrence, such as in the case of a trauma or cardiopulmonary arrest patient found in a cold environment. It's a common occurrence in a submersion or drowning patient.

Signs and symptoms

Some patients with hypothermia maintain a perfusing rhythm and only require rewarming. Others experience cardiopulmonary arrest and require resuscitation as well as rewarming. If appropriate equipment is available, rescuers in the field should assess core temperature (tympanic or rectal) because rewarming techniques vary based on the severity of the hypothermia.

Management

If the patient has maintained a perfusing rhythm:
- Remove wet clothing, insulate the patient, and protect him from wind.
- Transport the patient to the hospital, carefully avoiding any rough movement that may precipitate VF.
- Monitor core temperatures and cardiac rhythm. (Needle electrodes may be needed if adhesive electrodes won't function on very cold skin.)
- Provide additional supportive measures as needed (gently), such as intubation, while continuing to monitor cardiac rhythm.

ACLS concerns

If the patient has cardiopulmonary arrest, institute standard ACLS procedures with some modification within the algorithm. (See *Treating hypothermia,* page 254.)

Airway and breathing

After securing an airway, assess for breathing for 30 to 45 seconds (extra time is necessary because respiratory efforts may be difficult to detect). If the patient isn't breathing, initiate rescue breathing immediately and provide warmed humidified oxygen (108° to 115° F [42.2° to 46.1° C]) when possible.

Circulation

Assess for a pulse for 30 to 45 seconds because peripheral vasoconstriction and bradycardia may make the pulse difficult to detect. If the patient has profound bradycardia or no detectable pulse, initiate chest compressions immediately.

Treating hypothermia

Severe hypothermia is associated with reduced cerebral blood flow and oxygen requirement, decreased cardiac output, and reduced arterial blood pressure. Patients with hypothermia can appear dead because of diminished brain function. Therefore, hypothermia treatment requires special consideration. Initial treatment for all patients with hypothermia includes removing wet garments, protecting the patient against heat loss, avoiding rough movement and unnecessary activity, monitoring core temperature and cardiac rhythm, and maintaining the patient in a supine position.

Assess responsiveness, breathing, and pulse.

If pulse and breathing are present

If the patient's core temperature is 93.2° to 96.8° F (34° to 36° C), initiate passive rewarming and active external rewarming.

If the patient's core temperature is 86° to 93° F (30° to 38.9° C), initiate passive rewarming and active external rewarming of truncal areas only.

If the patient's core temperature is less than 86° F, initiate active internal rewarming by warming I.V. fluids (110° F [43.3° C]); administering warm, humidified oxygen (108° to 115° F [42.2° to 46.1° C]); performing peritoneal lavage; using extracorporeal rewarming; and inserting esophageal rewarming tubes.

Continue internal rewarming until core temperature is higher than 95° F (35° C) or spontaneous circulation returns or resuscitative efforts cease.

If pulse or breathing are absent

- Initiate cardiopulmonary resuscitation (CPR).
- Defibrillate ventricular fibrillation (VF) or pulseless ventricular tachycardia (VT) with up to a maximum of three shocks.
- Secure the patient's airway.
- Ventilate with warm, humidified oxygen (108° to 115° F).
- Establish I.V. access, and infuse warm normal saline solution (110° F).

If the patient's core temperature is less than 86° F, continue CPR, withhold I.V. medications, and transport patient to hospital.

If the patient's core temperature is greater than 86° F but less than 95° F, continue CPR, administer I.V. medications spaced at longer-than-standard ACLS intervals, and repeat defibrillation for VF or VT as core temperature rises.

Defibrillation

As soon as a defibrillator is available, assess the cardiac rhythm. Attempt defibrillation if VT or VF is present. Deliver up to three shocks. If this is unsuccessful, withhold additional shocks until the patient has been rewarmed.

Differential diagnosis

Underlying disorders and coinciding conditions need to be addressed while treating hypothermia. These situations may include drug overdose, alcohol use, and associated trauma, which also will present challenges to the rescuer.

Supportive therapy

Rewarming should be instituted for any patient with a core temperature lower than 93° F (33.8° C). A conscious patient with mild or moderate hypothermia can be managed with passive and active rewarming procedures.

Passive rewarming

In passive rewarming, the patient is placed in a warm room and wrapped in blankets.

Active external rewarming

In active external rewarming, heating devices, such as forced hot air, warm bath water, or warm packs, are carefully employed.

If the core temperature is 86° to 93° F (30° to 33.9° C), limit active external rewarming to neck, armpits, or groin areas. Use of these techniques in peripheral areas can contribute to a continued drop in core temperature as cold blood from the periphery is mobilized.

Active internal rewarming

For patients with severe hypothermia — that is, a core temperature less than 86° F — active internal rewarming is required. Follow this procedure:
- Administer humidified oxygen that has been warmed to between 108° and 115° F (42.2° and 46.1° C).
- Centrally administer I.V. fluids warmed to 110° F (42.2° to 43.9° C) at 150 to 200 ml/hour.
- Perform peritoneal lavage with potassium-free fluid, 2 L at a time, that has been warmed to 110° F (43.3° C).
- Perform pleural lavage with warm normal saline instilled into the patient's chest tube.
- Use extracorporeal blood warming with partial bypass, if available.
(*Note:* Esophageal rewarming tubes, used extensively in Europe, may soon be available in North America.)

Patients who are hypothermic for greater than 45 to 60 minutes have additional concerns that need to be addressed during the rewarming process. Fluid administration is needed because of expansion of the vascular space that occurs during vasodilation in rewarming procedures. Monitor heart rate and hemodynamic levels because of increased fluid requirements and the patient's response to rewarming techniques. Monitor serum potassium levels carefully because significant hyperkalemia may develop. Manage high serum potassium levels with I.V. calcium chloride, sodium bicarbonate, glucose, and insulin. Sodium polystyrene sulfonate (Kayexalate) enemas may also be necessary. More aggressive treatments include dialysis or exchange transfusion.

Additional considerations

In severe hypothermia, bradycardia may be physiologic, and the heart may not respond to artificial pacing. (Pacing isn't indicated unless bradycardia persists after rewarming.)

Drug metabolism is reduced in hypothermia, so increased intervals between doses are indicated once the core temperature is higher than 86° F (30° C). Drugs are commonly withheld if core temperature is lower than 86° F.

Toxicologic emergencies

Though exposure to poisons is common, poisoning rarely causes cardiac arrest. If you suspect poisoning is the cause of cardiac arrest, base your treatment on the specific poison involved.

Precipitating events

Poisoning can be accidental or intentional. In all cases, it's helpful to know the drug or substance involved, the approximate amount ingested, and the time elapsed since the poisoning occurred.

Signs and symptoms

The symptoms of poisoning vary with the individual agent taken.

Management

Gastric lavage is recommended only for patients who have ingested a potentially lethal amount of drug or toxin and present within 1 hour of ingestion. If a comatose patient requires gastric lavage, intubate before beginning the gastric lavage procedure.

Bear in mind that standard protocols for critically poisoned patients may not result in optimal outcomes. Remember the following considerations:
- Avoid high-dose epinephrine in cases of sympathomimetic poisoning.
- More prolonged resuscitation attempts are warranted in poisoned patients. If these are unsuccessful, organ donation may still be an option.
- The usual criteria for brain death aren't valid during acute toxic encephalopathy and can be used only after drug levels are no longer toxic.

Key points

Toxicologic emergencies
- Know drug or substance used, approximate amount, and time of the toxic reaction
- Various signs and symptoms depending on the agent
- ACLS procedures for all cases
- Frequent assessment of airway and breathing performance because of the potential for rapid deterioration
- Maintenance and support of circulation
- Toxic agent removed and reversed, if applicable
- Gastric lavage only recommended with potentially lethal amounts and within 1 hour of ingestion
- Avoidance of high doses of epinephrine with sympathomimetic poisoning
- Prolonged resuscitation attempts warranted
- Usual brain death criteria not valid during acute toxic encephalopathy; criteria can only be used after drug levels no longer toxic

Combating drug toxicity

Drug classes produce varying signs of toxicity that require different treatment measures. This table shows the signs of toxicity for various drug classes and their treatment options.

Drug class	Signs of toxicity	Treatment options
Anticholinergics diphenhydramine doxylamine	■ Cardiac arrest ■ Impaired conduction ■ Shock ■ Supraventricular and ventricular arrhythmias ■ Tachycardia	■ Administer physostigmine.
Beta-adrenergic blockers atenolol propranolol	■ Bradycardia ■ Cardiac arrest ■ Impaired conduction ■ Shock	■ Administer glucagon. ■ Administer a mixed alpha-beta agonist. ■ Apply external pacemaker or insert temporary pacemaker. ■ Administer insulin.
Calcium channel blockers diltiazem nifedipine verapamil	■ Bradycardia ■ Cardiac arrest ■ Impaired conduction ■ Shock	■ Administer a mixed alpha-beta agonist. ■ Infuse calcium I.V. ■ Administer insulin. ■ Apply external pacemaker or insert temporary pacemaker.
Cardiac glycosides digoxin foxglove oleander	■ Bradycardia ■ Bronchospasm ■ Cardiac arrest ■ Impaired conduction ■ Pulmonary edema ■ Shock ■ Ventricular arrhythmias	■ Administer digoxin immune Fab (ovine). ■ Infuse magnesium I.V. ■ Apply external pacemaker or insert temporary pacemaker.
Cholinergics carbamates organophosphates nerve agents	■ Bradycardia ■ Cardiac arrest ■ Impaired conduction ■ Shock ■ Supraventricular and ventricular arrhythmias	■ Administer atropine. ■ Administer pralidoxime. ■ Administer obidoxime.
Opiates heroin fentanyl methadone	■ Bradycardia ■ Hypotension ■ Slow, shallow respirations	■ Administer naloxone. ■ Administer nalmefene.
Sympathomimetics amphetamines cocaine methamphetamine phencyclidine	■ Acute coronary syndromes ■ Cardiac arrest ■ Hypertensive crisis ■ Impaired conduction ■ Shock ■ Supraventricular and ventricular arrhythmias ■ Tachycardia	■ Administer alpha-adrenergic blocker. ■ Administer benzodiazepines. ■ Administer lidocaine. ■ Administer sodium bicarbonate.
Tricyclic antidepressants amitriptyline desipramine nortriptyline	■ Bradycardia ■ Cardiac arrest ■ Impaired conduction ■ Shock ■ Tachycardia ■ Ventricular arrhythmia	■ Administer sodium bicarbonate. ■ Administer a mixed alpha-beta agonist or an alpha agonist. ■ Administer lidocaine (procainamide is contraindicated).

ACLS concerns

In all toxicologic emergencies, follow ACLS procedures.

Airway and breathing

Assess airway and adequacy of breathing frequently because the poisoned patient's status can deteriorate quickly, depending on the type and amount of drug ingested. Support and maintain circulation. Also try to remove and reverse the toxic agent, if applicable.

Circulation, defibrillation, and differential diagnosis

After ensuring adequate circulation, determine further treatment based on the type of drug taken or the effects of the drug on the patient. Also consider specific therapies based on the cardiopulmonary effect of the poisoning agent.

Torsades de pointes can occur with exposure to many drugs. Treatment includes correcting contributing factors such as hypoxemia and electrolyte abnormalities. Magnesium supplementation is recommended even if the serum magnesium concentration is normal, and potassium supplementation may be considered even with normal serum concentrations.

Electrical overdrive pacing (100 to 120 beats/minute) or pharmacologic overdrive pacing with isoproterenol can also be effective.

Supportive therapy

Consider specific therapies as indicated by the drug or toxin ingested. Many agents have antidotes, or specific therapies may be recommended. (See *Combating drug toxicity,* page 257.)

Consult a medical toxicologist or certified regional poison information center for unusual poisoning cases. Receiving specific information quickly will help you treat the patient as effectively and efficiently as possible.

Near-fatal asthma

Severe exacerbation of asthma, with signs and symptoms developing in less than 2½ hours, can lead to sudden death. Most often this occurs due to asphyxia from severe bronchospasm and mucus plugging.

Precipitating events

Arrest can result from hypoxia-induced cardiac arrhythmias and tension pneumothorax. Auto-PEEP (positive end-expiratory pressure) can also induce cardiac arrest by causing a gradual buildup of pressure resulting in air trapping. This occurs due to mechanical ventilation and can result in decreased blood flow and blood pressure.

The patient's outcome can be affected by:

■ whether the patient has true active asthma or another severe condition

■ preexisting conditions such as cardiac disease, pulmonary disease, acute allergic bronchospasm or anaphylaxis, and pulmonary embolism or vasculitis (Churg-Strauss syndrome)

■ medications the patient is taking or abusing (Beta-adrenergic blockers can cause bronchospasm, as can cocaine and opiates.)

■ discontinuation of long-term corticosteroid therapy, which may result in adrenal insufficiency and other problems.

Signs and symptoms

An asthma attack may begin dramatically with simultaneous onset of many symptoms or insidiously with gradually increasing shortness of breath. It typically includes progressively worsening shortness of breath, cough, wheezing, and chest tightness or some combination of these signs or symptoms. Cyanosis, confusion, and lethargy indicate the onset of respiratory failure.

Management

The goal of management is to aggressively treat the severe asthmatic crisis before it deteriorates to full arrest. The patient should be administered oxygen and transported to a health care facility as soon as possible.

ACLS concerns

The asthmatic patient may have difficulty maintaining an adequate airway secondary to bronchospasm and mucus plugging. If respiratory or cardiac arrest does occur, the rescuer uses standard ACLS procedures.

Airway and breathing

Oxygen is administered to achieve a partial pressure of arterial oxygen greater than or equal to 92 mm Hg. In an asthmatic crisis, intubation is indicated for:

■ obtundation

■ profuse diaphoresis

■ poor muscle tone as a clinical sign of hypercarbia

■ severe agitation, confusion, and fighting against the oxygen mask as clinical signs of hypoxemia.

It should be noted that an elevated partial pressure of arterial carbon dioxide doesn't indicate severity of the asthmatic episode. Treat the patient according to clinical symptoms, not numbers.

Circulation, defibrillation, and differential diagnosis

Hypoxia resulting from a severe asthma attack may result in cardiac arrhythmias and cardiac arrest. Assess the patient experiencing an asthmatic attack for adequate perfusion and circulation. If a cardiac arrhythmia does occur, treat according to ACLS protocol. Attempt to identify the trigger for an acute asthma attack.

Key points

Near-fatal asthma

■ Severe exacerbation can lead to sudden death

■ Outcome affected by the presence of true active asthma (instead of another severe condition), preexisting conditions, medications taken or abused, and discontinuation of long-term corticosteroid therapy

■ Oxygen to achieve a PaO_2 of greater than or equal to 92 mm Hg

■ Beta-agonists

■ Subcutaneous epinephrine or terbutaline (Brethine) if patient doesn't respond to albuterol

■ Corticosteroids administered early in the treatment

■ Nebulized anticholinergics typically administered with albuterol

■ Aminophylline as second-line therapy

■ If no response to inhaled adrenergics and corticosteroids, magnesium sulfate perhaps helpful

■ Ketamine may be helpful when intubating a patient with severe asthma

■ Heliox (80% helium and 20% oxygen) to delay intubation by decreasing breathing effort

Supportive therapy

Medications for treatment of acute asthma include:

■ A beta-agonist, such as nebulized albuterol (salbutamol), is the standard treatment for an acute asthma attack. Give 2.5 to 5 mg every 15 to 20 minutes up to three times in 1 hour; the maximum dose is 7.5 to 15 mg/hour.

■ Epinephrine (subcutaneous [S.C.]) may be used if the patient doesn't respond to albuterol or is in a life-threatening situation. Administer 0.01 mg/kg divided into three doses at 20-minute intervals, or terbutaline (Brethine) 0.25 mg S.C. every 30 minutes up to three doses.

■ Corticosteroids should be initiated early and are usually administered after oxygen and beta-agonist therapies have been initiated. Give either methylprednisolone 125 mg I.V. or an equivalent dose of hydrocortisone (between 40 and 250 mg).

■ Nebulized anticholinergics, such as ipratropium (0.5 mg), have a delayed onset of about 20 minutes. These agents are usually given in combination with albuterol, which acts immediately.

■ Aminophylline is a bronchodilator that can enhance effects of beta-agonists and corticosteroids. It's considered second-line, supportive therapy. I.V. aminophylline is given as a loading dose of 5 mg/kg over 30 to 45 minutes and is generally followed by an infusion at 0.5 to 0.7 mg/kg/hour. Give half of the loading dose or only the maintenance dose if the patient already takes theophylline.

■ Magnesium sulfate (I.V.) may be helpful in the patient who isn't responding to inhaled adrenergics and corticosteroids. Administer 2 to 3 g at rates of up to 1 g/minute.

■ Ketamine is an anesthetic agent that's considered helpful when intubating a patient with severe asthma because of its bronchodilating effects. The usual dose is a 0.5- to 1.5-mg/kg bolus repeated in 20 minutes or an infusion of 1 to 5 mg/kg/hour. Atropine 0.01 mg/kg should be administered along with ketamine because of the increase in bronchial secretions caused by ketamine.

■ Heliox is a mixture of helium and oxygen (80% helium and 20% oxygen) given to delay intubation while other medications are taking effect. It decreases the resistance to air flow to the bronchial branches by 28% to 48%, thereby decreasing the work of breathing and allowing time for other administered medications to take effect.

Additional considerations

Bilevel positive airway pressure can help reduce the work of breathing and can help delay or prevent the need for intubation. However, in some patients with severe asthma, oxygenation and ventilation can occur only after the patient is sedated with general anesthesia, given muscle paralytics, and intubated with an endotracheal tube.

Anaphylaxis

Anaphylaxis is a hypersensitivity reaction mediated by immunoglobulin E (IgE) and IgG4 antibodies. Reexposure to an antigen causes a reaction. The most important mediators are histamine, leukotrienes, prostaglandins, thromboxanes, and bradykinins. These mediators are activated in the body and produce the clinical signs of anaphylaxis: signs of hypotension, bronchospasm, and angioedema.

Precipitating events

The most common causes of anaphylaxis are insect stings, drugs, contrast media, and some foods. Latex-associated anaphylaxis, exercise-induced anaphylaxis, and even idiopathic anaphylaxis have been reported.

Signs and symptoms

The sooner a reaction occurs after exposure, the more likely it is to be severe. Signs and symptoms include:

- upper and lower airway edema
- cardiovascular collapse due to vasodilation and increased capillary permeability
- urticaria, rhinitis, conjunctivitis
- abdominal pain, vomiting, diarrhea
- sense of impending doom.

Management

The patient with anaphylaxis may exhibit various signs and symptoms, depending on the reaction, which can vary in intensity and severity over time. Intubate early if airway swelling is present and the patient doesn't rapidly respond to pharmacologic interventions. Oxygen should be delivered at high flow rates as appropriate.

Epinephrine is given to treat shock, airway swelling, or difficulty breathing. It's administered I.M. in 0.3- to 0.5-mg doses and can be repeated after 5 to 10 minutes if no improvement is seen.

Administer epinephrine 0.1 to 0.5 mg I.V. over 5 minutes only in profound, immediately life-threatening situations. In an arrest situation, progress rapidly to high-dose epinephrine I.V.

Scrape away any insect parts at the site of a sting (don't squeeze a venom sac that's intact). Then apply ice to the area to slow absorption.

Transport the patient to a health care facility as quickly as possible.

ACLS concerns

The following are modifications to standard ACLS treatments of airway, breathing, and circulatory support.

Key points

Anaphylaxis
- Hoarseness, lingual edema, and posterior or oropharyngeal swelling indicating early intubation
- Tracheal intubation and cricothyrotomy difficult, if not impossible
- Paralytic agents administered for intubation can have lethal consequences (patient deprived of any spontaneous breathing attempt)
- Alternative methods of oxygenation and ventilation: fiber-optic tracheal intubation, digital tracheal intervention, needle cricothyrotomy followed with transtracheal ventilation, and cricothyrotomy for the patient with massive neck swelling
- 2 to 4 L of isotonic crystalloid and high-dose epinephrine for rapid volume expansion to support circulation
- Other measures: administering antihistamines and steroids and following the appropriate algorithm for arrhythmias

Airway

The patient experiencing anaphylaxis requires close observation during drug therapy. Early intubation is indicated if hoarseness, lingual edema, and posterior or oropharyngeal swelling occur.

Individuals with angioedema are at especially high risk for rapid deterioration. Patients with hoarseness, lingual edema, and posterior or oropharyngeal swelling are at high risk for respiratory compromise.

Breathing

Deterioration of the patient is evident with stridor, severe dysphonia or aphonia, laryngeal edema, massive lingual swelling, facial and neck swelling, and hypoxemia. These symptoms can occur within 30 minutes or up to 3 hours.

Tracheal intubation and cricothyrotomy can be difficult if not impossible. Measures can result in increased laryngeal edema, bleeding, and further narrowing of the glottic opening. Agitation causes hypoxia to worsen.

Paralytic agents given to attempt intubation may prove lethal as the patient is deprived of any spontaneous breathing attempt.

Alternative methods of oxygenation and ventilation include fiber-optic tracheal intubation, digital tracheal intervention (using the rescuer's fingers and a smaller [less than 7-mm diameter] endotracheal tube), needle cricothyrotomy followed by transtracheal ventilation, and cricothyrotomy for the patient with massive neck swelling.

Circulation

Circulatory support includes rapid volume expansion through administration of 2 to 4 L of isotonic crystalloid solution and high-dose epinephrine. Other measures include administering antihistamines and steroids and following the appropriate algorithm for arrhythmias (usually PEA or asystole). In addition, prolonged resuscitation has been shown to be effective in young patients with healthy hearts. Support is essential to maintain oxygen delivery and circulation until the effects of anaphylaxis have resolved.

Defibrillation and differential diagnosis

The patient experiencing anaphylaxis may deteriorate to hypoxia, resulting in myocardial ischemia and arrhythmias. Defibrillate if appropriate. While treating the patient, the underlying cause should be investigated and identified for the patient.

Supportive therapy

Isotonic crystalloid I.V. solutions, such as normal saline, should continue to be administered for hypotension that doesn't respond promptly to epinephrine. I.V. solutions are generally rapidly infused from 1 to 2 L, and up to 4 L may be required for circulatory support.

The following medications may be given to patients with an anaphylactic reaction:

■ Antihistamines, such as diphenhydramine (Benadryl), are given slowly I.V. or I.M. in 25-mg doses.

■ Histamine blockers, such as cimetidine (Tagamet), can be given orally, I.M., or I.V. in 300-mg doses.

■ Inhaled albuterol may be given if bronchospasm is significant. If the patient is hypotensive, epinephrine should be given prior to inhaled albuterol to prevent a drop in blood pressure. Inhaled ipratropium may be helpful for patients taking beta-adrenergic blockers.

■ High-dose I.V. corticosteroids are administered slowly or may be given I.M. for a severe attack, especially in an asthmatic patient. The effect won't be evident for 4 to 6 hours.

■ Consider giving glucagon to patients unresponsive to epinephrine, especially to those taking beta-adrenergic blockers. The dosage is 1 to 2 mg every 5 minutes I.M. or I.V.

Additional considerations

Observe the patient for up to 24 hours because signs and symptoms of anaphylaxis may recur in 1 to 8 hours despite effective initial treatment.

Test your knowledge

Take the following quiz to test your knowledge of ACLS procedures in special situations.

1. The risk of stroke is increased in patients with a history of:

    A. atherosclerosis.
    B. multiple sclerosis.
    C. rheumatic arthritis.
    D. hypotension.

Correct answer: A

A patient with a history of atherosclerosis is at increased risk for stroke.

2. Which assessment tool helps with rapid assessment and recognition of stroke symptoms?

    A. Glasgow Coma Scale
    B. Cincinnati Pre-Hospital Stroke Scale
    C. Lumbar puncture
    D. Hunt and Hess Scale

Correct answer: B

Use the Cincinnati Pre-Hospital Stroke Scale in the primary survey to help determine if the patient is experiencing a stroke.

3. Supportive therapy for all stroke patients includes:

    A. fibrinolytic therapy within the first 3 hours on symptom onset.
    B. surgical clipping or coiling of an aneurysm.
    C. maintenance of airway and adequate oxygenation.
    D. administration of the appropriate antihypertensive agent.

Correct answer: C

Always maintain a patent airway and adequate oxygenation in the patient experiencing a stroke. The tongue is a common cause of airway obstruction.

4. A pregnant patient experiencing a cardiac arrest requires:

    A. displacement of her uterus to the left when in a supine position.
    B. placement on her right side.
    C. raising of her head 30 to 45 degrees.
    D. being kept in a supine position during chest compressions.

Correct answer: A

The large uterus presses on vital blood vessels and needs displacement to the side. The patient may also be slightly tilted to her left to assist with this measure.

5. Which of the following is an early sign of deterioration in a trauma patient?

    A. Change in level of consciousness
    B. Pupillary changes
    C. Increased heart rate
    D. Vomitus in the airway

Correct answer: A

A change in the level of consciousness is an early indication that the patient is experiencing neurologic compromise or cardiorespiratory failure.

6. When examining a patient, you detect an open pneumothorax. Immediate treatment for this involves:

    A. insertion of a chest tube.
    B. surgical exploration.
    C. needle decompression.
    D. sealing of the wound with occlusive dressing.

Correct answer: D

The open pneumothorax must be sealed to prevent atmospheric air from entering the chest cavity.

7. When treating a patient for submersion or drowning:

    A. clear the patient's airway of water before initiating rescue breathing.
    B. initiate ABCD survey while the patient is still in the water.
    C. consider the patient to have a spinal cord injury.
    D. administer abdominal thrusts.

Correct answer: C

Consider the patient to have a head or neck injury unless proven otherwise.

8. Primary respiratory arrest following electric shock or lightning strike can occur from which of the following?

    A. Paralysis of respiratory muscles during shock
    B. Pneumothorax from injury
    C. Contraction of respiratory muscles
    D. Ventricular fibrillation

Correct answer: C

Tetanic contraction of respiratory muscles occurs during the passage of the electric current and can result in respiratory arrest.

9. After initiating airway, breathing, and circulation in a hypothermic patient, the next priority is:

    A. administering defibrillations for VF.
    B. warming the patient.
    C. administering I.V. medications according to protocol.
    D. initiating I.V. therapy.

Correct answer: A

If there's a shockable rhythm on the monitor, attempt up to three defibrillations.

10. Which of the following is the standard initial therapy for near-fatal asthma?

    A. Immediate intubation and oxygenation
    B. Nebulized albuterol
    C. Epinephrine
    D. Corticosteroids

Correct answer: B

The initial standard therapy is albuterol or salbutamol, which may be given in 2.5- to 5-mg doses every 15 to 20 minutes up to three times in 1 hour. If this doesn't work, use epinephrine as an alternative. In an asthmatic crisis, intubation is indicated for obtundation, profuse diaphoresis, poor muscle tone, or severe agitation.

CHAPTER
TEN

Megacode review

The megacode review found in this chapter incorporates the basic ACLS principles and discusses the roles and expectations of the team members. This chapter uses a case study approach to present a realistic picture of what occurs in a code situation.

Roles of the team members

The megacode station in an ACLS class provides the learner with a dress rehearsal to help team members organize their roles when involved in a real code situation. Generally speaking, a team leader needs to direct care activities during a cardiac resuscitation. Everyone takes a turn being team leader. The other three members of the team take on the following responsibilities: airway management, cardiopulmonary resuscitation (CPR), and I.V. access and drug administration.

Team leader
During the megacode, the team leader performs the defibrillation role. However, in a real code situation, there may be someone else to defibrillate, allowing the team leader to lead or manage the activities. Although the team leader is the one designated to put the whole picture together, this person needs to understand that he's also a team member.

Teamwork
The word *teamwork* applies fully in a cardiac arrest. There are so many different activities occurring simultaneously that the team leader needs to be open to suggestions from other team members. For example, the person administering drugs may notice that 3 minutes have passed since the last dose of epinephrine was administered, or the person who intubated the patient may realize that breath sounds haven't been checked.

The ACLS megacode station gives the student a glimpse into those situations, as well as a turn at performing the various roles. Also, before testing day, the student is given the opportunity to practice with the equipment and to become familiar with the techniques.

Algorithms
Within the megacode, algorithms serve as guides to patient care, pointing the team in a unified direction. However, they shouldn't be used as a re-

placement for a team's assessment skills. Remember that research findings may alter the current recommendations, so a team must keep current and be aware of changes in standards of practice to ensure that the best possible care will be given to the patient.

Megacode testing

At Megacode testing stations, the ACLS instructor will give you a brief patient scenario. The areas typically will include any equipment the situation demands.

Some instructors try to set up the stations and scenarios that apply to the student's likely work situation. For example, if the student is a critical care nurse, the patient situation may occur in an intensive care setting. If the student is a dental hygienist, the situation may occur in a dental office.

It may be helpful to line up the equipment as you intend to use it or in an order you find most comfortable. You may use the equipment to remind yourself about what has occurred during the testing scenario. For example, you might place epinephrine nearer to the patient's I.V. site as a reminder that one dose has been given.

When presented with the patient situation, you may sometimes find that you need additional information in order to take an action or make a sound decision. Don't be afraid to ask for that information. For example, the instructors may have neglected to give the patient's weight. This information will be needed to calculate drug dosages or to choose the appropriate size or type of endotracheal tube. If you ordered an arterial blood gas analysis, you might need to ask if results have arrived. This information is helpful if adjustments in oxygenation seem indicated.

The instructor, in turn, may also ask you for information that's appropriate to the situation. For example, the instructor may ask if an alternate drug could be used during a particular algorithm, or he may remind you that there's currently no I.V. line for administration of epinephrine (or that the team is trying to insert a line). The instructor won't be trying to trick you, but rather he'll be trying to determine if you're thinking along the correct route or if you're simply guessing. Remember that there are alternative medications as well as alternative routes for giving certain medications.

Sometimes a student becomes so nervous that she forgets what was done and what's left to do. A seasoned instructor can differentiate an unprepared student from a nervous one and will provide guidance to redirect her back to the algorithm.

Sample megacode scenarios

Here are two megacode simulations that may help you bring together the principles of ACLS. In addition, they may help prepare you for the megacode section of the ACLS examination.

In the megacode scenarios, the instructor describes the patient's situation and each major change in the patient's condition. The megacode team leader then calls out instructions to the team, if appropriate. Each major action by team members is described, followed by rationales in bullet format. Try to think of the next step yourself before proceeding. This way, you'll get to test yourself and boost your confidence. However, only look at the scenario from the perspective of one team member at a time — trying to think about every single responsibility may prove overwhelming.

Scenario #1

> INSTRUCTOR: *A 66-year-old male is involved in a car accident in which his vehicle hit a telephone pole. He complains of pain in his chest, and he's pale and diaphoretic. A bystander at the scene calls 911.*

■ Promptly calling 911 is one of the most important actions in cases of suspected cardiac injury.

> INSTRUCTOR: *While waiting for help, the patient becomes unconscious. Bystanders initiate CPR.*

■ The acronym taught to all participants of CPR classes is ABCD (Airway, Breathing, Circulation, and Defibrillation). Cardiac compressions have been shown to maintain adequate perfusion pressures, and this contributes to cerebral resuscitation. Controversy remains about whether a layperson should actually perform mouth-to-mouth resuscitation, but the step is still recommended and taught.

> INSTRUCTOR: *The first person to arrive is a police officer. He has an automated external defibrillator (AED) and applies the patches. The machine instructs him to push the SHOCK button. One shock is delivered and the patient has a carotid pulse and spontaneous breathing but remains unconscious.*

■ After entry into the emergency medical service, defibrillation is perhaps the single most important step. If an AED is available, it should be used. The most common initial rhythm in cardiac arrest is ventricular fibrillation (VF), and the treatment to correct it is defibrillation.
■ The goal of the American Heart Association isn't only to have AEDs available in public places for all first responders to use but also to have first responders trained in their proper use. The more timely the defibrillation

after the loss of a pulse, the more likely that the defibrillation will be successful.

INSTRUCTOR: *The paramedics arrive. The patient is now conscious and complaining of chest pain. It's noted that the steering wheel is bent. They call into the dispatcher and begin the secondary ABCD survey; airway secured, breathing adequate, circulation available (including insertion of I.V.s), and differential diagnosis made. The patient is conscious and the airway is patent. A cervical collar is applied. Oxygen is delivered at 4 L/minute by nasal cannula.*

■ When someone complains of chest pain, the possibility of a myocardial infarction (MI) is the priority until ruled out. *Note:* In this situation, it needs to be determined whether the chest pain started before or after the accident.

■ The cervical spine needs to be supported until neck and spinal cord injury is ruled out by X-ray.

■ Oxygen reduces ST-segment elevation for some patients and helps to correct hypoxemia. (Hypoxemia and respiratory insufficiency can impede a diminished cardiac output and lead to an increase in infarction size.)

INSTRUCTOR: *I.V. access is obtained.*

■ Although some medications can be given by endotracheal tube, I.V. access is more desirable. (The patient complaining of signs of an acute MI has a greater possibility of cardiac arrest, so I.V. access is appropriate).

INSTRUCTOR: *A 12-lead electrocardiogram (ECG) is performed (if possible).*

■ The 12-lead ECG is crucial in differentiating one diagnosis from another; however, a normal ECG reading doesn't exclude the possibility of an ischemic event. If the reading indicates an acute MI, certain criteria can be applied to confirm the diagnosis so that time can be used efficiently.

INSTRUCTOR: *The patient is transported to the emergency department (ED).*

■ Rapid transport is desirable because the sooner treatment can begin for a trauma patient as well as for a patient with acute MI, the better the chance of survival and positive long-term outcomes.

INSTRUCTOR: *The patient arrives in your ED and is attached to a monitor. He has normal saline solution infusing I.V., and oxygen is being administered at 4 L/minute. The patient rates his chest pain as 5 on a scale of 0 to 10, with 0 being "no pain" and 10 being "unbearable pain." A 12-lead ECG is repeated. The patient's wife arrives in the ED. The paramedics report that the chest pain started after the accident occurred and that the patient hit the steering wheel with enough force to bend it. Vital signs are: blood pressure 126/82 mm Hg, pulse 88, respiration 22. His monitor strip shows the following rhythm:*

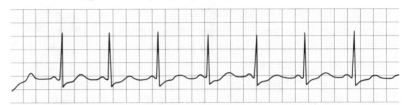

INSTRUCTOR: *His 12-lead ECG shows no ST-segment elevation. Now, all eyes turn to you for direction. Please describe your next action as team leader.*

TEAM LEADER: *I would quickly assess the patient for injury related to the accident as well as obtain a past medical history.*

■ The trauma patient needs rapid assessment to identify any life-threatening conditions that would impede airway, oxygenation, ventilation, or circulation.

INSTRUCTOR: *Medical history is benign. The patient isn't on any medications. However, he suddenly complains of difficulty breathing and then becomes unconscious.*

TEAM LEADER: *I would direct a team member to assess for breathing and check for a pulse. I would also check the monitor for a rhythm.*

INSTRUCTOR: *The patient isn't breathing and there's no palpable pulse. The monitor continues to show normal sinus rhythm.*

■ Pulseless electrical activity (PEA) is defined as the absence of a detectable pulse with a rhythm on the monitor. It's commonly associated with clinical states that can be reversed. Rapid identification and prompt treatment of these states improve the chance of survival.

TEAM LEADER: *I would direct the team members to begin CPR, including intubation. The I.V. access is already established. I would order the I.V. fluids to be run wide open, and I would assess for a reversible cause of PEA.*

■ The trauma patient who suffers cardiopulmonary deterioration may do so secondary to many causes. The mechanism of injury needs to be considered. The potential causes of reversible PEA that may be associated with trauma include:

– hypoxia secondary to pneumothorax or respiratory arrest.
– hypovolemia caused by injury to vital structures resulting in hemorrhage.
– cardiac tamponade causing diminished cardiac output.
– drug usage that may be the underlying cause of the accident.

Other frequent causes of PEA include acidosis, hyperkalemia, hypokalemia, and coronary or pulmonary thrombosis.

■ I.V. fluids run wide open may help reverse hypovolemia, which is the most common cause of PEA.

> INSTRUCTOR: *Intubation is complete and the patient is receiving 100% O_2. Pulse oximetry is 97%.*

> TEAM LEADER: *I would check for a pulse.*

■ If hypoxemia is the cause of PEA, then it may be reversed with adequate ventilation and the administration of O_2.

> INSTRUCTOR: *There's no pulse.*

> TEAM LEADER: *I would direct team members to continue CPR. I would assess breath sounds bilaterally.*

■ Tension pneumothorax diminishes cardiac output and should be considered a potential cause of PEA because this patient suffered a blunt trauma to the chest area.

> INSTRUCTOR: *The patient has equal bilateral breath sounds.*

> TEAM LEADER: *I would then order pericardiocentesis to relieve cardiac tamponade.*

■ This patient suffered a blunt chest trauma strong enough to bend the steering wheel, making cardiac tamponade a potential cause of PEA.

> INSTRUCTOR: *Pericardiocentesis is complete; 20 ml of blood was obtained.*

> TEAM LEADER: *I would check for a pulse while checking the rhythm on the monitor.*

> INSTRUCTOR: *You check the monitor and this rhythm appears on the screen:*

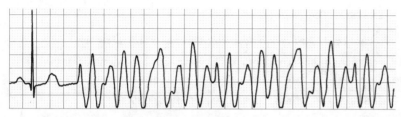

> TEAM LEADER: *I would ask for a pulse check.*

■ Confirmation of VF would indicate a pulseless rhythm.

> INSTRUCTOR: *Pulse absent.*

TEAM LEADER: *I would instruct a team member to place gel pads on the patient's chest.*

■ A conductive medium is necessary for proper defibrillation.

TEAM LEADER: *I would place the defibrillator paddles appropriately and announce "all clear," while looking around to confirm that all team members are clear from the patient.*

■ Team members may be so involved in their role that they don't always hear what doesn't specifically affect their job. Safety of the team is as important as caring for the patient.

TEAM LEADER: *I would defibrillate at 200 joules.*

■ Defibrillation is a Class I action for VF.

TEAM LEADER: *I would check the monitor for rhythm assessment. If there was no change, I would defibrillate at 300 joules.*

■ Joules need to be increased with successive defibrillations to decrease transthoracic impedance. It's also important to glance at the cardiac rhythm after confirming that everyone is out of the way to ensure that the rhythm is still VF.

TEAM LEADER: *I would check the monitor again for rhythm assessment. If there was still no change, I would defibrillate at 360 joules.*

■ Three successive stacked shocks are the ACLS standard before the pulse is checked again. It's always important to glance at the cardiac rhythm after confirming that everyone is out of the way to ensure that the rhythm is still VF before defibrillation.

INSTRUCTOR: *No change in rhythm.*

TEAM LEADER: *I would ask for a carotid pulse check.*

■ After the stacked defibrillations have been completed, a pulse check should be done.

INSTRUCTOR: *None present.*

TEAM LEADER: *I would do another secondary ABCD survey.*

■ Even though the secondary ABCD survey has been done before, it's done again, taking into account any treatment of the patient.

INSTRUCTOR: *A team member is performing CPR.*

TEAM LEADER: *I would tell a team member to administer 1 mg of epinephrine I.V. push.*

■ Epinephrine's actions have been previously discussed (see page 90); it's a Class I action in ACLS. The patient has I.V. lines in place from admission, so this route may be used if patent.

INSTRUCTOR: *Epinephrine is administered I.V. according to protocol.*

■ A fluid bolus accompanies infusion of the epinephrine, and the patient's arm is raised; both of these actions facilitate the drug's entrance into the venous system.

TEAM LEADER: *I would direct the team to continue CPR.*

■ Compressions are needed to circulate the administered drug.

INSTRUCTOR: *A team member is still performing CPR. The patient has a femoral pulse with chest compressions.*

■ Compressions should be effective enough to produce a palpable femoral pulse.

TEAM LEADER: *After a few minutes of CPR, I would again defibrillate the patient at 360 joules.*

■ After administering medications that can enhance defibrillation, wait a few minutes, and then try again to defibrillate.

TEAM LEADER: *I would announce "all clear" again and visually confirm that all team members are clear of the patient.*

INSTRUCTOR: *The patient is defibrillated according to protocol. The monitor still shows VF.*

TEAM LEADER: *I would check the carotid pulse.*

■ Confirm cardiac rhythm on the monitor by checking the patient.

INSTRUCTOR: *There's no carotid pulse; the cardiac monitor is unchanged.*

TEAM LEADER: *I would tell a team member to administer 300 mg of amiodarone I.V. rapid infusion diluted in a volume of 20 to 30 ml of saline solution or dextrose in water.*

■ Amiodarone's actions have been previously discussed (see page 107); it's indicated in VF unresponsive to epinephrine.

INSTRUCTOR: *Amiodarone infusion is initiated.*

TEAM LEADER: *I would direct the team in continuing CPR.*

■ CPR helps circulate the drug.

INSTRUCTOR: *CPR continues.*

TEAM LEADER: *I would defibrillate the patient again at 360 joules after a few minutes of CPR.*

■ The course of treatment is drug-defibrillate-drug-defibrillate. When the patient isn't being defibrillated, the leader should confirm that CPR is continued in the interim.

TEAM LEADER: *I would announce "all clear" again and visually confirm that all team members are clear from the patient.*

INSTRUCTOR: *The patient is defibrillated according to protocol. The monitor is unchanged after defibrillation.*

TEAM LEADER: *I would confirm cardiac rhythm on the monitor and check the carotid pulse.*

■ The cardiac rhythm should always be verified on the monitor.

INSTRUCTOR: *The carotid pulse is checked; none present.*

TEAM LEADER: *I would direct a team member to administer 40 units of vasopressin by I.V. push.*

■ Vasopressin or another dose of epinephrine may be administered (this would be the second dose). Either medication would be appropriate at this point. Vasopressin's actions have been previously discussed (see page 94) and are indicated in this situation.

INSTRUCTOR: *Vasopressin is administered according to protocol.*

TEAM LEADER: *I would continue CPR for a few minutes and then defibrillate the patient again at 360 joules.*

■ CPR promotes adequate circulation of the drug.

INSTRUCTOR: *CPR is continued for a few minutes.*

TEAM LEADER: *I would announce "all clear" again and visually confirm that all team members are clear of the patient.*

INSTRUCTOR: *The patient is defibrillated according to protocol. The monitor is unchanged after defibrillation.*

TEAM LEADER: *I see that the monitor still indicates VF, and I check the carotid pulse.*

■ Always confirm pulse check with the patient.

INSTRUCTOR: *There's no carotid pulse.*

TEAM LEADER: *I would tell a team member to administer 1.5 mg/kg of lidocaine by I.V. push and direct the team to continue CPR.*

■ Most instructors don't make you calculate the actual bolus, but if they do, reconfirm the patient's weight, ask if there is a calculator, and if no calculator is available, ask for pen and paper if you need them. Therefore, 1.5 mg $\times$ 70 kg = 105 mg or a 100-mg bolus.

INSTRUCTOR: *Lidocaine is administered; CPR continues.*

TEAM LEADER: *I would defibrillate the patient again at 360 joules, making certain that all team members are clear of the patient.*

INSTRUCTOR: *The patient is defibrillated according to protocol. The following rhythm appears on the monitor:*

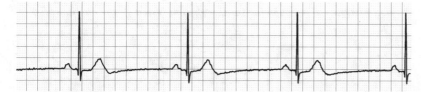

TEAM LEADER: *I see there's a rhythm change; it appears to be sinus bradycardia. I would then check for a pulse.*

■ Any time there's a rhythm change or a change in the patient's condition, always check for a pulse and reanalyze the rhythm.

INSTRUCTOR: *There's a pulse with this cardiac rhythm.*

TEAM LEADER: *I would reassess secondary ABCD.*

■ Again, a change in condition warrants a reassessment. Go through reassessment for airway, breathing, circulation, and differential diagnosis.

INSTRUCTOR: *The rest of the assessment is unchanged; the patient remains unconscious.*

TEAM LEADER: *I would direct a team member to apply a transcutaneous pacemaker with a rate of 80 stimulated beats/minute.*

■ The patient continues with symptomatic bradycardia. If a transcutaneous pacemaker isn't available, you may need to consider atropine; however, given the recent VF, you probably wouldn't want to rush on this therapy. A transcutaneous pacemaker allows you to bring up the rate without using a drug with potential adverse effects.

INSTRUCTOR: *A transcutaneous pacemaker is being applied to the patient.*

TEAM LEADER: *I would direct a team member to begin a lidocaine drip at 2 mg/minute I.V.*

■ Remember, after a ventricular event, a maintenance infusion should be ordered. The right drug to use is the bolus drug that terminated the rhythm. In this situation, lidocaine was the last drug used and is indicated for the maintenance infusion.

INSTRUCTOR: *Lidocaine drip is initiated.*

TEAM LEADER: *I would ask a team member for the patient's vital signs (blood pressure, pulse, respirations).*

■ Remember that you can always ask for information during the megacode.

INSTRUCTOR: *Blood pressure 70/20 mm Hg, pulse 80, respiration 20 with bagging. The following cardiac rhythm is seen on the monitor after TCP is started:*

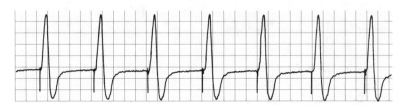

TEAM LEADER: *The monitor shows a ventricular paced rhythm with capture.*

■ Just because a pacemaker is turned on, it doesn't mean the ventricular tissue will capture the electricity and cause the myofibrils to shorten.

TEAM LEADER: *I would check the carotid pulse.*

■ A pulse check confirms that the captured pacing rhythm is perfusing the patient.

INSTRUCTOR: *Pulse is present with this rhythm.*

TEAM LEADER: *I would direct the team to run an I.V. infusion of normal saline solution wide open for a few minutes, and I would recheck the blood pressure.*

■ You could order dopamine right away, but given the fact that the patient just converted from a VF and had a bradycardia, he may need just a few minutes to have the pacer improve the heart rate; therefore, the blood pressure should be rechecked. Again, if you can use a therapy that doesn't require a drug, try it first. You don't want to infuse too much I.V. fluid and risk heart failure. A few minutes should help to make your differential diagnosis of the blood pressure problem.

INSTRUCTOR: *An I.V. infusion of normal saline solution is run wide open for a few minutes. Blood pressure and other vital signs are unchanged.*

TEAM LEADER: *I would direct a team member to begin a dopamine drip at 5 mcg/kg/minute, titrated to maintain a systolic blood pressure of 90 mm Hg. I would then direct the team to reassess vital signs.*

■ Dopamine's actions have been previously discussed (see page 93). The rate of infusion needs to stimulate an increase in blood pressure. The patient's vital signs need to be reassessed with any change in treatment to determine the effect of the drug. ABCD survey may also be redone at this time .

>INSTRUCTOR: *The dopamine infusion is started. Systolic blood pressure is maintained at 90 mm Hg with initiation of the infusion.*

>TEAM LEADER: *I would then complete the trauma assessment. When that was finished, I would transfer the patient to the intensive care unit.*

This scenario followed the algorithm for adult cardiac arrest, PEA, VF, and bradycardia.

Scenario #2

>INSTRUCTOR: *A patient arrives in your ED complaining of palpitations and mild dizziness. She's visibly anxious and crying. Vital signs are blood pressure 98/50 mm Hg, pulse 210, respiration 24. You attach her to the monitor; which shows this rhythm:*

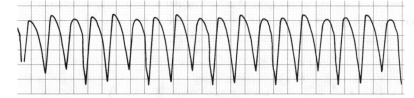

>TEAM LEADER: *The rhythm on the monitor appears to be ventricular tachycardia (VT). I would perform a primary ABCD survey.*

■ Primary assessment needs to be initiated to ascertain airway, breathing, and circulation.

>INSTRUCTOR: *The primary assessment indicates that the patient is conscious and breathing with a palpable pulse.*

>TEAM LEADER: *I would perform a secondary ABCD survey.*

■ Airway: Patient is spontaneously breathing.
■ Breathing: Ventilation is adequate; patient is receiving O_2 at 4 L/minute.
■ Circulation: I.V. access is established.
■ Differential diagnosis is being considered.
■ 12-lead ECG is ordered.
■ This is a wide-complex tachycardia; because the patient's condition is stable, the goal is to interpret the rhythm correctly.

>INSTRUCTOR: *Airway is natural; oxygen is in place by nasal cannula. An I.V. line is started and a 12-lead ECG is performed. A diagnosis of stable VT is made.*

TEAM LEADER: *I would direct a team member to administer 150 mg of amiodarone I.V. over 10 minutes.*

■ Amiodarone's actions have been previously discussed (see page 107).

INSTRUCTOR: *Amiodarone infusion is started. Blood pressure 70/20 mm Hg, patient has become more restless. Patient is arousable but unable to answer questions.*

TEAM LEADER: *I would check the carotid pulse.*

INSTRUCTOR: *The carotid pulse is present with this rhythm.*

TEAM LEADER: *I would direct a team member to place gel pads on the patient's chest. After announcing "all clear" and visually confirming that team members are clear of the patient, I would perform synchronized cardioversion at 100 joules.*

■ Patient is becoming unstable and cardioversion is indicated. Synchronization is critical in a rhythm with a pulse so that the joules aren't delivered during the vulnerable period of ventricular repolarization. When choosing to synchronize, confirm that the defibrillator is in the "synch" mode, usually by pushing an indicated button.

INSTRUCTOR: *Patient converts to this rhythm after cardioversion:*

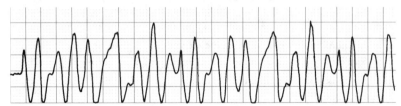

TEAM LEADER: *I would check the carotid pulse.*

INSTRUCTOR: *The carotid pulse is checked and is found to be absent.*

TEAM LEADER: *I would then defibrillate the patient at 200 joules.*

■ The crucial point here is that the synchronization is no longer applied. Some machines automatically lose the synchronization when the cardioversion joules are delivered. Some machines require the operator to physically push the SYNC button again to disable the command. The key is to look at the defibrillator and know whether the "sync" command is on or off and whether the patient's condition requires it on or off.

INSTRUCTOR: *The monitor is unchanged.*

TEAM LEADER: *I would then defibrillate the patient at 300 joules.*

INSTRUCTOR: *There's no change on the monitor.*

TEAM LEADER: *I would then defibrillate the patient at 360 joules, followed by a check of the carotid pulse.*

INSTRUCTOR: *The carotid pulse is absent with no change in rhythm.*

TEAM LEADER: *I would direct the team to intubate the patient and administer 1 mg of epinephrine by I.V. push.*

■ The ABCD survey is performed because the patient has experienced a change in condition. An airway needs to be secured and the patient requires epinephrine. Epinephrine's actions have been previously discussed (see page 90).

TEAM LEADER: *I would direct the team to begin CPR.*

■ Compressions are needed to circulate the drug.

INSTRUCTOR: *Endotracheal tube is placed and confirmed with breath sounds. Epinephrine is administered and CPR is in progress.*

TEAM LEADER: *I would defibrillate the patient at 360 joules after a few minutes of CPR. After defibrillation, I would check the carotid pulse and cardiac rhythm.*

INSTRUCTOR: *The patient is defibrillated and there's no change on the monitor. There's no change in the carotid pulse.*

TEAM LEADER: *I would direct a team member to administer amiodarone 300 mg I.V. rapid infusion diluted in a volume of 20 to 30 ml of saline solution or dextrose in water.*

■ Amiodarone's actions have been previously discussed (see page 107).

INSTRUCTOR: *Amiodarone is administered.*

TEAM LEADER: *I would defibrillate the patient again at 360 joules after a few minutes of CPR.*

INSTRUCTOR: *The patient is defibrillated.*

TEAM LEADER: *I would check carotid pulse and rhythm on the monitor.*

INSTRUCTOR: *There's no change in pulse or cardiac rhythm.*

TEAM LEADER: *I would direct a team member to administer 40 U of vasopressin by I.V. push.*

■ Vasopressin or a second dose of epinephrine may be given. Vasopressin's action has previously been discussed (see page 94).

INSTRUCTOR: *Vasopressin is administered.*

TEAM LEADER: *I would defibrillate the patient again at 360 joules after a few minutes of CPR.*

INSTRUCTOR: *The patient is defibrillated.*

TEAM LEADER: *I would check the carotid pulse and rhythm on the monitor.*

INSTRUCTOR: *The patient has the following rhythm on the monitor:*

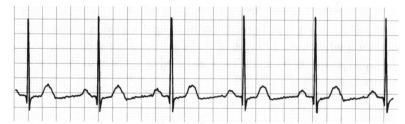

TEAM LEADER: *I would check the carotid pulse again.*

■ Confirm the patient has a pulse with this rhythm.

INSTRUCTOR: *Pulse is present.*

TEAM LEADER: *I would direct a team member to begin an amiodarone drip at 1 mg/minute.*

■ The last medication given is first administered as a drip if the rhythm is successfully converted.

INSTRUCTOR: *Amiodarone drip is initiated.*

TEAM LEADER: *I would reassess primary and secondary ABCD surveys and then admit the patient to the critical care unit.*

INSTRUCTOR: *Patient is stabilized and transferred to a monitored bed.*

This scenario followed the algorithm for stable VT, adult cardiac arrest, and VF.

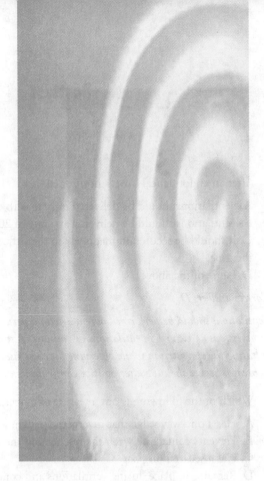

Posttest

Selected references

Index

Posttest

1. After an endotracheal tube is positioned:

    A. ventilations should be delivered in sync with chest compressions.
    B. ventilations should be delivered at a rate of 20 to 30 per minute.
    C. it should be secured immediately to the patient to prevent movement of the tube.
    D. None of the above.

Correct answer: D

Ventilations should be performed over a 2-second period asynchronously with chest compressions at 12 to 15 ventilations per minute. Assure proper placement by auscultating the epigastrium while observing for chest rise and fall with the first manual breath. Secure the tube after positive confirmation.

2. Which of the following is not a feature of a pocket face mask?

    A. Has a one-way valve that diverts the patient's exhaled gas
    B. Prevents contact between the rescuer and the patient
    C. Has a self-refilling bag
    D. Remains in place during ventilations and compression

Correct answer: C

The pocket face mask is a barrier device that has a one-way valve that diverts the patient's exhaled gas and prevents contact between the rescuer's and patient's secretions. It can be left in place during CPR. The self-refilling bag is a feature of the bag-valve unit.

3. After insertion of a Combitube and attachment of a bag-valve mask to the first (esophageal) lumen, ventilation doesn't cause a rise and fall in the chest and sounds are heard over the epigastrium. The next step is to:

    A. attach the bag-valve mask to the second (endotracheal) lumen and ventilate.
    B. inflate both cuffs to prevent the escape of oxygen.
    C. pull up on the tube so the printed ring is 2″ (5.1 cm) above the teeth.
    D. deflate both cuffs to allow epigastric area emptying.

Correct answer: A

The first lumen is in the esophagus if the device is inserted midline and to the depth of the printed ring at the level of the teeth. There's no chest expansion noted with bag-valve mask ventilations. The bag-valve mask is attached to the second lumen, which has endotracheal placement, and ventilates. Placement is confirmed and the device is secured.

4. While you're assisting with pericardiocentesis, it's most important to notify the practitioner:

    A. if the patient develops dyspnea.
    B. when blood enters the syringe.
    C. if jugular vein distention develops.
    D. if arrhythmias are noted.

Correct answer: D

During pericardiocentesis, arrhythmias may occur if the needle touches the myocardium. An alligator clamp attached to electrocardiograph lead V should be attached to the needle in order to quickly detect an arrhythmia.

5. Emergent treatment of tension pneumothorax includes which procedure?

    A. Needle thoracentesis
    B. Pericardiocentesis
    C. Emergency thoracotomy
    D. Intubation

Correct answer: A

Immediate needle thoracentesis is indicated for the patient with tension pneumothorax to allow air to escape and organs to return to their original position.

6. Death occurs from tension pneumothorax due to:

    A. compression of the organs in the thoracic cavity.
    B. massive hemorrhage into the pleural space.
    C. increased venous return.
    D. collapse of the lungs.

Correct answer: A

Organs in the thoracic cavity are compressed, resulting in decreased ventricular filling and decreased cardiac output. Death will occur if the condition isn't treated.

7. Which of the following is the most common initial rhythm in sudden cardiac arrest?

    A. Ventricular tachycardia
    B. Atrial fibrillation with rapid ventricular response
    C. Bradycardia
    D. Ventricular fibrillation

Correct answer: D

The most common rhythm seen with sudden cardiac arrest is ventricular fibrillation. The only effective treatment is defibrillation.

8. Which of the following wouldn't be an indication for cardiac pacing?

A. Hemodynamically unstable bradycardia
B. Malignant ventricular tachycardia
C. Cardiac arrest due to drug overdose
D. Premature atrial contractions

Correct answer: D

Premature atrial contractions aren't considered to be dangerous or life-threatening.

9. Which statement regarding the precordial thump technique is accurate?

A. Until it's administered, delayed use of an available defibrillator is acceptable.
B. It should be used in a witnessed arrest when a defibrillator isn't readily available and the patient is pulseless.
C. It's a highly successful technique.
D. It may be used for atrial arrhythmias.

Correct answer: B

The precordial thump technique should be used only when it's a witnessed arrest and the patient is pulseless; use of this technique should never delay defibrillation.

10. The P wave represents which event?

A. Atrial repolarization
B. Atrial depolarization
C. Ventricular depolarization
D. Ventricular repolarization

Correct answer: B

The impulse spreading across the atria generates a P wave.

11. To gather information about impulse conduction from the atria to the ventricles, which reading should be studied?

A. P wave
B. PR interval
C. ST segment
D. QRS complex

Correct answer: B

The PR interval measures the interval between atrial depolarization and ventricular depolarization. A normal PR interval is 0.12 to 0.20 second.

12. The period when myocardial cells are vulnerable to extra stimuli begins with the:

A. end of the P wave.
B. start of the R wave.
C. peak of the T wave.
D. peak of the QRS complex.

Correct answer: C

The peak of the T wave represents the beginning of the relative, although not the absolute, refractory period when the cells are vulnerable to stimuli.

13. For a patient with symptomatic sinus bradycardia who is experiencing a myocardial infarction, appropriate nursing interventions include establishing I.V. access to administer which agent?

A. atropine
B. Anticoagulant
C. Calcium channel blocker
D. Thrombolytic

Correct answer: A

Atropine is the standard treatment for symptomatic sinus bradycardia.

14. Treatment for symptomatic atrioventricular block includes which of the following?

A. Beta-adrenergic blockers
B. Ventilatory support
C. Pacemaker insertion
D. Fluid administration

Correct answer: C

A pacemaker is commonly used to maintain a steady heart rate in patients with symptomatic heart block.

15. Beta-adrenergic blockers, such as metoprolol and atenolol, and calcium channel blockers, such as verapamil, are commonly used to treat which sinus node arrhythmia?

A. Sinus bradycardia
B. Sinus tachycardia
C. Sinus arrest
D. Sinus block

Correct answer: B

Beta-adrenergic blockers and calcium channel blockers are commonly used to treat sinus tachycardia.

16. In atrial flutter, the key consideration in determining treatment is:

A. atrial rate.
B. ventricular rate.
C. configuration of the flutter waves.
D. configuration of the fibrillatory waves.

Correct answer: B

If the ventricular rate is too fast or too slow, cardiac output will be compromised. A rapid ventricular rate may require immediate cardioversion.

17. Carotid sinus massage is used to:

A. prevent the continual development of premature atrial contractions.
B. increase the ventricular rate in atrioventricular (AV) block.
C. convert paroxysmal atrial tachycardia to sinus rhythm.
D. treat ventricular tachycardia.

Correct answer: C

Carotid sinus massage triggers atrial standstill by inhibiting firing of the sinoatrial (SA) node and slowing AV conduction. This allows the SA node to reestablish itself as the primary pacemaker. In atrial flutter, the technique may increase the block and slow the ventricular rate, but it won't convert the rhythm.

18. The inherent rate for the atrioventricular (AV) junction is:

A. 20 to 40 beats/minute.
B. 40 to 60 beats/minute.
C. 60 to 80 beats/minute.
D. 80 to 100 beats/minute.

Correct answer: B

The normal, or inherent, rate for the AV junction is 40 to 60 beats/minute.

19. If the ventricles are depolarized first in a junctional rhythm, the P wave will:

A. appear before the QRS complex.
B. appear within the QRS complex.
C. appear after the QRS complex.
D. not be present.

Correct answer: C

Junctional rhythms originate in the atrioventricular junction. Impulses generated in this area cause the heart to be depolarized in an abnormal way, and P waves will be retrograde or inverted.

20. A patient with rapid supraventricular tachycardia develops ventricular fibrillation after delivering a synchronized cardioversion shock. What is the treatment of choice for a patient with ventricular fibrillation?

A. Defibrillation
B. Transesophageal pacing
C. Synchronized cardioversion at the same rate
D. Synchronized cardioversion at a higher rate

Correct answer: A

Patients with ventricular fibrillation are in cardiac arrest and require defibrillation.

21. A patient with a slow idioventricular rhythm that doesn't respond to atropine should receive which treatment?

A. lidocaine
B. dobutamine
C. Transcutaneous pacing
D. Another dose of atropine

Correct answer: C

Transcutaneous pacing is a temporary way to increase the rate and ensure adequate cardiac output. Neither lidocaine nor dobutamine are indicated for a slow idioventricular rhythm.

22. Which agent is commonly given with albuterol for the asthmatic patient?

A. methylprednisolone
B. ipratropium
C. aminophylline
D. epinephrine

Correct answer: B

Ipratropium is a nebulized anticholinergic that has a delayed onset of 20 minutes. It's usually given in combination with albuterol, a beta-adrenergic agonist that has an immediate action.

23. The patient with anaphylaxis should initially receive which agent?

A. Corticosteroids
B. epinephrine
C. Antihistamines
D. Histamine-2 blockers

Correct answer: B

Epinephrine is the drug of choice for the patient in anaphylactic shock. Oxygen at a high flow rate should also be given.

24. Airway, breathing, and circulation modifications for the patient with hypothermia include:

    A. assessing for breathing and pulse for 30 to 45 seconds.
    B. administering warming techniques immediately.
    C. withholding defibrillation until the patient is warmed.
    D. providing standard BLS and ACLS support.

Correct answer: A

Detecting breathing and a pulse in a patient with hypothermia can be difficult because of the markedly reduced oxygen requirements and decreased cardiac output associated with the condition.

25. Vigorous warming of the patient with hypothermia and aggressive care techniques may result in:

    A. successful resuscitation of the patient.
    B. ventricular fibrillation.
    C. aggravation of hypotension.
    D. no particular effect.

Correct answer: B

The patient is susceptible to ventricular fibrillation. Be careful to avoid initiating this rhythm with a treatment that's too aggressive.

26. As a hypothermic patient rewarms, concerns for the patient include:

    A. monitoring serum electrolytes.
    B. providing humidified oxygen.
    C. assessing for underlying conditions.
    D. carefully monitoring fluids to prevent hypertension.

Correct answer: A

Hyperkalemia may develop due to metabolic changes occurring during rewarming and should be monitored for and treated promptly.

27. Gastric lavage is recommended for:

    A. all patients who have ingested lethal amounts of drugs, regardless of time.
    B. overdose of antiarrhythmic agents.
    C. patients who present within 1 hour of ingestion.
    D. comatose patients.

Correct answer: C

Gastric lavage is indicated for patients who have ingested a potentially lethal amount of drug or toxin and present within 1 hour of ingestion.

28. Which of the following is a common arrhythmia that can occur as a complication of many drugs?

    A. Tachycardia
    B. Bradycardia
    C. Ventricular fibrillation
    D. Torsades de pointes

Correct answer: D

Torsades de pointes can occur with exposure to many drugs.

29. Which agent is used to treat torsades de pointes in patients who overdose?

    A. magnesium
    B. calcium chloride
    C. glucagon
    D. epinephrine

Correct answer: A

Magnesium can suppress the arrhythmia by reducing the amplitude after depolarizations thought to cause torsades de pointes.

30. Near-fatal asthma can result in sudden death from which complication?

    A. Asphyxia from severe bronchospasm
    B. Hypoxia
    C. Diminished blood flow and blood pressure
    D. Unresolved preexisting problems

Correct answer: A

Bronchospasm and mucus plugging—both common complications—can result in asphyxia.

31. In the patient with asthma, intubation is indicated by which sign?

    A. Elevated Pa_{CO_2}
    B. Tachycardia
    C. Confusion
    D. Wheezing

Correct answer: C

Confusion is a clinical sign of hypoxia that requires intubation. Other signs of hypoxia include obtundation, profuse diaphoresis, poor muscle tone, and severe agitation.

32. A patient who has been electrocuted may have which sign?

    A. Hypotension
    B. Heart block
    C. Myocardial infarction
    D. Tachycardia

Correct answer: D

Tachycardia, hypertension, and nonspecific electrocardiograph changes can occur as well as myocardial necrosis due to autonomic nervous system stimulation.

33. A 72-year-old patient is experiencing the sudden onset of mental status change, including slurred speech and vision changes. The patient should be immediately evaluated for:

    A. alcohol level.
    B. blood glucose level.
    C. neurologic impairment.
    D. history of diabetes.

Correct answer: C

The patient is experiencing the early signs of stroke. Immediate evaluation and treatment improves patient outcome.

34. Which of the following tools is useful in rapid neurologic examination of a trauma patient?

    A. Glasgow Coma Scale
    B. Hunt and Hess scale
    C. Cincinnati Prehospital Stroke Scale
    D. NIH Stroke Scale

Correct answer: A

The Glasgow Coma Scale is used to assess the patient's verbal and motor responses if a neurologic condition is suspected.

35. Which of the following are appropriate antihypertensive agents to administer to the patient who has experienced a stroke?

    A. labetalol or nitroprusside sodium
    B. nifedipine or nitroglycerin
    C. mannitol or diazepam
    D. lorazepam or thiopental

Correct answer: A

Nitroprusside sodium should be administered at 0.5 mg/kg/minute for patients with a diastolic blood pressure over 140 mm Hg. Give labetalol 10 mg I.V. push over 1 to 2 minutes; repeat every 10 minutes (or double the dosage) to a maximum dosage of

150 mg for patients with a systolic blood pressure over 220 mm Hg, a diastolic blood pressure from 121 to 140 mm Hg, or a mean arterial pressure over 130 mm Hg.

36. Which measure can rapidly lower increased intracranial pressure (ICP) in the case of impending herniation?

A. Elevation of the head of the bed 20 to 30 degrees
B. Intubation and hyperventilation
C. Hyperosmolar therapy
D. Barbiturates

Correct answer: B

Intubation and hyperventilation can rapidly lower ICP in the case of impending herniation by reducing carbon dioxide level and constricting blood vessels.

37. When considering the administration of defibrillation to a pregnant patient, you should know:

A. to administer half the amount of joules initially.
B. shocks are contraindicated in pregnancy due to the developing fetus.
C. to remove the fetus by emergency cesarean delivery before defibrillating the patient.
D. the requirements are unchanged.

Correct answer: D

Defibrillation hasn't been shown to harm a developing fetus.

38. Physiologic considerations of the pregnant patient in cardiac arrest include:

A. decreased cardiac output and a normal heart rate.
B. increased systemic and pulmonary vascular resistance.
C. increased blood volume and oxygen consumption.
D. increased pulmonary functional capacity.

Correct answer: C

The pregnant patient will have increases in blood volume, oxygen consumption, cardiac output, and heart rate.

39. Which of the following is the priority in treating the trauma patient who has decreased responsiveness, facial trauma, and possible spinal cord injury?

A. Application of a cervical collar and spinal immobilization equipment
B. Assessment of neurologic status
C. Removal of blood from the mouth and use of the jaw-thrust maneuver to open the airway
D. Determination of circulatory efficiency

Correct answer: C

Ensuring patency of the airway and assessment for breathing is essential. The spine should be kept immobilized by another rescuer until immobilization equipment can be applied.

40. Extreme tachycardia and arrhythmias in a patient with trauma may be due to which condition?

A. Myocardial contusion
B. Tension pneumothorax
C. Hypovolemia
D. Neurologic changes

Correct answer: A

Myocardial contusion is due to blunt chest trauma and may result in tachycardia and arrhythmias as well as ST-T wave changes.

41. Which term is used for a victim of a water incident who requires support in the field followed by transportation to a facility for observation and treatment?

A. Water rescue
B. Submersion
C. Drowning
D. Near-drowning

Correct answer: B

A victim of submersion requires assessment and intervention as well as further treatment and observation at a facility.

42. Which consideration is true regarding ACLS treatments and the patient with hypothermia?

A. Standard ACLS procedures are followed.
B. I.V. medications are given at longer standard intervals.
C. The patient must be warmed until the core temperature is greater than 86° F (30° C) before basic life support can be initiated.
D. Automatic external defibrillation isn't indicated until the patient's temperature is greater than 86° F.

Correct answer: B

Medications are withheld until the temperature increases in a patient with severe hypothermia. If moderate hypothermia is present, I.V. medications may be given at longer intervals.

43. Treatment of pulseless electrical activity (PEA) involves which treatment measure?

    A. Immediate defibrillation
    B. Administration of atropine
    C. Treatment of the underlying causes
    D. Use of an external pacemaker

Correct answer: C

Hypovolemia, hypothermia, cardiac tamponade, and tension pneumothorax are potential causes of PEA that require reversal.

44. Which statement about the administration of thrombolytics and acute coronary syndromes is true?

    A. It should be considered for patients with ST-segment elevation on the electrocardiogram (ECG).
    B. It should be considered for patients with ST-segment depression on the ECG.
    C. It should be considered for patients with T-wave inversion on the ECG.
    D. It should be considered for patients with bundle-branch block on the ECG.

Correct answer: A

Thrombolytics are a consideration for therapy when the 12-lead ECG indicates ST-segment elevation or new left bundle-branch block.

45. Which statement regarding acidosis in the patient with cardiac arrest is true?

    A. It's unrelated to metabolic factors.
    B. It may be due to inadequate ventilation.
    C. It's treated with bicarbonate.
    D. It must be treated with fluids.

Correct answer: B

Acidosis may be due to respiratory and metabolic factors and is initially corrected with adequate perfusion and ventilation.

46. During defibrillation, delivery of the current is expected to increase when:

    A. using lighter paddle pressure.
    B. using the lowest shock energy.
    C. using stacked countershocks.
    D. not using a conductive medium.

Correct answer: C

Transthoracic resistance will decrease with consecutive countershocks.

47. A dopamine infusion administered at 20 mcg/kg/minute will result in:

    A. constriction of the peripheral vessels.
    B. decreased cardiac output.
    C. dilation of the great vessels.
    D. renal arterial vasodilation.

Correct answer: A

Dopamine administered at this rate will result in peripheral arterial vasoconstriction.

48. Which is the drug of choice to reverse a verapamil overdose?

    A. atropine
    B. calcium chloride
    C. potassium chloride
    D. amiodarone

Correct answer: B

Calcium chloride is used for the patient in unstable calcium channel blocker overdose or beta-adrenergic blocker overdose.

49. A patient converts from pulseless ventricular tachycardia to sinus rhythm after defibrillation. Which agent should the patient then receive?

    A. epinephrine
    B. dopamine
    C. lidocaine
    D. atropine

Correct answer: C

The patient should be placed on a lidocaine drip unless a more successful agent was administered prior to the successful defibrillation.

50. Asystole sometimes can be mistaken for which type of arrhythmia?

    A. Idioventricular rhythm
    B. Pulseless ventricular tachycardia
    C. Fine ventricular fibrillation
    D. Complete heart block.

Correct answer: C

In some cases, ventricular fibrillation masquerades as asystole; however, the more common cause of a false report of asystole is operator error. Asystole should be verified in two leads.

Selected references

Alexander, J.H., et al. "Prophylactic Lidocaine Use in Acute Myocardial Infarction: Incidence and Outcomes from Two International Trials," *American Heart Journal* 137(5):799-805, 1999.

American Heart Association. *Guidelines 2000 for CPR and ECC by American Heart Association.* Philadelphia: Lippincott Williams & Wilkins, 2000.

Antman, E.M., et al. "Enoxaparin Prevents Death and Cardiac Ischemic Events in Unstable Angina-Non–Q-Wave Myocardial Infarction: Results of the Thrombolysis in Myocardial Infarction (TIMI) 11B Trial," *Circulation* 100(15):1593-1601, 1999.

Aufderheide, T., et al. *Heartsaver AED for the Lay Rescuer and First Responder.* Dallas: American Heart Association, 1999.

Babar, S.I., et al. "Vasopressin Versus Epinephrine During Cardiopulmonary Resuscitation: A Randomized Swine Outcome Study," *Resuscitation* 41(2):185-92, 1999.

"The Clinical Presentation of Acute Asthma in Adults and Children," in *Emergency Asthma.* New York: Marcel-Dekker, 1999.

Cobb, L.A., et al. "Influence of Cardiopulmonary Resuscitation Prior to Defibrillation in Patients with Out-of-Hospital Ventricular Fibrillation," *JAMA* 281(13):1182-88, 1999.

Davis, E.A., et al. "Institution of a Police Automated External Defibrillation Program: Concepts and Practice," *Prehospital Emergency Care* 3(1):60-65, 1999.

Eisenburger, P., and Safar, P. "Life Supporting First Aid Training of the Public: Review and Recommendations," *Resuscitation* 41(1):3-18, 1999.

Emergency Nurses Association. *Trauma Nursing Core Course,* 5th ed., 2000.

"The Era of Reperfusion: Part 7: Section 2: Acute Stroke," *Circulation* 102(suppl I):I-204-16, 2000.

Erbel, R., and Heusch, G. "Coronary Microembolization: Its Role in Acute Coronary Syndromes and Interventions," *Herz* 24(7):558-75, 1999.

Fahmy, F.S., et al. "Lightning: The Multisystem Group Injuries," *Journal of Trauma* 46(5):937-40, 1999.

Gibbs, N.A., et al. "State of the Art: Therapeutic Controversies in Severe Acute Asthma," *Academic Emergency Medicine* 7:800-15, 2000.

Gilbert, M., et al. "Resuscitation from Accidental Hypothermia of 13.7° C with Circulatory Arrest," *The Lancet* 355(9201):375-76 (letter), 2000.

Gliner, B.E., and White, R.D. "Electrocardiographic Evaluation of Defibrillation Shocks Delivered to Out-of-Hospital Sudden Cardiac Arrest Patients," *Resuscitation* 41(2):133-44, 1999.

Hallstrom, A., et al. "Cardiopulmonary Resuscitation by Chest Compression Alone or with Mouth-to-Mouth Ventilation," *New England Journal of Medicine* 342(21):1546-53, 2000.

Handley, J.A. "Four-Step CPR: Improving Skill Retention," *Resuscitation* 36(1):3-8, 1998.

Hazinski, M., et al., eds. *2000 Handbook of Emergency Cardiovascular Care for Healthcare Providers.* Dallas: American Heart Association, 2000.

Iserson, K.V. *Pocket Protocols for Notifying Survivors About Sudden Unexpected Deaths.* Tucson, Ariz.: Galen Press, Ltd., 1999.

Ishoo, E., et al. "Predicting Airway Risk in Angioedema: Staging System Based on Presentation," *Otolaryngology — Head and Neck Surgery* 121(3):263-68, 1999.

Kaye, W., et al. "Factors Associated with Survival from In-Hospital Cardiac Arrest: A Pilot of the National Registry of Cardiopulmonary Resuscitation," *Circulation* 100 (suppl I):I-313, 1999.

Kothari, R., et al. "Acute Stroke: Delays to Presentation and Emergency Department Evaluation," *Annals of Emergency Medicine* 33(1):3-8, 1999.

Kothari, R.U., et al. "Cincinnati Prehospital Stroke Scale: Reproducibility and Validity," *Annals of Emergency Medicine* 33(4):373-78, 1999.

Krismer, A.C., et al. "Cardiopulmonary Resuscitation During Severe Hypothermia in Pigs: Does Epinephrine or Vasopressin Increase Coronary Perfusion Pressure?" *Anesthesia and Analgesia* 90(1):69-73, 2000.

Kudenchuk, P.J., et al. "Amiodarone for Resuscitation After Out-of-Hospital Cardiac Arrest Due to Ventricular Fibrillation," *New England Journal of Medicine* 341(12):871-78, 1999.

Langhelle, A., et al. "Airway Pressure with Chest Compressions Versus Heimlich Maneuver in Recently Dead Adults with Complete Airway Obstruction," *Resuscitation* 44(2):105-08, 2000.

Mancini, M.E., and Kaye, W. "AEDs: Changing the Way You Respond to Cardiac Arrest," *AJN* 99(5):26-30, 1999.

Mayo, P., and Radeos, M.S. "The Severe Asthmatic: Intubated and Difficult to Ventilate," in *Emergency Asthma.* Edited by Brenner, B.E. New York: Marcel-Dekker, 1999.

Medical Services and First Aid. OSHA Standard 1910:151.

Morrison, L.J., et al. "Mortality and Prehospital Thrombolysis for Acute Myocardial Infarction: A Meta-Analysis," *JAMA* 283(20):2686-92, 2000.

National Safety Council. *1999 Injury Facts,* 1999 ed. Itasca, Ill.: National Safety Council, 1999.

National Safety Council and American Heart Association. *Heartsaver FACTS.* Sudbury, Mass.: Jones & Bartlett Pubs., 1999.

"Near-Fatal Asthma," *Circulation* 102(suppl I):I-237-40, 2000.

Niemann, J.T., and Cairns, C.B. "Hyperkalemia and Ionized Hypocalcemia During Cardiac Arrest and Resuscitation: Possible Culprits for Postcountershock Arrhythmias?" *Annals of Emergency Medicine* 34(1):1-7, 1999.

Nursing Procedures, 3rd ed. Springhouse, Pa.: Springhouse Corp., 2000.

Nursing2001 Drug Handbook. Springhouse, Pa.: Springhouse Corp., 2001.

Plaisance, P., et al. "Inspiratory Impedance During Active Compression-Decompression Cardiopulmonary Resuscitation: A Randomized Evaluation in Patients in Cardiac Arrest," *Circulation* 101(9):989-94, 2000.

Project Team of the Resuscitation Council. "Emergency Medical Treatment of Anaphylactic Reactions," *Journal of Accident and Emergency Medicine* 16(4):243-47, 1999.

Sadowski, Z.P., et al. "Multicenter Randomized Trial and a Systematic Overview of Lidocaine in Acute Myocardial Infarction," *American Heart Journal* 137(5):792-98, 1999.

Schellinger, P.D., et al. "A Standardized MRI Stroke Protocol: Comparison with CT in Hyperacute Intracerebral Hemorrhage," *Stroke* 30(4):765-68, 1999.

Solomonov, E., et al. "The Effect of Vigorous Fluid Resuscitation in Uncontrolled Hemorrhagic Shock After Massive Splenic Injury," *Critical Care Medicine* 28(3):749-54, 2000.

"Special Challenges in ECC: Section E," *Circulation* 102(suppl I):I-229-56, 2000.

Stewart, C.E. "When Lightning Strikes," *Emergency Medical Services* 29(3):57-67, 2000.

Thiemann, D.R., et al. "Lack of Benefit for Intravenous Thrombolysis in Patients with Myocardial Infarction Who Are Older Than 75 Years," *Circulation* 101(19):2239-46, 2000.

Tintinalli, J.E., ed. *Emergency Medicine: A Comprehensive Study Guide,* 5th ed. New York: McGraw-Hill Book Co., 2000.

"Toxicology in ECC: Section 2," *Circulation* 102(suppl I):I-223-28, 2000.

Vilke, G.M., et al. "Are Heroin Overdose Deaths Related to Patient Release After Prehospital Treatment with Naloxone?" *Prehospital Emergency Care* 3(3):183-86, 1999.

Voelckel, W.G., et al. "Effect of Small-Dose Dopamine on Mesenteric Blood Flow and Renal Function in a Pig Model of Cardiopulmonary Resuscitation with Vasopressin," *Anesthesia and Analgesia* 89(6):1430-36, 1999.

Wassertheil, J., et al. "Cardiac Arrest Outcomes at the Melbourne Cricket Ground and Shrine of Remembrance, Using a Tiered Response Strategy: A Forerunner to Public Access Defibrillation," *Resuscitation* 44(2):97-104, 2000.

Wenzel, V., et al. "Vasopressin Decreases Endogenous Catecholamine Plasma Levels During Cardiopulmonary Resuscitation in Pigs," *Critical Care Medicine* 28(4):1096-100, 2000.

Whitten, M., and Irvine, L.M. "Postmortem and Perimortem Caesarean Section: What Are the Indicators?" *Journal of the Royal Society of Medicine* 93(1):6-9, 2000.

Index

i refers to an illustration

i refers to an illustration

i refers to an illustration

i refers to an illustration

i refers to an illustration

i refers to an illustration

i refers to an illustration

i refers to an illustration

i refers to an illustration

i refers to an illustration

i refers to an illustration